The
Journal of Infectious Diseases

Published by the John McCormick Institute for Infectious Diseases

Volume 58
1936

Chicago, 1936

Composed and Printed by
George Banta Publishing Company
Menasha, Wisconsin, U. S. A.

OPSONINS FOR DIPLOCOCCUS MORBILLORUM AND FOR STREPTOCOCCUS SCARLATINAE IN CONVALESCENT MEASLES SERUM, CONVALESCENT SCARLET FEVER SERUM AND PLACENTAL EXTRACT

RUTH TUNNICLIFF

CHICAGO

On account of the favorable reports on the use of convalescent measles serum and placental extract in the prevention and modification of measles and on the use of convalescent scarlet fever serum in the prevention and cure of this disease, it seemed worth while to determine whether these materials had a high opsonin content for S. scarlatinae and D. morbillorum.[1]

Weaver and Tunnicliff[2] demonstrated that antitreptococcus horse serums of high opsonic content for streptococci rapidly lose their opsonic power, which may for sometime be largely restored by the addition of fresh human or guinea pig serum, and that guinea pigs are protected by such serums against fatal doses of streptococci so long as they can be reactivated by fresh serum. This may be for at least two years. The immunity in guinea pigs produced by the injection of immune serum persisted for about eight days. Serums with low opsonic content did not protect guinea pigs.

In cases of streptococcus infection in man several times fresh serum of the individual was still able to reactivate antistreptococcus horse serum even though the patient's blood had less opsonic effect on streptococci than normal blood.

Tunnicliff[3] obtained similar results when using the serum of a sheep immunized with hemolyzing scarlet fever streptococci. This serum had a high opsonin content, was specific and protected mice against streptococci from scarlet fever, but not against those from other sources such as erysipelas, mastoiditis and influenza. This immune serum rapidly lost its opsonic and protective power, which was restored by the addition of fresh normal sheep serum.

Received for publication, May 1, 1935.

From the John McCormick Institute for Infectious Diseases.

1. After having called the green producing diplococcus of measles D. rubeolae (J. Infect. Dis. **52:** 39, 1933), I was advised by Dr. A. R. Prévot, member of the International Commission on Nomenclature, against this designation on account of rubeolae in Latin meaning "German measles." Therefore, I withdraw the proposed name and substitute D. morbillorum, as suggested by Doctor Prévot.
2. J. Infect. Dis. **9:** 130, 1911.
3. J. A. M. A. **75:** 1339, 1920.

Serum of high opsonic content from goats[4] and from a horse[5] immunized with D. morbillorum protected mice against a fatal dose of this organism. The immune goat serum prevented the measles reaction produced in rabbits by infective material from measles. Normal goat serum had no such effect. These immune serums with high opsonic content were also effective in preventing or modifying measles in susceptible human beings.

It has been known that the serum of patients during recovery from scarlet fever[6] and measles[7] show a marked increase in opsonin for their respective cocci, but so far as I know reactivation experiments have not been made on aged serums collected from these diseases after recovery, so-called convalescent serum.

In the following experiments serum from an adult who had never had either scarlet fever or measles, was used as the control. Serum from an adult, who had suffered from both diseases years previously, and presumably protected against them (immune adult serum), and specific serum from a horse immunized with scarlatinal streptococci were included for comparison. Normal horse serum was the control for the immune horse serum. The immune horse serum which is both antibacterial and antitoxic was obtained from Dr. Elliott S. Robinson, director of the Massachusetts Antitoxin and Vaccine Laboratory. The convalescent measles and scarlet fever serums were furnished by Dr. William Thalhimer from the Samuel Deutsch Serum Center at Michael Reese Hospital, Chicago. One convalescent scarlet fever serum was provided by Dr. Paul S. Rhoads from the Cook County Hospital. The placental extract was obtained through Dr. John F. Anderson from E. R. Squibb and Sons.

The strains of S. scarlatinae I used, produce slightly granular conical colonies which do not color heated blood agar, while a recently isolated strain of D. morbillorum forms depressed conical colonies and turns both heated and unheated blood agar green.

The method of reactivation used in studying the opsonic content of stored serum was employed. Equal parts of normal guinea pig blood and 2 per cent sodium citrate solution in salt solution (citrated blood) are mixed and supply the leukocytes as well as the agents for reactivation. If the serum contains antiseptic, it and its control must be diluted 1:5 or 1:10 depending on the amount of antiseptic, on account of its inhibiting effect on phagocytosis. Equal parts of serum, citrated blood and bacterial suspension are mixed in capillary pipets, incubated 25 minutes at 36 C. Smears are made on glass slides and stained with a blood stain. For comparison both the number of cocci ingested per leukocyte in 100 polymorphonuclear leukocytes and the number of such cells taking part in phagocytosis are noted. The two methods give similar results.

Heparin was tried as an anticoagulant as described by Boener and Mudd.[8]

---

4. Tunnicliff R., and Hoyne, A.: J. A. M. A. **87:** 2139, 1926.
5. Tunnicliff, R. and White, B.: Boston M. & S. J. **197:** 272, 1927.
6. Tunnicliff, R.: J. Infect. Dis. **4:** 304, 1907; **8:** 302, 1911.
7. Tunnicliff, R.: J. Infect. Dis. **22:** 462, 1918.
8. Am. J. M. Sc. **89:** 22, 1935.

The opsonic indexes were the same as with sodium citrate although there was slightly more phagocytosis in the heparin specimens.

On account of not having a normal serum collected at the same time as the placental extract, normal serum, placental extract, pooled convalescent scarlet fever serum, and measles serum were heated at 56 C. for one half hour to get rid of normal opsonins and then reactivated. The relations were the same as with unheated materials although the figures were higher. The opsonic indexes in this article represent the mean of four experiments.

TABLE 1.—*Opsonic Index*

	Opsonic Index to	
	S. scarlatinae	D. morbillorum
Anti-scarlatinal streptococcus horse serum	5.2	0.7
Pooled convalescent scarlet fever serum (26)	4.6	2.6
Pooled convalescent measles serum (10)	1.8	6.1
Serum from adult immune to measles and scarlet fever	2.2	3.4
Placental extract	2.2	3.0

Serums from 6 persons convalescing from scarlet fever varied in their opsonic content for S. scarlatinae, some showed high opsonic indexes (3.8–5.2), some showed indexes only slightly higher than normal (1.3–1.7). The mixture of 26 specimens gave an index of 4.6 and indicates the value of a pooled serum. This index was a little lower than that of immune scarlet fever horse serum (5.4) and higher than that of an immune adult serum (2.2) and that of placental extract (2.2). The pooled scarlatinal serum showed an opsonic index of 1.6 for S. erysipelatis and one of 2.6 for D. morbillorum. Three of the 5 single specimens contained an increased amount of opsonin for D. morbillorum. The increased index for S. erysipelatis and for D. morbillorum probably meant that some of the persons had suffered from erysipelas and measles previously.

The pooled serum from 10 individuals convalescing from measles showed a high opsonic index to D. morbillorum (6.1). Individual serums had indexes ranging from 2.2–7.1. The opsonic index for this organism of the serum of an immune adult was 3.4 and that of placental extract 3.0. The pooled measles serum did not contain any opsonin for S. erysipelatis but showed an increased opsonic index (1.8) for S. scarlatinae due to the high indexes for this organism of four of the serums. Other single specimens had a low opsonic content for S. scarlatinae.

McKhann and Chu[9] have shown that the protein material obtained from the human placenta by salt extraction contains substances, presumably antibodies, which may blanch scarlet fever rashes and prevent or modify measles. I find that the specimen of placental extract examined has an opsonic index for S. scarlatinae of 2.2 and for D. morbillorum of 3.0 which is equal to the opsonic content of immune adult serum, but not so high an index for the measles coccus as pooled convalescent measles serum or so high an index for S. scarlatinae as pooled convalescent scarlet fever serum and immune horse serum. This specimen contained no increase in opsonin for S. erysipelatis, S. aureus, S. viridans and Type I pneumococcus.

9. J. Infect. Dis. **52**: 268, 1933.

The placental extract diluted 1:5 with salt solution on account of antiseptic, was absorbed 3 times with S. scarlatinae and D. morbillorum. The scarlatinal streptococcus absorbed the opsonin for the homologous and an heterologous scarlet fever streptococcus, but not the opsonin for D. morbillorum, Type I pneumococcus and S. viridans. The measles coccus absorbed the opsonin for this coccus but not for S. scarlatinae, Type I pneumococcus and S. viridans.

CONCLUSIONS

Pooled convalescent measles serum may have a high opsonic content for D. morbillorum and about the same amount of opsonin for S. scarlatinae as placental extract and serum from a person who had measles and scarlet fever years previously (immune adult serum). Pooled convalescent scarlet fever serum may give a higher opsonic index to S. scarlatinae than pooled measles serum but not so high an index as immune horse serum. It may have an opsonic index for D. morbillorum about equal to that of immune adult serum and placental extract. Placental extract also may give a high opsonic content for both S. scarlatinae and D. morbillorum, equal to that of immune adult serum.

The results of these experiments indicate that the high opsonic content of convalescent measles and scarlet fever serum and of placental extract for D. morbillorum and S. scarlatinae may account for some of their protective and curative power in measles and scarlet fever.

THE DEMONSTRATION OF CAPSULES ABOUT HEMOLYTIC STREPTOCOCCI WITH INDIA INK OR AZO BLUE

E. M. BUTT
C. W. BONYNGE
AND
R. L. JOYCE
LOS ANGELES, CALIFORNIA

Gins[1] was perhaps the first to employ India ink for outlining bacterial capsules and organisms that are stained with difficulty. Since his paper there have been several articles about the use of India ink for similar purposes, notably those by Rulison,[2] Gozóny[3] and Baker.[4] However, in none of these reports is there a consideration of the action of diluents used in the suspension of the organisms that influence the size of the capsular zone. Such factors, we have found, are of considerable importance in obtaining the maximum zone about encapsulated bacteria in India ink.

It is well known that most of the direct and indirect methods for visualizing bacterial capsules, described in text books and in the current literature are of dubious value for the demonstration of capsules of hemolytic streptococci. Furthermore the employment of India ink for such purposes without regard to the necessary details give poor results. When properly used, India ink is of great value for the demonstration of bacterial capsules. The improved India ink technique is given in detail and also a new method for the use of azo blue instead of India ink.

INDIA INK

The choice of India ink is important. We use Peliken ink #541 (Manufactured by Gunther Wagner, New York); the Higgins waterproof ink will prove satisfactory providing it is centrifuged until the coarse particles are thrown down.

Capsule development and characteristic colony formation is favored by growth in medium containing ascitic fluid. Strains to be studied for these characteristics are streaked on agar plates of veal infusion agar p_H 7.2 to which has been added 5 per cent defibrinated sheep blood and 20 per cent ascitic fluid. Incubation is carried on at 35 C. for 6–8 hours, preferably in moist atmosphere maintained by water in an open pan in the incubator.

Received for publication, May 3, 1935.

From the Departments of Pathology and Experimental Medicine, University of Southern California School of Medicine.

1. Centralbl. f. Bakt. (Abt. 1) **52:** 620, 1909.
2. J. A. M. A. **54:** 1426, 1910.
3. Centralbl. f. Bakt. **68:** 594, 1913.
4. Brit. J. Exper. Path. **1:** 127, 1920.

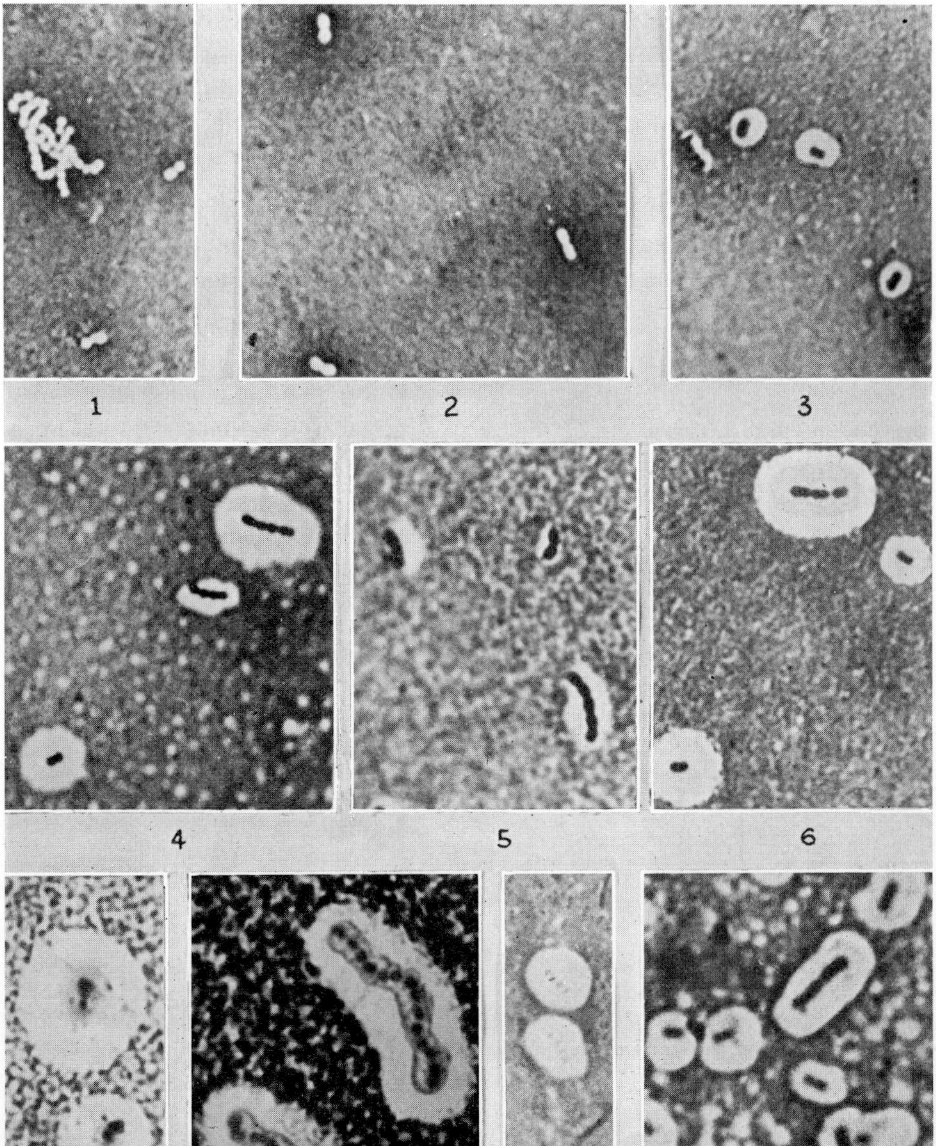

Fig. 1.

Cultures are usually made in the morning and are ready for study about 4:00 o'clock in the afternoon. With some strains better results have been obtained by placing the cultures in the icebox overnight and incubating at room temperature the next morning for three or four hours.

A drop of 6 per cent dextrose is placed on a meticulously clean slide and sufficient organisms are added to make a thin suspension. A small drop of India ink is evenly mixed with the suspension and is spread over the slide in a thin film using the edge of a glass slide as in the preparation of a blood film. The film is allowed to dry and then counterstained with equal parts of stock methylene blue solution and methyl alcohol. If other counterstains are preferred the film is first fixed with methyl alcohol, then stained with an aqueous solution of the dye of choice. The excess stain is washed off with water and the slide is allowed to air dry without blotting.

If exudates are to be examined for encapsulated organisms, the ink is mixed with the exudate, then diluted with 6 per cent dextrose solution and quickly spread over the slide. If the exudate is first diluted with dextrose solution, a gelatinous mass is obtained that is difficult to handle and causes a partial precipitation of the ink.

A 6 per cent dextrose-diluted ink gives much larger zones than ink diluted with water or normal salt solution. In fact many of the "capsulated" strains of hemolytic streptococci do not produce zones at all in India ink diluted with water.

The methyl alcohol acts to fix the film so that subsequent washing with water fails to disturb the background of ink.

AZO BLUE TECHNIQUE

A one per cent solution of azo blue in 6 per cent dextrose is used in essentially the same manner as India ink. A thin suspension of the organisms is made in a drop of the dye which is thinly smeared with the edge of a slide and allowed to dry. The bodies of the organisms appear as pale silver bodies

---

Fig. 1—Photomicrographs × 1500

1. "Noncapsulated" beta hemolytic streptococci in India ink, unstained.
2. Beta hemolytic streptococci (Streptococcus epidemicus) in India ink diluted with water, unstained.
3. Beta hemolytic streptococci (Streptococcus epidemicus) in India ink diluted with normal salt solution, counterstained with methylene blue.
4. Beta hemolytic streptococci in India ink diluted with 6 per cent dextrose, counterstained with methylene blue.
5. Pneumococcus (S strain of type III) in India ink diluted with normal salt solution counterstained with methylene blue.
6. Pneumococcus (S strain of type III) in India ink diluted with 6 per cent dextrose, counterstained with methylene blue. Note the delicately outlined inner zone.
7. Pneumococcus (S strain of type III) from an exudate counterstained with methyl violet. India ink diluted with 6 per cent dextrose.
8. Pneumococcus (S strain of type III) in India ink counterstained with methylene blue over which has been superimposed a thin film of Higgin's waterproof vermillion ink.
9. Beta hemolytic streptococci (Streptococcus epidemicus) in azo blue, without counterstain.
10. Pneumococcus (S strain of type III) in azo blue counterstained with methylene blue.

in very large clear zones that are oval and for the most part free of particles of dye. If counterstaining is desired, a methyl-alcohol solution of methylene blue is employed. The smear is stained for a few seconds with the solution and the excess dye is quickly washed off with undiluted methyl alcohol. The preparation is then quickly dried.

The zones of hemolytic streptococci in azo blue are larger than in dextrose-diluted ink but the background is less pleasing because of its coarseness. However, the dye is cheap and easy to obtain.

Azo blue (obtainable from Coleman and Bell, Norwood, Ohio) is a blue-black powder soluble in water, giving a violet colored solution. The aqueous solution turns red upon the addition of sodium hydroxide and a purple color is formed on the addition of hydrochloric acid. Azo blue is an oxytetrazo dye, electronegative and differs from congo red, also a tetrazo dye, in that it gives only temporary protection against heat coagulation of serum and does not protect against precipitation of serum by mercuric chloride, while congo red acts as a good protective. The bacterial zones in congo red are very much smaller than in azo blue or dextrose-diluted ink. Some years ago Benians substituted congo red for India ink but it has not proved satisfactory in any of the modifications we have tried.

COMMENT

We have used the terms capsular spaces or zones only for descriptive purposes to indicate the large, clear, oval areas about "capsulated" bacteria in India ink or azo blue preparations. Furthermore, we have carefully avoided the term "capsules" in speaking of India ink zones because we are not convinced that they represent in their entirety the actual capsules. It is possible that the zones are evidences of surface tension or propulsion forces which may be initiated in the reaction of capsular material with the medium in which the India ink particles are suspended. The variation in the size of the clear spaces controllable by experimental procedures and the presence of a much smaller stainable capsule would suggest this possibility. These spaces may represent the "Aussenhülle" that Tonniessen[5] has called the zone outside the "ectoplasm," sometimes seen in preparations stained by direct methods or they may conform to "hülle" that Fürst[6] was able to develop in a dilute serum water containing dextrose. This phase will be considered more fully later.

It is of little importance, however, in the evaluation of these methods whether the zones are completely filled with capsular material, since "non-capsulated" bacteria do not produce zones in India ink in spite of the use of modifying procedures as outlined. This applies also to beta hemolytic streptococci. The greater number of these strains fail to show zones by the ink method. Streptococcus epidemicus of Davis and the beta streptococcus recovered from epidemic adenitis of the guinea pig produce by far the largest zones in India ink of any of the streptococci. There are other strains of beta streptococci such as those recovered from the throats of scarlet fever pa-

5. Centralbl. f. Bakt. (Abt. 1) **85:** 225, 1921.
6. Centralbl. f. Bakt. **56:** 97, 1910.

tients and other types of hemolytic streptococcus infections that will produce small zones in India ink but nothing comparable to the large zones about the Streptococcus epidemicus. We do not wish to indicate, however, that Streptococcus epidemicus is a disease specific organism as we have obtained typical strains from erysipelas, otitis media, mastoiditis and scarlatinal complications.

We have studied the pneumococcus (S strains of type III) and Klebsiella pneumoniae Friedländer under similar conditions and have found that the zones vary in size according to the methods used. In water-diluted India ink the zones are small while in dextrose-diluted India ink, the zones are large, in fact larger than those initiated by Streptococcus epidemicus.

SUMMARY

The size of the capsular zone about hemolytic streptococci in India ink is partly dependent upon the character of the fluid used in diluting the ink. The largest zone is obtained in India ink diluted with 6 per cent dextrose, while in water-diluted ink the capsular zone is small or not present. Azo blue may be substituted for India ink in the demonstration of bacterial capsules.

FAILURE TO INFECT MONKEYS WITH POLIOMYELITIS VIRUS THROUGH ISOLATED INTESTINAL LOOPS

EDWIN H. LENNETTE

AND

N. PAUL HUDSON

CHICAGO

The weight of evidence at the present time favors the nasopharynx as the portal of entry of the poliomyelitis virus in natural infections. Uncertainty of proof lies in the non-cultivability of the infectious agent and the technical difficulty in demonstrating the virus in this site. In spite of this handicap, it has occasionally been found in washings of the nasopharyngeal mucosa of patients and carriers, thus indicating the likely modes of distribution and infection. The theory is made complete by the experimental evidence that the olfactory tract acts in the monkey as the route of migration of the virus from the nasal mucosa to the brain and cord.

Evidence of a different kind, however, has suggested the gastrointestinal route as the portal of entry. A few outbreaks of poliomyelitis have been attributed epidemiologically to individual milk supplies. Water has also been incriminated. Even then, one may raise the question of contamination of the upper mucosal parts. If the unmedullated fibers of the cranial nerves I and XIII of the monkey are invaded by the virus, similar fibers of the submucous intestinal sympathetics might likewise be a pathway of the virus to the central nervous system. Attempts to obtain experimental evidence for this have generally been unsuccessful. Flexner and Lewis,[1] Landsteiner and Levaditi,[2] Leake,[3] Amoss,[4] Schultz,[5] Thompson,[6] Clark and his associates[7] and Jungeblut and Thompson[8] have failed to produce infection in monkeys or higher apes by administering the virus through a stomach tube or by mixing it with food.

Several investigators, on the other hand, have reported positive experimental results. Leiner and von Wiesner[9] produced the disease in 1 of 2 Macacus rhesus after preliminary injection of opium to reduce intestinal

---

Submitted for publication, May 9, 1935.

From the Department of Hygiene and Bacteriology, The University of Chicago.

1. J. Exper. Med. **12:** 227, 1910.
2. Compt. rend. Acad. d. sc. **149:** 1014, 1909; Compt. rend, Soc. de biol. **67:** 787, 1909; Ann. Inst. Pastuer **24:** 833, 1910.
3. Hyg. Lab. Bull. No. 111, p. 21. 1918.
4. Rivers, Thomas: Filterable Viruses, Baltimore, Williams & Wilkins, 1928, p. 174.
5. Proc. Soc. Exper. Biol. and Med. **26:** 632, 1929.
6. J. Exper. Med. **51:** 777, 1930.
7. Clark, P. F.; Schindler, J., and Roberts, D. J.: J. Bact. **20:** 213, 1930; Clark, P. F.; Roberts, D. J., and Preston, W. S., Jr.: J. Prev. Med. **6:** 47, 1932.
8. Immunität, Allergie u. Infektionskr. **3:** 1, 1930–1931.
9. Wien. klin. Wchnschr. **23:** 817, 1910.

motility. Demme[10] fed a monkey saponin before giving it virus and it developed poliomyelitis, while a control animal remained normal. M. cynomolgus was thought by Kling, Levaditi and Lepine[11] to be more susceptible than M. rhesus to virus given by mouth. They, as well as Saddington,[12] succeeded in infecting cynomolgus by this means. In a recent summary of results, Kling, Levaditi, and Hornus[13] reported that 10 of 19 monkeys of various kinds had succumbed to the experimental disease, and they suggested that the ingestion of contaminated materials should still be considered in the epidemiology of the disease.

In attempts to apply the virus more directly to the intestinal mucosa, the virus has been injected into the intestine after laparotomy. Postive results were obtained by Leiner and von Wiesner,[9] and Kling, Levaditi and Hornus,[13] but Clark, Roberts and Preston[7] were unsuccessful. Toomey[14] clamped off intestinal loops in M. rhesus and, after the disappearance of the pinch reflex, injected virus suspensions with positive results. He likewise obtained infection by subserosal injection of virus and concluded in general that the intestinal sympathetic fibers are susceptible to virus invasion.

In surveying the literature, it is clear the epidemiological evidence should not be disregarded and any experimental data obtainable would be of value in elucidating the problem. However, the experimental information so far adduced is entirely inconclusive. As a rule, either special procedures or severe manipulations are necessary to secure positive results. We thought it worth while to introduce a new method of approach in using the animal susceptible to nerve fiber invasion and in employing isolated loops of intestine. In this way, large amounts of virus could be applied to physiologically normal mucosa without the interference of intestinal contents. We were entirely unsuccessful in obtaining poliomyelitic infections.

EXPERIMENTAL

Bowel loops were preapred at various levels. In two monkeys a segment of ileum 20 to 25 cms. in length was isolated, the distal end being cut about 15 cms. from the ileo-cecal valve. The continuity of the bowel was re-established by an end-to-end anastomosis of the interrupted ileal segments. The blood and nerve supplies were left intact. The intestinal loop of one animal (T) was made into a pouch by closing the distal end and bringing the proximal end to the outside through a left rectus stab wound. In a second animal (TV), a Thiry-Vella fistula was made by bringing both ends of the isolated bowel out through stab wounds in the left rectus muscle.

Attempts to make fistulae at jejunal levels were unsuccessful owing to the tremendous loss of body salts and fluids from the loops, losses which we were unable to replace despite repeated blood transfusions and phleboclysis with Ringer's solution.

10. Deutsche Zschr. f. Nervenh. **116:** 156, 1930.
11. Bull. Acad. d. med., Paris **102:** 158, 1929; **105:** 190, 1931.
12. Proc. Soc. Exper. Biol. and Med. **29:** 838, 1932.
13. Bull. Acad. d. Med., Paris **111:** 1, 1934.
14. Proc. Soc. Exper. Biol. and Med. **31:** 680, 1934.

The remaining two monkeys in our series had been used in bacteriologic studies and had been prepared by Drs. G. M. Dack and E. Petran[15] of this department. The reader is referred to their article for a complete description of the operative technic, diagrams of the altered bowel loops and illustrations[1] of the prepared animals. One of these animals (TC) had a Thiry-Vella fistula of the colon. In the other (CP), the isolated bowel consisted of terminal ileum, ascending colon and transverse colon. The fecal stream was diverted to the descending colon by an end-to-side anastomosis of the proximal end of the ileum to the splenic flexure of the colon. Leakage of intestinal contents was prevented by turning in the cut end of the large gut.

The animals were quartered in a large outdoor cage for several months between operation and use and were in good condition when the experiment was begun.

In the first experiment monkeys T and TV (Thiry and Thiry-Vella fistulae of ileum) received in the bowel loops in seven daily instillations a total of 41 cc. and 44 cc., respectively, of 20 per cent virus-cord emulsion. A small rubber catheter (French No. 8) attached to a Luer syringe proved satisfactory for placing the inoculum into the loops. Each loop was first flushed out with 5 to 10 cc. of warm physiological saline solution to remove mucus and cellular detritus. The virus-cord emulsion was then injected slowly to avoid sudden distention of the bowel and consequent reverse peristalsis. Immediately after injection the animals were masked, according to the method of Dack and Woolpert,[16] to prevent manual and labial transfer of virus from the loops to the mouth. The animals quickly became accustomed to the masks. After a minimum period of 6 hours the masks were removed, the abdomen was scrubbed with soap and water and then washed with 70 per cent alcohol. A large dose of virus was thus given enterically over 7 days but at no time subsequently did we obtain any evidence of infection, as indicated by fever or symptoms.

The experimental conditions were not deemed entirely satisfactory, however, because some virus was always lost by leakage from the stomata and the avoidance of reverse peristalsis in the bowel segments was difficult. We then decided on the insertion of whole cord, either glycerolated or fresh. This method had the added advantage of permitting comparatively huge doses of infectious material to be introduced into the loops.

The following method was found to be the most satisfactory for placing the infected cord into the bowel segments. To one end of a block of cord, 5 to 8 cms. long, with the meninges still attached, a long piece of heavy thread was tied and the free end passed through a 10 cm. length of glass tubing. By gently pulling the thread the cord was drawn up into the tubing. One end of the tube was inserted into the orifice of the fistula and the cord was expelled by means of a glass rod whose diameter approximated that of the bore of the tubing employed. The injected material was forced farther into the loop by using a large catheter (French No. 16). The thread was permitted to hang outside the mouth of the fistula and served as a means of determining how

15. J. Infect. Dis. **54:** 220, 1934.
16. J. Prev. Med. **6:** 129, 1932.

rapidly the spinal cord was digested. A tight abdominal bandage kept the material in the loops and prevented the animals from licking and fingering the stomata of the fistulae. These bandages were removed on the third day, after which nothing recognizable as cord material could be recovered from the loops.

From the middle of October, 1933, to the middle of January, 1934, each of the 4 monkeys in our series received from 8 to 11 grams of whole glycerolated or fresh poliomyelitis spinal cords. Four administrations of preserved and 2 of fresh tissue were made. Here again, despite the huge amount of infectious material injected, there was no significant rise in temperature nor was any other sign of infection noted.

In a further attempt to induce infection by this route, recourse was had to the method that Schultz and Gebhardt[17] proposed for increasing the incidence of infections by the intranasal route. Accordingly, on February 1, 2 and 3, 1934, each monkey received 5.0 cc. of a 10 per cent crude virus-cord emulsion, each instillation of virus being preceded by a preliminary flushing out of the isolated loop with phosphate buffer solution of p_H 5.0. The animals were observed closely and no evidence of reaction to the virus was obtained. From these results it seems that an acid solution, which in our hands has increased the permeability of the nasal mucosa to the virus, had no effect on the invasion of virus through the intestinal mucous lining.

To determine if sufficient virus had been absorbed from the bowel to produce humoral neutralizing antibodies without antecedent evidence of infection, the blood serums obtained from these animals 44 days after the last instillation of virus were tested. Serum from all 4 animals failed to neutralize the virus. Histological examination of the cords of the test monkeys at several levels confirmed the diagnosis of experimental poliomyelitis.

The administration of large amounts of virus furnished the opportunity to test for the local production of neutralizing antibodies. The isolated bowel segments and the lymph nodes draining them were removed under ether anesthesia. Lymph nodes were separated from the bowel and mesentery, and extracted separately. Extracts were prepared by mincing each tissue specimen as finely as possible with scissors, washing with sterile saline several times to remove gross blood, and grinding with sand. After thorough grinding, 10 cc. sterile saline was added to each sample and extraction permitted to go on overnight in the refrigerator. Freezing 10 times in a carbon dioxide-alcohol mixture was performed the following day as a further means of releasing cell fluids.

Each extract was bacteriologically cultured before being used in the neutralization test. In several instances the presence of contaminating bacteria in large numbers necessitated passing the extracts through Berkefeld N filters.

The tests were carried out as above except that 0.25 per cent virus-cord emulsion was used instead of 1 per cent. The gut and lymph node extracts from every monkey failed to inactivate the virus. Furthermore, no virus was

17. Proc. Soc. Exper. Biol. and Med. **30:** 1010, 1933.

present in the two extracts tested, as determined by intracerebral injection of 2 cc. of material into normal monkeys.

The table summarizes the experimental work and results.

TABLE 1.—*Summary of Experiments on Intestinal Pathogenesis of Poliomyelitis*

Monkey	T	TV	CP	TC
Isolated part of gut	Ileum	Ileum	Cecum	Transverse Colon
Virus Administration	1. Daily administration of 20 per cent emulsion of viruscord for 7 days, totalling:			
	41 cc.	44 cc.		
	2. Four administrations of whole, glycerolated virus-cord Two administrations of whole, fresh virus-cord, totalling:			
	8.6 gms.	10.2 gms.	10.3 gms.	11.1 gms.
	3. Administration to each monkey of 5 cc. 10 per cent emulsion of virus-cord on 3 successive days after irrigation of isolated loops with phosphate buffer solution of p_H 5.0.			
Results	No infection	No infection	No infection	No infection
	Neutralization tests on undiluted serums taken 44 days after last administrations of virus were negative			
	Neutralization tests on extracts of isolated gut and regional lymph nodes			
	Gut: Negative*†	Negative	Negative	Negative*
	Nodes: Negative†	Negative	Negative*	Negative

* These extracts were passed through Berkefeld N filters to remove bacteria.
† These extracts injected in 2.0 cc. amounts intracerebrally into test animals to detect presence of virus; results negative.

SUMMARY

Suspensions of poliomyelitic spinal cords of monkeys were instilled repeatedly into loops of isolated bowel in 4 M. rhesus without producing infection. Attempts to induce poliomyelitis in these animals by administering whole virus-cord were likewise negative, despite the comparatively huge dosage employed. Subsequent efforts were preceded by a preliminary washing out of the loops with phosphate buffer solution, p_H 5.0, in an endeavor to increase the permeability of the intestinal mucosa. This method, found to be so useful in increasing the incidence of infection by the nasal route, was ineffective when applied to the bowel inasmuch as no evidence of infection was obtained.

Thus, while virus in one form or another was administered intensively over a period of 3 months, no poliomyelitis occurred at any stage of this prolonged experiment.

Neutralizing antibodies were not demonstrated in the serum 44 days after the last instillation of virus. Saline extracts of the isolated intestinal loops and of the regional lymph nodes draining them failed to inactivate the virus. The virus was not demonstrated in the two extracts tested.

We were unable to find experimental evidence that the poliomyelitis virus invades M. rhesus by the intestinal route, when large amounts of virus were applied to normal mucosa over long periods of time in the absence of the usual intestinal contents.

STUDIES ON THE BACTERICIDAL ACTION OF BOVINE WHOLE BLOOD AND SERUM TOWARDS BRUCELLA ABORTUS AND BRUCELLA SUIS

M. R. IRWIN
B. A. BEACH
AND
F. N. BELL*
MADISON, WISCONSIN

The presence of antibodies in normal serum has long been recognized, following the report of Nutall[1] in 1888. A general review of the work in this field has been published by Knorr.[2] References to later experiments may be found in more recent papers[3] and an excellent summary of many of the conflicting conclusions is given in a recent textbook.[4]

In a previous article[5] it was pointed out that studies on naturally occurring antibodies have in general been limited to analyses of differences between species. Mention in the literature is made occasionally of individual differences in the experimental material, but as yet no systematic study has been attempted, except in humans for the isoagglutinins, and for the results obtained by the Schick and the Dick tests.

It would be a matter of fundamental interest to determine whether or not the universally occurring individual reactions to bacterial infections within an animal species might be correlated with differences in antibody content. This is as yet an open question. Some evidence has been presented[5,6] that individuals naturally susceptible to certain infections can be defined with reasonable accuracy on the basis of the low bactericidal action of their whole blood against the specific pathogen. Conversely the blood of those naturally resistant was found for the most part to have an appreciable bactericidal power.

Received for publication, May 9, 1935.

From the Departments of Genetics (187), Veterinary Science, and Agricultural Bacteriology, Agricultural Experiment Station, University of Wisconsin, in cooperation with the Bureau of Animal Industry, U. S. D. A. Published with the approval of the Director of the Station.

* Now at Washington State College, Pullman, Washington.

1. Ztschr. f. Hyg. u. Infektionskr. **4:** 353, 1888.
2. Kolle, W.; Kraus, R., and Uhlenhuth, P.: Handbuch der pathogenen Mikroorganismen, Berlin, Urban & Schwarzenberg **2:** 663, 1929.
3. Mackie, T. J., and Finkelstein, M. H.: J. Hyg. **31:** 35, 1931; Mackie, T. J.; Finkelstein, M. H., and Van Rooyen, C. E.: J. Hyg. **32:** 494, 1932; Gordon, J., and Wormall, A.: J. Path. & Bact. **31:** 753, 1928; Irwin, M. R., and Bell, F. N.: J. Infect. Dis., **57:** 74, 1935.
4. Topley, W. W. C.: An Outline of Immunity, Baltimore, William Wood & Company, 1933.
5. Irwin, M. R., and Bell, F. N.: J. Infect. Dis., **57:** 74, 1935.
6. Irwin, M. R., and Hughes, T. P.: J. Immunol. **24:** 343, 1933; Malone, R. H.; Avari, C. R., and Naidu, B. P. B.: Indian J. M. Research **13:** 121, 1925.

The following experiments were initiated to test the technic in cattle to be subjected to infection with Brucella abortus. If the more susceptible members of a population might be determined before infection, the use of such animals would afford a more precise measure of the value of various therapeutic and curative agents than is possible in a random group of individuals.

MATERIALS AND METHODS

The animals from which blood for the tests was taken were of two classes. The first group ("recovered") consisted of 14 animals which had been given intra-stomachal infections[7] with Brucella abortus in 1928, from whose serums agglutinins had nearly, or entirely, disappeared, and whose milk did not contain the organism. Of these at first infection, 5 ("resistants") had produced normal calves, 9 ("susceptibles") had aborted. The other group was composed of 23 ("non-infected") females of varying ages.

A single strain of Br. abortus has been in principal use throughout the tests to be described. Numerous checks with two other cultures have given no results that could be ascribed to strain differences of the bacteria. We are indebted to Dr. I. F. Huddleson of Michigan State College, and to Dr. J. Traum, of the University of California, for the cultures of Br. abortus.

Blood was taken aseptically from the jugular vein, and collected in sterile tubes. For the tests using whole blood just sufficient anti-coagulant to prevent clotting for 24 hours, was placed in each tube. A uniform quantity (0.5 cc.) of whole blood, serum or plasma, was added to each of a series of small culture tubes into which had been placed 0.05 cc. of decimal dilutions of a 36- or 48-hour culture of a standardized saline suspension of the organism. In the majority of cases these samples were tested in duplicate. The tubes were incubated at 37.5 C. for 24–26 hours. The contents of each tube were then poured into a petri dish with fluid pork infusion agar, and incubated five or six days. For controls, 0.05 cc. of the different dilutions was mixed with the fluid medium and poured into petri dishes. Unless otherwise stated, the blood and serum samples were mixed with bacterial dilutions within a few hours after withdrawal.

EXPERIMENTAL

Bactericidal effect of whole blood on Br. abortus.

A preliminary survey showed marked differences between individuals in the ability of their citrated whole blood to destroy the organism. Accordingly, at each day for testing, a representative of each of the "high" and the "low" groups as shown in table 1 was included in the animals bled, as a check on the uniformity of the results and as a measure of the relative bactericidal activity of various bloods. These tests extended over a period of 18 months prior to infection of the animals in September, 1933. Each animal was tested from 6 to 15 different times.

The number of bacterial colonies in the control plates, as given in table

7. Hart, E. B.; Hadley, F. B., and Hmuphrey, G. C.: Univ. Wis. Agric. Exper. Sta. Res. Bull. no. 112, 1932.

1, is an average of actual counts for the two highest dilutions (−7 and −6) during these experiments. The variation is given by the standard deviation (σ). The estimates for the lower dilutions are based upon the mean numbers in the two highest dilutions.

TABLE 1.—*Bactericidal Action of Ox Whole Blood on Brucella Abortus*

	Colonies in controls and in blood-bacterial mixtures				
Bacterial Dilutions	−3	−4	−5	−6	−7
Controls	10^5*	10^4*	10^3*	113 (σ =66)	10 (σ =7)
Blood reactions					
High	+(10–200)	f.c. (0–50)	0	0	0
Intermediate	++	+, (5–300)	f.c. (0–100)	0	0
Low	C	+++	++	f.c. (2–60)	f.c. (0–10)

* Estimated average number.
Symbols. C =confluent growth, equal to control; +++ =abundant growth; ++ = less abundant growth; + = scattered colonies, 50 to 300; f.c. =few colonies, number in parentheses.

It was found that there were three grades of bactericidal activity for the "whole blood" of the 37 animals at test. Those bloods which consistently destroyed more than 1000 organisms per 0.5 cc. were placed in the "high" group, slightly less (>100 and <1000), in the "intermediate," and markedly less, in the "low" group. No differences between cultures were noted on several parallel tests employing three different strains of the organism. The division of the "recovered" and "non-infected" animals according to the bactericidal activity of their whole blood is given in table 2.

TABLE 2.—*Classification of Animals According to the Bactericidal Action of their Whole Blood*

Animal Groups	Bactericidal activity			Total
	High	Intermediate	Low	
"Non-infected"	4	18	1	23
"Recovered"				
Resistant	4	0	1	5
Susceptible	0	0	9	9
Total	8	18	11	37

The majority (18) of the non-infected animals were of the "intermediate" class, 4 were definitely in the "high," and only one in the "low" grouping. The status of the only member of the "low" class is doubtful, the previous history of this animal being unknown. No other instance of such a low bactericidal action has been found in tests on the blood of other cattle, presumably normal. The similarity by this test to the "low" group of the "recovered" animals would suggest a previous infection.

It is somewhat surprising that the "recovered" animals were either in the "high" or in the "low" group. The "resistants" with one exception showed "high" activity, and all those previously "susceptible" displayed a "low" reaction. On the basis that the blood of normal cattle usually will possess a much greater antibacterial action than was present in these previously "susceptible" individuals, it would seem that some disturbance in the antibody system of these particular animals had taken place, which reduced the activity of their whole blood. No satisfactory explanation of this condition can be made at present. The bactericidal action of the whole blood of the "recovered" in the "high" class was no more pronounced than that of the "non-infected" bloods of the same group. However, three years had elapsed since the infection of those "recovered," and any possible enhanced expression due to an acquired immunity might well have disappeared in that time.

Direct comparisons have been made of the relative activity of citrated and heparinized whole blood. Parallel tests on blood samples from several individuals, treated with each of the anti-coagulants, gave practically the same end-point of activity for each sample.

PLASMA-CELL MIXTURES

Of considerable interest are the activities of plasma and cells interchanged between bloods of the different groups, as summarized in table 3. For these tests, citrated blood was centrifugalized, the plasma pipetted off, the cells washed in physiological saline, and the various mixtures made as given in the table. Counts by one of us (F. N. B.) of the total red and white cells following these manipulations showed in general only a slight decrease in the number of leucocytes, rarely of more than one-fourth of the original number.

The results in the table show clearly that components of the plasma determined the antibacterial action of the mixture. Occasionally an effect was noted slightly less than that of the sample of the whole blood from which the plasma was obtained, but never a more pronounced activity. Cells alone, with saline added in volume equivalent to the serum displaced, had little or no destructive action on the bacteria; on the contrary, growth was noted in two cases.

Plasma which had been stored at 2–3 C. for varying periods of time and then was mixed with fresh cells showed a gradual decrease in bactericidal action. After 28 days, the action was reduced to little or nothing.

TABLE 3.—*The Bactericidal Action of Plasma-cell Mixtures*

Class of: Plasma	Class of: Cells	Results of bactericidal action: High	Intermediate	Low
High	High	6*	0	0
High	Intermediate	5	2	0
High	Low	5	7	0
Intermediate	High	0	5	0
Intermediate	Intermediate	0	3	0
Intermediate	Low	0	3	0
Low	High	0	0	10
Low	Intermediate	0	0	5
Low	Low	0	0	1
Stored Plasma:				
High[1]	High	2	3	0
High[2]	Low		1	1
High[3]	High			1
Cells only	High			2
	Low			1

[1] Stored at 2–3 C. for 7 days.
[2] Stored at 2–3 C. for 14 days.
[3] Stored at 2–3 C. for 28 days.
* The numbers refer to the different tests of each combination.

BACTERICIDINS IN SERUM

A summary is given in table 4 of the bactericidal effect of whole blood, of serum from defibrinated and clotted blood, and of plasma from citrated and heparinized blood. For convenience, this bactericidal activity is given by an index number, after Mackie.[3] In the table, each index is an exponent (base 10, see table 1) determined by the end-point of growth in the blood-bacterial, or serum-bacterial mixtures, as compared with the growth in the highest dilution in the control plates.

Plasma from citrated blood from animals of the "high" and "intermediate" groups displayed a uniformly greater bactericidal activity than was found in whole blood. The effect in the "low" group was variable, chiefly in the plasma from three "recovered" individuals. For the others of this group, the reaction was equal to that of the plasma of the other two groups in 14 of 17 tests.

TABLE 4.—*Bactericidins in Serum*

Activity of whole blood	C	H	D	S	Heated[1]	Citrated whole blood (from table 1)
High	>5	3, 4	3	4	0	3, 4
Intermediate	>4, 5	3, 4		4	0	2, 3
Low	0 (2)* 1(1)* $^{3}_{5}$(14)*	2(1) 3(1)		0.(1)* 2.(1)* 3.(5)*	0	0, 1

Symbols. C, H, D and S denote plasma from citrated and heparinized, and serum from defibrinated and clotted blood, respectively.
[1] Serum or plasma heated at 56 C. for 30 minutes.
The numbers represent the difference between the indices of the dilutions corresponding to the end points of growth of the serum-bacterial mixture and that of the control. For example, in table 1 the end point of growth for the control was at the dilution of −7, of whole blood of the "high" group at −4, the difference being 3. See Mackie et al.[3]
* Numbers in parentheses represent the number of different trials.

The antibacterial action of plasma from heparinized blood, and of serum from defibrinated and clotted blood was comparable in parallel tests on the same individuals, and was higher than that of the whole blood. Serum from representatives of the "low" class destroyed more organisms than did parallel samples of whole blood from the same animals. This effect was often less than that of citrated plasma. If an amount of sodium citrate was added to clotted serum proportionate to the volume used as an anti-coagulant (1 per cent), the effect was enhanced. Plasma from citrated blood probably should not be used to determine accurately the bactericidins in ox blood. This does not apply, however, to the use of citrated whole blood.

The bactericidal action was destroyed by heating either serum or plasma at 56 C. for 30 minutes, with a more variable effect after heating for 20 minutes. Serum or plasma stored at ice box temperature (2 to 3 C.) showed a slight loss in destructive action at 7 days, the activity decreasing gradually until after 28 days there was little or none. The addition of guinea pig complement to heated and/or to stored serum did not restore the bactericidal power to a point greater than that of the guinea pig serum per se. However, the activity was restored by the addition of beef serum complement. Further studies on the nature of the bactericidal mechanism will be given in another report.

BACTERICIDAL EFFECT ON BRUCELLA SUIS

Citrated whole blood of each of the 37 animals was assayed for bactericidal action towards a strain of Br. suis, of known pathogenicity for rabbits.[5]

These tests were always made concurrently with those on one or more of the strains of Br. abortus, as described above No appreciable destructive activity of whole blood for the porcine strain was shown in two different tests of each of the individuals. A single exception was noted, but a retest was in agreement with the results of the other samples. Succeeding trials on several bloods have been in accord. No differences have been found between citrated and defibrinated whole blood in their bactericidal effect toward this organism.

The mean number of colonies of the blood-bacterial mixture as compared with the average number in the controls is given in the insert, with symbols as in table 1.

	Bacterial dilutions				
	−3	−4	−5	−6	−7
Average number of colonies in controls	15.10^4	15.10^3	15.10^2	150	15
Colonies in blood-bacterial mixtures:					
(a) Citrated	C	+++	++	f.c. (33)	f.c. (3)
(b) Defibrinated	C	+++	++	f.c. (21)	f.c. (3)
Defibrinated Serum (0.5 cc.)	++	+	f.c. (0–10)	0	0

Serum (0.5 cc.) alone was capable of destroying between 100 and 1000 organisms, a marked contrast to the decided lack of bactericidal activity of the whole blood towards this strain.

Resistance and susceptibility to Brucella abortus.

The majority of the animals were infected in September, 1933. Two drops of a heavy suspension of Br. abortus were placed in the conjunctival sac of each, and later the contents of an aborted fetal stomach were fed. Details of the methods of infection will be given elsewhere; the immediate purpose is to give the correlation of the bactericidal action of the whole blood with the results following infection. These are given in table 5.

TABLE 5.—*Correlation of the Bactericidal Power of Whole Blood with Reaction to Infection*

	Resistant (Calved normally)	Susceptible (Aborted)	Totals
Non-infected animals			
High	2	1	3
Intermediate	3	11	14
Low	1	0	1
Total	6	12	18
Recovered animals			
High	3	1	4
Low	8	0	8
Totals	11	1	12
	17	13	30

The number of animals not previously infected whose blood possessed a high bactericidal power was not large enough to propose any significant difference following infection between them and the "intermediate" class. A comparison by percentages is very misleading because of the small numbers involved. The results then are no more than suggestive of the ability by such a technic to pick out the resistant and susceptible members of a population. It may be possible by refinements in the technic to detect other differences, and these attempts are in progress at present.

Attention should be called to the resistance displayed by the "non-infected" animal whose blood was of the "low" group. As previously mentioned, the early history is unknown and a previous infection is suggested by these reactions.

Only one of 12 "recovered" animals was susceptible on reinfection. At post mortem this individual was found to have diseased kidneys, possibly a contributing factor in breaking down the acquired immunity shown by the others of this group.

DISCUSSION

There are two points of view from which to consider the data that have been presented. The results of the tests of whole blood and of serum with strains of Br. abortus allow the deduction that normal ox whole blood and serum possess bactericidins in an appreciable amount against this pathogen. This is in accord with experiments of Mackie et al.[3] However, in our work it was found that serum or plasma produced a bactericidal effect appreciably greater than that of whole blood. Although the reactions of whole blood and of serum are not directly comparable, since equal amounts of each were used in the tests, later trials employing amounts of serum equivalent to 0.5 cc. of whole blood have shown the same relative bactericidal activity, i.e. greater in serum than in the presence of cells.

In our experiments these results were very marked within the group of "low" individuals, whose whole blood showed a minimum reaction, but whose serum destroyed more organisms than the whole blood of this group, and in most cases, more than the whole blood of the "high" group. The reciprocal interchange of serum and cells of these various classes would seem to eliminate any explanation of the results by ascribing peculiarities to the leucocytes of the "low" group. The explanation of these findings is not clear at present.

Another puzzling result is the departure from normal of the reactions of the whole blood found in the "low" group of the "recovered" animals. Lacking tests on these before their first infection, one can only assume that they show a reaction lower than was present before infection, since with but one exception, itself of doubtful status, all other uninfected animals in these tests and in others which have followed have given an appreciable bactericidal activity.

Fiessinger and Cattan[8] report a disappearance of bactericidal action of the whole blood in typhoid fever patients, a somewhat similar phenomenon except that for these animals in our experiments the active infection is past. Our results would be easily explainable if the animals were carriers; the evidence for this, however, is negative.

If these findings may be partly explained by the observations of Rous and Jones[9] concerning the protective action of leucocytes on bacteria against serum components, the question is still unanswered as to the reason for the differences displayed by the "recovered" animals.

---

8. Presse med. **36:** 1185, 1928.
9. J. Exper. Med. **23:** 601, 1916.

SUMMARY AND CONCLUSIONS

Bovine serum normally contains bactericidins for Brucella abortus. Whole blood shows a bactericidal effect slightly less than comparable amounts of serum alone.

Individual animals show uniformity in reaction at different times, with a difference between animals in bactericidal activity.

Certain animals, recovered from a previous infection of Br. abortus, showed a loss in bactericidal properties of the whole blood as compared to that of presumably normal animals.

Bovine whole blood exerted no bactericidal effect on Brucella suis; the reaction of serum for this organism was decidedly less marked than for Br. abortus.

NOTE ON THE SPONTANEOUS CONTAMINATION OF A BACTERIAL CULTURE BY AN ORGANISM RESEMBLING HARTMANELLA CASTELLANII

LAWRANCE E. SHINN

AND

PHILIP B. HADLEY

PITTSBURGH, PENNSYLVANIA

Castellani,[1] in reports published in 1930, has described an ameba found by him in cultures of Cryptococcus pararoseus. The organism in question was readily transplantable on glucose agar and essentially pure cultures (associated only with dead bacteria) could be obtained. Douglas,[2] working with the same material, came to the conclusion that this ameba had not been previously described and that it was a representative of the genus Hartmanella.

The motile cell was described as a small ameba ranging from 13.5 to 22.5 microns in diameter and possessing a single nucleus and one or two contractile vacuoles. The pseudopodia were of the blunt type but were often preceeded or accompanied by very fine hair-like micropseudopodia. The motility was said to be slight. Enzymes capable of liquefying gelatin or coagulated serum were reported.

The cysts varied in diameter from 9 to 12 microns and were roundish with a coarse granular cytoplasm and a well marked double contoured membrane; the outer surface of which had a distinctly crinkled appearance. A single nucleus was present. On the basis of the foregoing characterizations and in view of the nuclear structure, Douglas proposed the establishment of a new species with the name Hartmanella castellanii.

Van Rooyen,[3] working with the same material in 1932, made a very complete survey of the response of the ameba to its bacterial environment. He arrived at the conclusion that the clearing of cultures by this organism was the result of a simple phagocytic process and not caused by any lytic ferment. The ability of the amebic strain to ingest and thrive on a number of bacterial species was carefully investigated.

During the latter part of 1934 the present authors were engaged in a study of a variant form of Bact. pneumoniae (Friedländer's bacillus) which arose, as a very special type of colony on litmus lactose agar. This colony was characterized by raised, waxy, white ridges arranged in a radial pattern with bridges of the same nature arranged concentrically. It resembled a

---

Received for publication, May 11, 1935.

From The Western Pennsylvania Hospital, Institute of Pathology.

1. J. Trop. Med. Hyg. **33:** 160, 188, 221, 237, 1930.
2. J. Trop. Med. Hyg. **33:** 258, 1930.
3. J. Trop. Med. Hyg. **35:** 118, 1932.

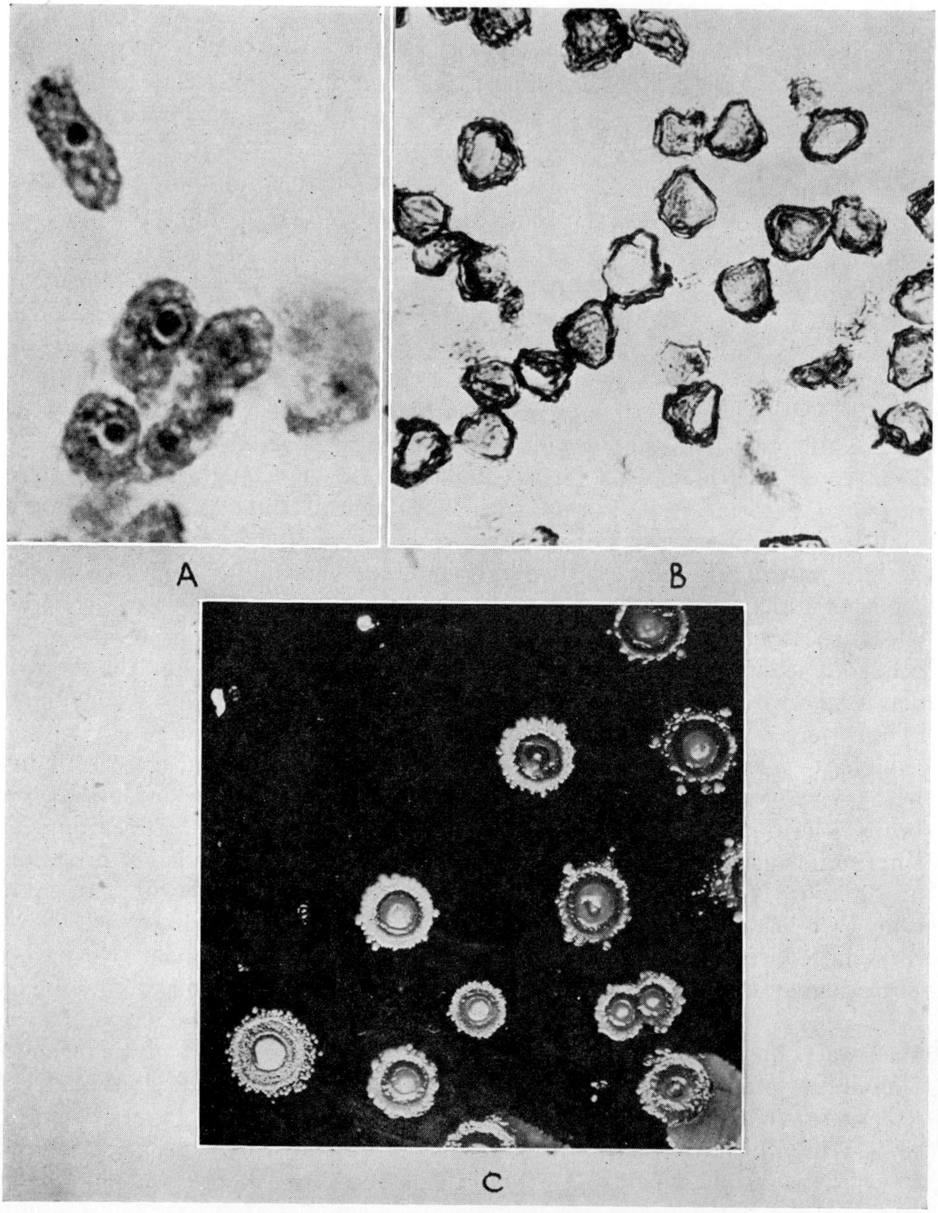

Fig. 1 A.—Amebas—paraffin section, stained with iron hematoxylin to show nucleus and karyosome.

B.—Encysted form—paraffin section, stained with Mallory's aniline blue. This stain gives a sky blue cyst wall and cherry red enclosed organism. The angular or polygonal nature of the cysts is to be noted. This is shown just as sharply in fresh mounts in saline or broth.

C.—Secondary colony formation by migrating amebae. Friedländer's bacillus.

highly fenestrated example of the usual mucoid colony. After the culture had been propagated on this medium in an unchanged condition for some weeks by serial, point inoculations, the specific colony form suddenly became transformed into an amorphous mass of growth. After two to three days, secondary colonies appeared in a halo formation some distance out on the plate from the original colony, while the central part of the old colony became markedly eroded. Microscopic examination of this central area disclosed a mass of closely packed amebic cysts and a number of actively motile amebas.

The active motile cells measured from 15 to 25 microns in diameter. The cytoplasm was clearly divided into a granular endoplasmic and a clear ectoplasmic zone. Motility was well maintained at 37°C. on the agar surface. The pseudopodia were short and thick but were usually preceded and accompanied by hair-like, filamentous micropseudopodia which often appeared to be branched. There was a single well defined nucleus and a large spherical karyosome. The clear space between the nuclear membrane and the karyosome often appeared to contain a large number of chromatin granules. There was usually only one contractile vacuole, but occasionally two.

The cysts measured from 9 to 15 microns in diameter and were composed of coarsely granular cytoplasm with a single nucleus and were surrounded by a double cyst wall; the outer wall being always much folded and crinkled. The cysts, judging both from the external wall and the enclosed protoplasmic mass, were typically polygonal in shape; in which respect they appeared to differ from those described by Castellani and by Douglas. As most frequently seen, they manifested a distinctly triangular appearance as contrasted with the cysts of Hartmanella castellanii which, both from the description and from the photographs presented by Castellani, appear clearly to be round. Whether this marks our form as a different species or even as a variant we do not feel competent to state. There are apparently no published statements, other than Douglas' report, on the differentiation of Hartmanella castellanii from Hartmanella hyalina. It would seem that both points need clarification by those interested in the classification of amebas.

To return to the description of our species; excystment has been observed in warm stage preparations on several occasions. In all cases, the ameba made its exit by way of one of the cyst angles where the wall seemed to have little or no thickness. On several occasions the enclosed ameba appeared to try two or three such points before finally utilizing one of them. Excystment, once begun, took place within two to three minutes and the cyst walls were apparently left intact. The vacuole began rhythmic action about 20 minutes before the ameba began to emerge; and in the typical instance was extruded last; the nucleus issuing first.

On agar plates, infected bacterial colonies usually gave a secondary halo formation as a result of viable bacteria being carried out and deposited at a distance. Within 24 hours, active amebas could be found over the entire plate, their outward extension occurring for the most part in radial lines from the central colony. However, if they did not find other bacterial growth suitable to their requirements they soon became encysted. At times, they even appeared to travel below the surface of the agar. The upper layer of agar, inhabited by large numbers of amebas, soon became spongy, either because of enzymatic action or mechanical undermining and tunnelling.

We have investigated the reaction of the amebas to a limited number of bacterial environments by permitting the migratory organisms to encounter colonies of various bacterial species on adjacent areas of agar. No cells of the originally associated species seemed to be carried, at least in a viable state, beyond the primary halo. Certain organisms were chosen from Van Rooyen's compilation for Hartmanella castellanii because of their clear cut positive or negative character. The results for our ameba are given in table I.

TABLE 1

Bacterial Species	Activity
B. pneumoniae S Friedländer	++
B. pneumoniae M Friedländer	+
E. coli	++
E. typhi	+
Salmonella	++
B. dysenteriae Shiga	++
B. dysenteriae Flexner	++
Pnuemococcus I	0
Pneumococcus III	0
S. aureus	+

The agreement between the results of this brief test and those reported by Van Rooyen lends confirmation to the apparent similarity of the organisms. One difference is noted; namely that in the reported data on H. castellanii the Shiga dysentery strain was shown to be susceptible in contrast to the Flexner Y which was not. We find no difference in the ease with which our amebas attack these two dysentery strains.

The results on Bact. pneumoniae will also bear comment. It was found that the mucoid phase was apparently much more resistant to the lytic action of the amebas than was the smooth phase, although not completely so. As an illustration of this we mention the repeated occurrence of the transformation of the smooth phase culture to the mucoid phase during the amebic invasion of the culture growth. With a smooth phase culture, the secondaries established by migrating amebas were usually destroyed, in their turn, except when a sudden transformation to the mucoid phase occurred. This was frequently the case. It is probable that the capsular substance exerted either a mechanical or chemical deterring action on the invading amebas. This may also operate in favor of the type III pneumococcus.

In view of the attempts on the part of several investigators, during the earlier years of inquiry into the nature of the phenomenon of the bacteriophage, to relate the observed lysis to the activity of amebas, it is perhaps pertinent to introduce a few words on this subject.

Unquestionably the activity of the amebae on plate cultures of several bacterial species produce appearances that possess superficial resemblances to the phenomenon of transmissible autolysis. The culture may be largely destroyed, the growth, if any, left on the plate shows a characteristic ragged or patchy appearance, and there eventually arise secondary colonies that may reveal a culture phase different from that of the original culture.

In all such cases of lysis, however, the presence of the free, motile, or of the encysted amebas can easily be observed on the plate, not only amidst the culture debris, but also on areas of the clear agar upon which no growth had occurred. Moreover, there were never observed in the culture growth under attack by the amebas any indication of a localized lytic action in any way resembling lytic plaques.

For this reason we believe there is slight possibility of confusion between the type of culture destruction produced by H. castellanii and the phenomenon of lysis effected by a typical sample of bacteriophage.

SUMMARY

An ameba resembling Hartmanella castellanii has been found as a spontaneous contaminant in a stock culture of the Friedländer bacillus.

Some minor differences in morphology between the cysts of this strain and those of Castellani's strain were observed.

The phenomenon of secondary colony formation, resulting from the transfer of viable bacteria across the agar surface by the amebas, is described.

Observations on the response of the amebas to a limited number of bacterial species gave results similar to those reported for Hartmanella castellanii.

Only superficial resemblance was found between the "lysis" of bacterial colonies produced by amebas and the type of colony lysis effected by the bacteriophage.

GROWTH STIMULATING FACTORS FOR MICROÖRGANISMS

MELVILLE SAHYUN*
PAUL BEARD
E. W. SCHULTZ
J. SNOW
AND
E. CROSS
STANFORD UNIVERSITY, CALIFORNIA

INTRODUCTION

In 1901 Wildiers[1] reported the discovery of a growth stimulating factor for yeast. He termed it "Bios." Since that time the question of growth factors has been one of the most interesting and widely discussed subjects of biological research. In 1925 Tanner[2] presented a comprehensive review of the "Bios" question, and more recently (1933) Peskett[3] contributed another survey of the literature on growth factors. It is therefore unnecessary to present herein another review on this subject other than to summarize in brief some of the most recent contributions that bear some connection to this investigation.

The concepts of growth factors are not sharply defined. Hormones are essential to growth, vitamins, certain essential amino acids and certain inorganic salts, so that anyone of these constituents may be considered a growth factor. Rhan[4] considers growth as essentially a chemical synthesis, but growth also involves both processes of catabolism and anabolism. Whether or not the organism is unicellular or multicellular, certain catalytic agents are essential in order that the living organism might be able to carry on its various processes of metabolism and cell division. In our opinion such an organic catalytic agent that enables the living system not only to metabolize its food but to proliferate may be considered as a growth factor or an "activator."

In an investigation on the growth of staphylococci Hughes[5] reported that these microörganisms require an "activator" and in his opinion this factor

---

Received for publication, May 17, 1935.

From the Department of Bacteriology and Experimental Pathology, Stanford University, California.

* Biochemical Research Laboratory, Frederick Stearns & Company, Detroit, Michigan.

This work was supported in part by a grant from Eli Lilly and Company, Indianapolis, Indiana.

1. Cellule **18:** 313, 1901.
2. Chem. Rev **1:** 397, 1925.
3. Biol. Rev. **8:** 1, 1933.
4. Quart. Rev. Biol. **8:** 77, 1933.
5. J. Bact. **23:** 437, 1932.

was characterized as belonging to a chemical group of "natural bases." Hughes described the general properties of his "activator" as resembling those of vitamin B. Since Hughes' factor possesses the properties of "natural bases," it seems quite unusual that it should be "heat stable" in acid solution and heat unstable in alkaline solutions. Should this factor truly possess basic characteristics, upon isolation in a pure state, it would constitute a distinct growth factor different from the other factors reported by others.

Knight and Fildes[6] reported an "activator" for B. sporogenes. They ascribed to it the following characteristics: acidic, ether soluble, the barium salts are soluble in aqueous alcohol, does not contain N, S or halogens, easily oxidized by potassium permanganate and hydrogen peroxide and upon oxidation its physiological functions are destroyed. These properties resemble to a considerable extent those of "auxin" the plant growth factor, previously reported by Kögl.[7]

Mueller and coworkers[8] described another growth factor for the diphtheria bacillus, the properties of which were not thoroughly investigated. However, they reported it to be non-basic, not precipitable by any of the usual precipitants and highly insoluble in alcohol and water.

Tatum and collaborators[9] reported the presence of a growth stimulating factor in various plants such as potatoes, oranges, lettuce, etc., that greatly stimulates the fermentation of corn-starch by certain butyric acid bacteria. The properties of this growth stimulant were not described.

Upon analysis of these reports one finds a considerable variation in the chemical properties of growth activators as described by different investigators. Thus (a) Hughes' activator differs from the others in possessing basic properties; (b) Knight and Fildes' activator is acidic, ether soluble and very readily oxidizable. This might indicate that this factor might be an unsaturated fatty acid. (c) Mueller's activator on the other hand, may or may not be identical with that of Knight and Fildes. (d) As regards Tatum's factor, we are not in a position to say whether or not he was dealing with one or more factors, as Tatum and collaborators were more interested in studying the effect of this unknown growth stimulant on the growth of butyric acid bacteria.

In this investigation an attempt was made to isolate one of the growth factors for microörganisms which henceforth will be referred to as "activator." Unforeseen events prevented us from bringing this work to completion. We, therefore, report on the following:

The method pursued in isolating this activator.

The effect of the activator on the growth of certain pathogenic organisms.*

The effect of the activator on the growth of the colon bacillus and a possible method of standardizing the activator.

6. Brit. J. Exper. Path. **14:** 112, 1933.
7. Die Umschau, Frankfurt-a-M., No. 40, 1932; Naturwissenschaften **21:** 17, 1933.
8. J. Bact. **25:** 59, 1933.
9. J. Bact. **27:** 207, 1934.

* The effect of the activator on pathogenic organisms will be presented in a later publication.

The effect of certain amino acids on the growth of the colon bacillus.

A comparison between the effects of certain amino acids and the activator on the growth of the colon bacillus.

PREPARATION OF THE ACTIVATOR (MELVILLE SAHYUN)

Two different procedures were followed in preparing the activator in a concentrated form so that the associated nitrogenous impurities have been considerably reduced.

Alcohol Extraction.

Acid Hydrolysis.

ALCOHOL EXTRACTION

This procedure was found suitable in removing a large amount of nitrogenous impurities from semi-hydrolyzed proteins such as peptones. Peptone was selected for our experimental work due to the fact that it is widely used as a laboratory medium for the culturing of a large number of microörganisms.

Difco peptone was used in this experiment. The general procedure is as follows:

The desired amount of dry peptone is dissolved in the smallest amount of hot water and 5 times its volume of hot 95 per cent ethyl alcohol is added, thoroughly mixed and allowed to stand for 24 hours or more. The supernatant liquid is decanted and the residue is extracted with 80 per cent ethyl alcohol. Extraction of the residue with 80 per cent alcohol is repeated two or three times. The clear alcoholic extracts are collected and acidified with 1 N sulfuric acid to approximately p_H 5.4, whereupon a precipitate is formed. This mixture is allowed to stand for a few hours and filtered through a buchner filter. Filtration is rapid. The alcohol is removed by distillation under vacuum and the aqueous residue is concentrated. The color is dark brown. A considerable amount of nitrogenous impurities may be removed by filtration through charcoal. The solution should be hot and acid, otherwise the coloring matter is not adsorbed. Adsorption of the activator on charcoal will be discussed later. The charcoal filtrate is almost colorless. This fraction is termed A E P: alcoholic extract of peptone.

The A E P fraction is next treated with 30 per cent phosphotungstic acid dissolved in 5 per cent sulfuric acid. A white heavy precipitate is formed. Enough of this precipitant is added until no further precipitate forms. In order to avoid the addition of an excess of the phosphotungstic acid reagent, precipitation of the activator is best carried on in two steps. The two crops of the precipitates are collected together and washed with 5 per cent sulfuric acid. The precipitate is best separated by centrifugation. Since all the active ingredient is found in the phospho-tungstic precipitate the filtrates may be discarded. The phospho-tungstic acid is removed quantitatively by barium hydroxide in the usual manner. In order to insure the absence of barium ions from the final solution, filtration is carried out through either a Chamberland filter or a Mandler filter. The p_H of the solution should be slightly acid to litmus. This fraction is termed A E P/P; the phospho-tungstic acid precipitate of the alcoholic extract of peptone. It is almost colorless.

Butyl Alcohol Extraction.—A sample of the A E P/P fraction is extracted with twice its volume of butyl alcohol. Extraction may be carried out under a reflux condenser for two or three hours. The mixture is next transferred into a separatory funnel and allowed to stand for 24 hours. The butyl alcohol fraction may thus be removed and the aqueous residue is reextracted in a similar manner. The butyl alcohol fractions are brought together and the alcohol is distilled under vacuum. The residue is brought to dryness, dissolved in 80 per cent ethyl alcohol, filtered and brought to dryness once more. The dry residue is finally taken up in the original amount of water and sterilized by filtration through a sterile Chamberland L3 candle.

The aqueous residue of the butyl alcohol fraction is treated in a similar manner.

Each of the two fractions were tested and found to contain growth stimulating effect on microörganisms.

Ultrafiltration.—A description of the apparatus used in this investigation is reported by McBain and Kistler.[10] Number 600 cellophane membrane is used. When this membrane is

10. J. Gen Physiol. **12:** 187, 1928.

soaked in water for a few hours and used for ultrafiltration, molecules up to the size of a trisaccharide were found to be ultrafiltrable.[11] Each of the various fractions described above was ultrafiltered and the ultrafiltrates of the various fractions were collected separately, sterilized and tested. It was found that all the active ingredients were present in the ultrafiltrates. It becomes obvious from this experiment that the molecular size of the activator cannot be larger than that of a trisaccharide.

SUMMARY
OF THE CHEMICAL PROPERTIES OF PEPTONE ACTIVATOR

Peptone appears to contain at least two growth activators: A butyl soluble and a non-butyl soluble activator. The following are some of the properties studied:

BUTYL SOLUBLE ACTIVATOR

It is soluble in butyl alcohol, in water, in 80 per cent ethyl alcohol and insoluble in ether.

Its growth activation is destroyed by prolonged boiling in strong acids or alkalis.

It is precipitated by phospho-tungstic acid in acid solution.

Upon treatment with alkaline phospho-tungstate it imparts a blue color, the intensity of which is increased upon heating. Whether or not this is a specific reaction for the activator was not determined. Epinephrine and other compounds are known to produce such a reaction.

The following tests are negative: Ferric chloride, Biuret, and Sullivan. This indicates that probably it is not a ring compound, does not have a biuret linkage and does not contain a SH group. Test for sulphur is negative also.

Its nitrogen content is not a measure of its growth stimulating effect, so that in all probability the nitrogen compounds associated with it are impurities.

It is ultrafiltrable.

BUTYL INSOLUBLE ACTIVATOR

It is soluble in water, in 80 per cent alcohol but insoluble in butyl alcohol and in ether.

Its growth stimulating effect is partially destroyed by prolonged boiling in strong acids and in alkalis. This indicates that there might be more than one factor.

Adsorption experiments show that one fraction is adsorbed on charcoal in acid solution and possibly another in alkaline solutions.

Other properties are as reported above.

ACID HYDROLYSIS

In following this procedure red blood corpuscles were used as a source for the preparation of growth activator. The blood corpuscles may be hydrolyzed with either sulfuric or hydrochloric acid. In this investigation, hydrochloric acid was preferred to sulphuric acid in order to avoid the expense of using large quantities of barium hydroxide that would be required for the removal of the sulphate.

To every liter of blood corpuscles 500 cc. of concentrated hydrochloric acid is added shaking well during the addition. The mixture is heated on a boiling water bath shaking at intervals for two or three hours until the precipitated blood proteins are redissolved. The acid mixture is then boiled on a sand bath under a reflux condenser for 24 hours, transferred to an evaporating dish over a boiling water bath. By concentrating the hydrolysate in this manner to one fourth the volume, adding distilled water and reconcentrating, a considerable amount of the hydrochloric acid may be removed. To the concentrated dark mass 40 per cent sodium hydroxide is added with constant stirring until the reaction is slightly acid to litmus. It is allowed to stand over night whereupon it is filtered through a buchner filter and the precipitate thoroughly washed with boiling distilled water. The filtrates are collected and concentrated over a water bath and neutralized to litmus. After standing overnight they are filtered again and the second crop of precipitate washed as formerly. The various precipitates may be kept and large amounts of amino acids may be recovered in a crystalline state if so desired. The active principle is in the filtrate. 96 per cent alcohol is gradually added until no further precipitate forms and the

11. Sahyun, M.: J. Biol. Chem. **94:** 253, 1931.

alcoholic mixture is placed overnight in a ice box or in a refrigerator. The crystalline mass is filtered and washed carefully with cold 80 per cent alcohol. The alcoholic filtrates are collected and concentrated, the alcohol being removed under vacuum. The aqueous residue is rendered alkaline and 96 per cent ethyl alcohol is added in a similar manner to the above procedure. Another crop of crystals is recovered. The alcoholic filtrates are acidified before distilling the alcohol. The aqueous residue is transferred to an evaporating dish and concentrated over a water bath until crystals are formed, upon cooling the addition of small amounts of alcohol increases the yield. In the process of crystallization the adjustment of p_H is necessary, for it is well known that different amino acids have different isoelectric points. The removal of the various amino acids in a crystalline state by the above manipulation is repeated 6 to 7 times. (No attempts were made to identify the various amino acids recovered, but each fraction was recrystallized several times from alcohol and the filtrates added to the mother liquor. The pure amino acids thus recovered did not show any marked growth effect.) When no further amino acid crystals separate out, the residue is made up to a volume of 200 cc. It possesses a golden brown color. It is acidified to litmus and treated with activated charcoal (10 grams approximately), thoroughly stirred and placed in a refrigerator overnight. It is then filtered over a buchner filter and the charcoal washed with distilled water. The filtrate is almost colorless and very active. Nevertheless a considerable quantity of the activator is adsorbed on charcoal along with the coloring matter. The charcoal left in the buchner filter is transferred into a 400 cc. beaker and treated with hot 0.1 N sodium hydroxide until the washing is perfectly colorless. The adsorbates recovered are slightly colored pale straw and are very active. Both the adsorbates and the filtrates appear to have the same properties. When added together and concentrated to 100 cc. and tested for their growth effect a dilution of 1/1,000,000 had a remarkable effect on growth.

The butyl alcohol experiment was tried on the final extract, but no activator was found in the butyl alcohol layer. Treatment with phospho-tungstic acid showed that the activator is completely precipitated with this reagent. The addition of alkaline phospho-tungstate imparts a blue color. Oxidation with the well known oxidixing reagents completely destroys the activity of the activator. Upon ultrafiltration the activator is found in the ultrafiltrates. Other chemical and physical properties that were observed indicated that the activator of the blood hydrolysate was similar to that fraction of peptone that is insoluble in butyl alcohol.

THE EFFECT OF THE ACTIVATOR ON THE GROWTH AND METABOLISM OF COLON BACILLUS (MELVILLE SAHYUN, PAUL BEARD, E. W. SCHULTZ AND J. SNOW)

It has been recognized that colon bacillus grows readily in simple synthetic mediums. This peculiar characteristic of this microörganism lies in the fact that it has the ability to synthesize its own growth factor. Robertson[12] has shown that the filtrate of a synthetic medium in which the colon bacillus had been grown for 68 generations permitted the continued growth of yeast. As it will be shown in this investigation the growth of this microörganism is slow for at least the first 36 hours. This lag period may be explained on the grounds that a sufficient amount of the growth factor or activator has to be first produced by the microörganism before a rapid growth is attained.

In this section we shall deal with the effect of the activator on:

The rate of growth of the colon bacillus.

The carbohydrate metabolism of the colon bacillus.

The growth of the colon bacillus after it had reached its maximum population in a peptone medium.

A suggested method for the standardization of the activator.

The production of an activator by the colon bacillus.

12. J. Infect. Dis. **34:** 395, 1924.

PROCEDURE

Technic of Inoculation.—Strain No. 142 of colon bacillus (secured from the bacteriophage laboratory of this department), was used throughout. This microörganism was first cultured on an agar slant and incubated for 18 hours before using it in our various experiments. Cultures were removed by means of a straight platinum rod and introduced into sterile tubes containing 10 cc. of 0.5 per cent saline. The contents of the tube were thoroughly mixed and 1 cc. of this inoculum was transferred into another sterile test tube containing 10 cc. of saline. The object of this was to wash the organisms and to introduce the same amount of inoculum in each instance.

Bacterial Count.—The results of the various experiments in this and the following section are in terms of viable plate counts and not relative turbidity. A viable plate count was made on each flask before and after incubation at the intervals of time indicated in each experiment.

Medium.—The medium finally selected contained the following ingredients and was termed No. 12. An improvement was made in the medium used in the last few experiments and will be discussed later. The ingredients were of the purest chemicals available.

MEDIUM NO. 12

Ammonium sulfate	4.716 grams
Glucose	2.000 grams
....	
Sodium chloride	5.000 grams
M/5 $KH_2 PO_4$	100.0 cc.
1 N NaOH	16.4 cc.
0.5 per cent Mixture of $MgCl_2-FeCl_2-CaCl_2$	1.0 cc.

Final Volume = 1 liter
*p*H = 7.6
Nitrogen = 1 mg. per 1 cc.

Whenever a nitrogen free medium was used, the ammonium sulfate was entirely omitted.

In preparing the medium the ammonium sulfate, glucose and sodium chloride were first dissolved in ammonia free distilled water to make up a volume of 600 cc. The remaining ingredients were then slowly added while shaking the container, and made up to a volume of 1 liter. It was then filtered and sterilized by autoclaving.

Activator.—The activator was prepared as previously described in section I. Additional data on nitrogen content of the various fractions are found in this paper.

The determination of glucose and total nitrogen were according to Sahyun's[13] and Cole's[14] methods, respectively.

EXPERIMENTAL

Exper. 1.—In this experiment the nitrogen content of the various fractions of the peptone activator are presented. Each of the data reported represent the average of three analyses.

	Total Nitrogen percent
Difco Peptone (Theoretical value)	16.520
Difco Peptone (Actual analysis)	16.404
A E P/P: Phospho-tungstic acid Precipitate of the alcoholic extract of peptone	0.825
Ultrafiltrate of A E P/P	0.720
A E P/P After filtration through activated charcoal (Norit) at *p*H 5.8	0.420
Butyl soluble fraction of A E P/P	0.150
Butyl insoluable fraction A E P/P	0.660

13. Unpublished.

14. Practical Physiological Chem., 8th Edition, 386. Cole, S. W., Heffer & Sons, Ltd. publishers, Cambridge, England.

Exper. 2.—In this experiment a comparative study of the effect of the various fractions of the peptone activator and that of peptone on the growth of the colon bacillus was investigated. The amount of each fraction added into 100 cc. of the synthetic medium No. 12 contained approximately 1 mg. N. The purpose of this is to show that the stimulation of growth is not due to the nitrogenous content of the various fractions of the activator. Peptone was used as a standard and the amount of peptone was based on its nitrogen content. A control containing 100 cc. of the synthetic medium and the microörganisms was performed. The results are found in table 1.

TABLE 1.—*The Effects of the Various Fractions of the Peptone Activators and of Peptone Based on their Respective Nitrogen Contents on the Growth of the Colon Bacillus. Each Flask Contained 100 cc. of Medium No. 12 Containing 1 mg. N. per 1 cc. The Initial Number of Microörganisms was 100,000 per 1 cc.*

Sample No.	Material	Activator Nitrogen	Total Nitrogen	Population of the colon bacillus at 24 hours
1	Control	—	100	350,000
2	$\frac{AEP}{P}$	1	101	550,000,000
3	Butyl soluble	0.15	100.15	450,000,000
4	Butyl insoluble	0.7	100.7	500,000,000
	Acid Charcoal Filtrate of $\frac{AEP}{P}$	1.0	101	470,000,000
6	Acid Charcoal Adsorbate $\frac{AEP}{P}$	1.0	101	510,000,000
7	Ultrafiltrate of $\frac{AEP}{P}$	1.0	101	450,000,000
8	Peptone	1.65	101.65	200,000,000
In the following 100 cc. of 0.5 per cent saline was substituted for medium No. 12.				
9	A E P	1.64	1.64	10,000,000
10	Peptone	1.65	1.65	40,000,000

Exper. 3.—The data from the foregoing are further supported in this experiment and the ability of the activating substance to maintain effect over a long period of time is demonstrated. The "constant flow chamber" described by Cleary, Beard and Clifton[15] provides for continual renewal of food from a reservoir into culture chamber and the simultaneous elinimation of an equal amount of fluid from the chamber, thus holding to a minimum the accumulation of metabolites. This device was set up in duplicate, using 1.0 per cent peptone as medium, labeled A and B, and their populations allowed to reach a stable level. Activator to the amount of 10.0 cc. per liter was added to one reservoir and its effect watched by population counts. At intervals the position of the reservoirs was changed, A reservoir to B culture flask, or the reverse as the case might be. The rise and fall of the populations following the change demonstrate the accelerating effect. The data follow.

TABLE 2.—*Constant Flow Experiment Duplicate Culture Flasks A and B Inoculated 5/3/34*

Date	Bacteria per cc. "A"	"B"
5/7	1,130,000,000	1,140,000,000
5/7 Activator added to "A" 10 cc. per liter.		
5/9	1,730,000,000	1,010,000,000
5/10	2,980,000,000	980,000,000
After count of 5/10 reservoir "A" changed to "B" position and "B" to "A".		
5/12	1,460,000,000	1,400,000,000
5/17	1,000,000,000	2,480,000,000
5/19	720,000,000	2,720,000,000
5/21	750,000,000	2,590,000,000
After count of 5/21 "A" and "B" returned to original positions.		
5/24	2,150,000,000	750,000,000
5/24 After count rate of flow decreased from 3 drops to 1 drop per minute.		
5/28	2,130,000,000	540,000,000*
5/29	2,030,000,000	670,000,000

* Effect of metabolites resulting from decreased rate of flow probably explains low level of populations.

15. J. Bact. **29:** 205, 1935.

Exper. 4.—Herein we demonstrate the effect of the activator on the growth of the colon bacillus with particular reference to its carbohydrate and nitrogen metabolism. Immediately after the addition of the activator A E P/P in the various dilutions as shown in the table and inoculation, samples were removed, filtered through a sterile Chamberland L-3 candle and glucose and nitrogen determinations were performed on the filtrate in duplicate sets. Each flask contained 100 cc. of the medium No. 12. To a control flask 1 cc. of the inoculum was added to 100 cc. of the medium. The results are as follows:

TABLE 3.—*The Effect of the Activator A E P/P on the Growth and Glucose and Nitrogen Metabolism of the Colon Bacillus*

No.	Activator: Amount cc.	Activator: Time days	Total: Nitrogen per 100 cc. mg	Total: Glucose per 100 cc. mg	Population of the colon bacillus per 1 cc.
	1.0	0	97.4	195	60,000
		1	92.7	6	1,000,000,000
		2	92.0	—	650,000,000
2	0.2	0	98.8	194	60,000
		1	95.4	50	650,000,000
		2	95.4	—	240,000,000
3	0.1	0	97.4	195	60,000
		1	93.3	65	450,000,000
		2	93.3	—	340,000,000
4	Control (none)	0	99.0	195	60,000
		1	99.5	194	160,000
		2	99.0	190	1,100,000

STANDARDIZATION OF THE ACTIVATOR

The following method is suggested for the determination of the strength of the unknown activator in solution. If the activator is contaminated with large amounts of impurities, the method is not suitable. As a standard any well known medium might be used, but it would be preferable to adopt a standard medium, a standard synthetic medium and a standard microorganism. In this experiment, Martin's broth was selected since in the laboratory this medium is used for the standardization of bacteriophage and is prepared in large lots of uniform strength. Martin's broth is prepared and sterilized in tubes containing 9 cc. each. For our purposes, the synthetic medium No. 12 containing 1 mg. nitrogen as ammonium sulphate per 1 cc. and colon bacillus strain No. 142 were taken as the other standards. The synthetic medium was also prepared and sterilized in tubes containing 9 cc. each.

Procedure.—One cc. of the unknown activator is introduced into 9 cc. of the synthetic medium and thoroughly mixed by means of a sterile pipette. The first tube is, therefore, dilution 1:10. One cc. of this dilution is removed by the same pipette and introduced into another 9 cc. of the same medium. The pipette is discarded and another sterile pipette is used for mixing. The second tube contains the activator in dilution 1:100. The same procedure is continued until the desired final dilution is reached. Next, the washed microörganisms are introduced as quantitatively as possible (approximately 1,000,000 bacteria per test tube). Martin's broth is treated in a similar manner using medium No. 12 for dilutions. The tubes are incubated and readings are taken at 2, 6, 12 and 24 hours after incubation. The turbidity of the standard was used as basis for judging the relative rate of growth. The unknowns referred to in table 4 consist of the peptone activator A E P/P and the final filtrate of the blood hydrolysate (see section I). The scale for measuring the turbidity due to the growth of colon bacillus is as follows:

4 plus .... heavy growth
3 plus .... very good growth
2 plus .... good growth
1 plus .... fair growth
(*d*) .... doubtful
— .... no growth

Standardization of the Activator

Material for Standardization	Time in hours	Dilutions 1	10^{-1}	10^{-2}	10^{-3}	10^{-4}	10^{-5}	10^{-6}	10^{-7}
Martin's (Standard)	2	—	—	—	—	—	—	—	—
	4	+++	++	+	—	—	—	—	—
	6	+++	+++	++	++	—	—	—	—
	12	+++	+++	+++	++	+	—	—	—
	24	++++	+++	+++	++	++	—	—	—
Peptone activator $\frac{AEP}{P}$	2		—	—	—	—	—	—	—
	4		+++	+++	++	+	—	—	—
	6		+++	+++	++	+	—	—	—
	12		++++	++++	+++	+	—	—	—
	24		++++	++++	+++	++	+	—	—
Blood hydrolysate activator	2		++	+	(*d*)	—	—	—	—
	4		++++	+++	+++	++	(*d*)	—	—
	6		++++	++++	+++	++	+	—	—
	12		++++	++++	++++	+++	++	+	—
	24		++++	++++	++++	+++	++	++	—

ISOLATION OF THE COLON BACILLUS ACTIVATOR

The following is a description of the method used for the isolation of the colon bacillus:

A flask containing the improved synthetic medium was inoculated with the washed microorganisms and incubated for 10 days. At the end of that time the organisms were removed by filtration through a Chamberland filter. The volume of the colon bacillus filtrate was concentrated to about 50 cc. under reduced pressure. By so doing the development of a brown color was avoided. The concentrated filtrate was next treated with activated charcoal and kept in a refrigerator over night. The following day it was filtered and the charcoal was washed with cold distilled water. The charcoal remaining in the filter was next treated with hot 0.1 N sodium hydroxide and filtered while hot. It was washed several times with the hot dilute alkali. The charcoal filtrates were collected and concentrated under reduced pressure. Five times the volume of the concentrate of 96 per cent ethyl alcohol was added and the mixture was slightly acidified until no further precipitate could be formed. After standing for a few hours filtration becomes very rapid. The alcoholic filtrate of the adsorbate was brought to dryness under vacuum and then taken up with distilled water, filtered and sterilized. The final solution contained most of the activator.

The following results demonstrate the effect of the various fractions of the colon bacillus filtrate on its growth in a synthetic medium.

TABLE 4.—*The Effect of the Various Fractions of the Colon Bacillus Filtrate on its Growth*

Material	Amount used cc.	Time hrs.	Population of Colon Bacillus per 1 cc.
Concentrate*	1	0	150,000
The colon bacillus filtrate		18	540,000,000
Charcoal filtrate of 1	1	0	150,000
		18	60,000,000
Charcoal adsorbate of 1	1	0	150,000
		18	600,000,000
Alcohol soluble fraction of the adsorbate 3	1	0	150,000
		18	590,000,000
Precipitate of the alcoholic extract of the adsorbate 3	1	0	150,000
		18	950,000

* The original amount of the filtrate after 10 days incubation was 500 cc. This was concentrated to 50 cc. In each succeeding step, the amount was kept at 50 cc.

DISCUSSION

The behavior and properties of a growth activating substance isolated from peptone have been described, and a method of evaluating it quantitatively developed. The substance has been obtained in a relatively pure form, but has probably not yet been prepared in its ultimate state of purity.

Various fractions based upon butyl alcohol solubility, precipitability by phospho-tungstic acid and ability to be adsorbed on activated carbon have been studied. These fractions differ in their nitrogen content but show no real difference in their effect on bacterial growth.

Marked effects upon early rates of growth in synthetic mediums, and somewhat less pronounced effects on rates in routine peptone media have been observed, and it is further shown that these are not due to utilization of the active principle as nutritive substance. The difference in purity of the various fractions is shown by the difference in bacterial growth when portions of activator are presented to the colon bacillus as sole sources of nitrogen. The activating effect is not destroyed by growth in mediums containing the activator. On the contrary it is shown that the microörganism actually synthesizes the substance and that it can be demonstrated to occur in increased amount in a synthetic medium devoid of amino acids. It can be isolated from the filtrate of such mediums by procedures similar to those employed for isolation from peptone.

THE EFFECT OF CERTAIN AMINO ACIDS ON THE GROWTH OF THE COLON BACILLUS (MELVILLE SAHYUN, PAUL BEARD, E. W. SCHULTZ, J. SNOW AND E. CROSS)

Simultaneously with our studies on the growth stimulating factors for microörganisms and their influence on the rate of growth, if was found desirable to consider the influence of certain amino acids on the growth of the colon bacillus.

In 1919, Koser and Rettger[16] studied comprehensively the effect of a large number of amino acids on the growth of microörganisms and reported that there was no marked difference in the availability of the different amino acids to the microörganisms they investigated. Since then several investigators have added valuable contributions to this subject. In 1926, Gordon and M'Leod[17] classified the amino acids they studied into three groups, with respect to their effect on the growth of certain bacteria: (a) Those indifferent towards growth, (b) those favoring growth and (c) those that are inhibitory. The results of these investigators may be objected to on the basis that fairly large amounts of amino acids were used and that peptone and not a simple synthetic medium was employed. Recently Mueller, Klise, Porter and Graybel[18] reported that tryptophane and cystine were apparently essential for the growth of a certain strain of the diphtheria bacillus. In an investigation on the nitrogen requirements of B. typhosus Fildes, Gladstone and Knight[19] reported that tryptophane was probably essential to the growth of these microorganisms. Burrows[20] studied the requirements of Cl. botulinum and found

16. J. Infect. Dis. **24:** 301, 1919.
17. J. Path. & Bact. **29:** 13, 1926.
18. J. Bact. **25:** 59, 1933.
19. Brit. J. Exper. Path. **14:** 189, 1933.
20. J. Infect. Dis. **54:** 164, 1934.

that tryptophane and cystine possessed growth stimulating effect. Prior to Burrows investigation, Hosaya and Kishino[21] had reported that they were able to grow Cl. botulinum on a gelatin medium which contained no tryptophane.

The effect of amino acids on the growth of microörganisms may be due to three factors: (a) The availability of the nitrogen and carbon of the amino acids, (b) the inability of the organisms to synthesize a certain amino acid which is essential to its protein constituent and (c) the influence of a certain group of amino acids on growth. In an investigation on infusoria (paramecium and ameba) Hammet[22] reported that sulfhydryl compounds stimulate the rate of cell division, but that the oxidation products of these compounds such as the sulfoxide, sulfonate and sulfinate retard growth.

In this investigation we report our findings on the influence of certain amino acids on the growth of the colon bacillus in a simple synthetic medium and present also a comparison between the influence of certain amino acids and that of the growth activator on growth.

GENERAL PROCEDURE

The synthetic medium No. 12 employed contains the same ingredients as the one described in the preceding section. Whenever a nitrogen free medium was required the ammonium sulfate was entirely omitted. It was sterilized by autoclaving. The same strain of the colon bacillus was used and the technic of inoculation and bacterial count are as previously described.

All the amino acids studied are of Eastman's products. Amino acids that are sparingly soluble in water were first dissolved in either 0.1 N HCl or 0.1 N NaOH. Sterilization of solutions of amino acids was accomplished by filtration through a sterile Chamberland candle L-3. Heat sterilization of the amino acids such as boiling or autoclaving was avoided for fear that some of the amino acids might undergo a chemical change as is the case with cystine and tryptophane.

EXPERIMENTAL

Exper. 1.—In this experiment the effect of amino acids on the growth of the colon bacillus was investigated. Flasks of approximate size (capacity 200 cc.) containing 50 cc. of the sterile medium were employed. Two synthetic mediums were used: One contained 1 mg. N as ammonium sulfate and the other was ammonium sulfate nitrogen free but identical in every other respect. Bacterial count was performed immediately after inoculation and at 16 and 24 hours, respectively, after incubation. In some experiments 3 day old cultures of the colon bacillus were used. The results are recorded in order to show the difference between the use of an 18 hour culture and an old culture. Old cultures are unreliable and in this we confirm the earlier findings of Koser and Rettger.[16] Some of the amino acids that were observed to produce a considerable influence on the rate of growth of the colon bacillus were studied separately and the results are reported in tables 7 and 8. The results of this experiment are found in table 5.

About 100,000 organisms per 1 cc. were introduced into each flask.

Exper. 2.—A reference has been made to the improved medium No. 12. During the course of this investigation it was observed that the addition of a special phosphate buffer to the synthetic medium already prepared brought about a higher population. The special phosphate consisted in neutralizing 5 cc. of concentrated phosphoric acid (C. P.) with 2 N sodium hydroxide and incorporating it in two liters of medium No. 12 (this phosphate is additional to the buffer already found in the medium). The effect of this special phosphate on the increased population of the colon bacillus is clearly demonstrated in the following table, where not only the effect of amino acids but that of the activator also were studied on the rate of growth of the colon bacillus.

---

21. Scient. Rep. Gov. Inst. Infect. Dis. **4:** 123, 1925.
22. Protoplasma **7:** 297, 1929.

The effect of certain amino acids on the rate of growth of the colon bacillus in a buffered medium with and without nitrogen. The nitrogen in the medium is in the form of ammonium sulfate—1 mg. N per 1 cc. 50 cc. of the medium were used for each test.

TABLE 5.—*The Effect of Amino Acids on the Growth of the Colon Bacillus*

Amino acids	Amount per 100 cc.	Time	Age of culture	Population Medium No. 12	
				No ammonium sulfate nitrogen	Nitrogen as ammonium sulfate
				Number of organisms per 1 cc.	Number of organisms per 1 cc.
	mg	hrs.	hrs.		
Glycine	40	16	18	125,000	1,800,000
		24		150,000	37,000,000
		16	72		100,000,000
		24			800,000,000
d-l Alanine	40	16	18	180,000	2,000,000
		24		300,000	11,000,000
		16	72		4,000,000
		24			100,000,000
d-l Leucine	40	16	18	600,000	5,000,000
		24		1,200,000	45,000,000
		16	72		60,000,000
		24			100,000,000
α-Amino-caproic	40	16	18	120,000	230,000
		24		50,000	330,000
α-Amino-isobutyric acid		16	18	100,000	3,000,000
		24		100,000	21,000,000
l-Proline	40	16	18	300,000	6,500,000
		24		450,000	480,000,000
		16	72		1,400,000
		24			45,000,000
d-l Valine	40	16	18	130,000	2,000,000
		24		180,000	25,000,000
Amino-phenyl Acetic acid	40	16	18		390,000
		24			1,200,000
Phenyl-alanine	40	16	18	180,000	430,000
		24		200,000	1,300,000
d-Arginine-hydrochloride	40	16	18	1,175,000	1,000,000
		24		1,150,000	21,000,000
Lysine-hydrochloride	40	16	18	900,000	3,000,000
		24		1,000,000	11,000,000
di-iodo tyrosine	40	16	18	30,000	1,500,000
		24		50,000	1,700,000
Amino-caprylic	40	16	18	67,000	2,000,000
		24		210,000	21,000,000
Amino-valeric acid	40	16	18	50,000	270,000
		24		340,000	3,000,000
Control	none	16	18		200,000
		24			400,000

Exper. 3.—In studying the effect of cystine on the rate of growth of the colon bacillus considerable difficulties were encountered on account of the extreme insolubility of this amino acid in water. In view of Hammet's conception of the influence of the SH group of certain organic compounds and that of its oxidation products on the rate of cell-division in the infusoria we investigated the effect of the following compounds on the rate of growth of the colon bacillus:

Cysteine	= R-S-H	Sulfhydryl
Cystine	= R-S-S-R	Disulfide
Cysteic acid	= $R\text{-}SO_2OH$	Sulfinate
Taurine	= $R\text{-}SO_2H$	Sulfonate

As we were unable to obtain satisfactory results with cystine without resorting to a considerable quantity of alkali to bring it into solution, it was decided to treat this amino acid in a small amount of 0.1 N NaOH and heat it to boiling until the crystalline material went into

TABLE 6.—*The Effect of a Special Phosphate Buffer on the Population of the Colon Bacillus. Each Flask Contained 50 cc. of the Medium*

Amino acids or activator	Amount	Time	Population	
			Special phosphate improved No. 12	Original No. 12
	mg.	hrs.	per 1 cc.	per 1 cc.
Glutamic acid	50	0	90,000	90,000
		24	660,000,000	94,000,000
Aspartic acid	50	0	90,000	90,000
		24	123,000,000	32,000,000
Asparagine	50	0	90,000	90,000
		24	230,000,000	185,000,000
Activator $\frac{AEP}{P}$	1 cc.	0	240,000	240,000
		16	1,000,000,000	720,000,000
		24	1,200,000,000	600,000,000
Control	(None)	0	90,000	90,000
		24	660,000	250,000

Note: The amino acids were chosen at random.

solution. In this connection may we bring into attention the fact that by so doing a certain amount of cystine is probably reduced to cysteine as was demonstrated by the investigation of Shimohara and Kilpatrick.[23] Bearing this in mind the stimulating effect of amino acid thus treated on the growth of the colon bacillus is probably due to its reduced form.

The results of the effect of these four related compounds are shown in the following table.

TABLE 7.—*The Effect of Cysteine, Cystine, Cysteic Acid and Taurine on the Growth of the Colon Bacillus in the Synthetic Medium No. 12*

Nature of compound	Amount per 50 cc.	Time hrs.	Population per 1 cc.
Cystine (Not boiled) (RS-SR)	20	0	150,000
		16	1,700,000
		24	1,600,000
Cystine (Boiled in 0.1 N NaOH for 15 minutes)	20	0	60,000
		16	5,000,000
		24	85,000,000
Cysteine (R-S-H)	20	0	40,000
		16	21,000,000
		24	230,000,000
Cysteic Acid ($R\text{-}SO_2OH$)	20	0	150,000
		24	550,000
Taurine ($R\text{-}SO_2H$)	20	0	100,000
		24	9,600,000

Exper. 4.—The following amino acids: Cysteine, glutamic acid, aspartic acid, asparagine, tryptophane, tyrosine and histidine, were investigated further with respect to the influence of the various amounts used in each on the rate of growth of the colon bacillus. The data presented in table 8 are self-explanatory.

Exper. 5.—Although we have shown the influence of the activator and that of the various available amino acids on the growth of the colon bacillus, a doubt might still exist as to what we call an activator. The effect of such an activator might be due to that of a mixture of amino acids on the growth of the microörganism in question. Therefore, in order to dispel any doubt lingering in our minds as to the true existance of an activator, a comparative study of the effects of the most suitable amino acids and of the activator on the rate of growth of the colon bacillus was undertaken. This was done with particular reference to the early logarithmic growth phase.

23. J. Biol. Chem. **105:** 241, 1934.

TABLE 8.—*The Influence of Various Amounts of each Amino Acid on the Rate of Growth of the Colon Bacillus. The Amounts Indicated are Mg. per 100 cc. of the Improved Medium No. 12. The Number of Microörganizms Introduced into each Flask of 100 cc. was Approximately 100,000 per 1 cc.*

Amino acid	Amount mg.	Time	Population at 24 hrs. per 1 cc.
Cysteine	10		20,000,000
	20		40,000,000
	40		90,000,000
	50		150,000,000
	100		10,000,000
	200		350,000
Glutamic acid	10		3,000,000
	20		5,000,000
	40		18,000,000
	60		45,000,000
	100		135,000,000
	200		200,000,000
Aspartic acid	10		36,000,000
	40		63,000,000
	100		75,000,000
	200		300,000,000
Asparagine	10		27,000,000
	20		60,000,000
	30		90,000,000
	40		100,000,000
	100		270,000,000
	200		400,000,000
Tryptophane	10		20,000,000
	20		38,000,000
	40		60,000,000
	100		100,000,000
Tyrosine	10		50,000,000
	40		120,000,000
	60		50,000,000
	100		30,000,000
Histidine	10		18,000,000
	40		60,000,000
	60		250,000,000
	100		400,000,000

The amino acids that showed the greatest stimulating effect on the growth of the colon bacillus were selected along with a few others in order to make the medium as comparable as possible to a protein hydrolysate. They are as follows: Alanine, arginine, histidine, glutamic acid, aspartic acid, tyrosine, tryptophane, asparagine, proline and cysteine. The amount of each amino acid added was as determined in experiment 4.

The details of the experiment are as follows:

A. Into a flask of 100 cc. of the sterile medium No. 12 containing 1 mg. N as ammonium sulfate the above mentioned amino acids were added.

A^1. Into another flask containing the same ingredients as in A, 1 cc. of the activator was introduced.

B. In this experiment the amino acids were introduced into the synthetic medium that did not contain any sulfate nitrogen.

B^1. In this experiment the same ingredients as in B were used and in addition 1 cc. of the activator.

C. The purpose of this control experiment was to show the slow rate of growth of the colon bacillus in the synthetic medium containing the ammonium sulfate nitrogen only.

C^1. The same ingredients as in C were used and in addition 1 cc. of the activator.

One cc. of the activator used in the above experiments contained approximately 1 mg. nitrogen.

A viable plate count was made immediately after inoculation, 1.5, 3, 5, 6, 7 and 8 hours respectively. The results are expressed in terms of $\log_{10}$ and are found in the accompanying figure.

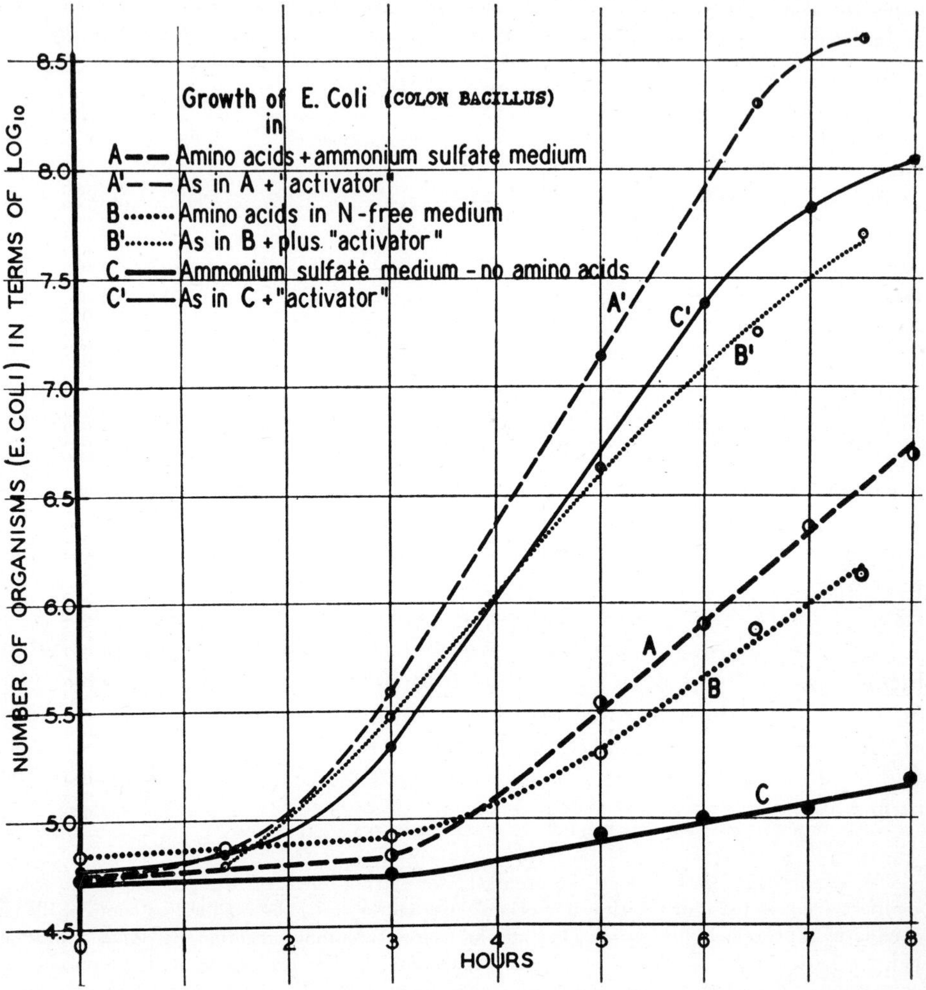

DISCUSSION

The ability of the colon bacillus to utilize 20 different amino acids with and without a supplementary source of nitrogen in the form of ammonium sulfate has been investigated.

There is obviously a wide diversity in the utilization of these as evidenced by the crop yields after equal time intervals. The rate of utilization of the individual amino acids is shown to vary greatly. This might be construed as evidence that the amino acid serves at least in some cases a function aside from that of a mere nitrogen source. It is also shown that the age of inoculum may be related to the rate of consumption of certain of the amino acids, i.e., some acids seemed to be taken up with greater avidity by old cultures than by young, in other instances the reverse was apparent.

These studies also indicate superior growth in an amino-acid-ammonium sulfate mixture than in mediums containing either animo nitrogen or ammonium sulfate nitrogen alone, even though the total nitrogen of the mediums were the same. This may be interpreted as evidence that certain of the amino acids are incorporated intact or partially intact into the protoplasmic synthesis, although as is known, synthesis of the full amino acid complement from strictly inorganic sources can be effected.

Further when the activator, previously described, was added to any of these three mediums in amounts of 1.0 cc. of activator to 100 cc. of medium (1.0 mg. N/cc. activator) striking accelerations of growth were demonstrable in every instance. This again demonstrates the rôle of activator in the growth of the colon bacillus. The enormous effect on the rate of protoplasmic synthesis can hardly be accounted for on a basis of nutrition from the 1.0 mg. of nitrogen included in the activator material.

It is also brought out that while in most instances crop yield was increased with increase of amino nitrogen, there were critical concentrations for maximum growth with the acids cysteine and tyrosine. Growth steadily increased up to this threshold but dropped so sharply beyond this limit as to suggest a toxic effect.

This is of particular interest in considering the reports concerning the rôle of the SH group in certain compounds on cell division. These studies have indicated that cysteine (R-S-H) is responsible for the stimulating effect. Taurine, cysteic acid, and cystine failed to exhibit any such effect.

During the progress of these studies a new type of phosphate buffer formed by the neutralization of phosphoric acid with sodium hydroxide was developed and demonstrated to have a decidedly superior effect over that of the conventional phosphate type of buffer. More rapid rates of growth and greater crop yields were observed when this was used in addition to the buffer already present.

SUMMARY

Two different methods are described for the preparation of a growth stimulating factor for microörganisms from organic materials such as peptone and blood.

Extraction with 80 per cent alcohol.—By following this method the growth stimulating factor or activator (as it is termed by the authors), appeared to contain two principles, (1) a butyl soluble fraction and (2) a butyl insoluble fraction. Both fractions were observed to be ultrafiltrable through cellophane membrane No. 600, which allows molecules up to the size of a trisaccharide to pass through only. This is an indication that the molecular size of the growth factor investigated cannot be larger than that of a trisaccharide.

Acid hydrolysis.—The second procedure was based on hydrolyzing the blood in 25 per cent hydrochloric acid for 19 hours. The amino acids were then removed by repeated crystallization. The final product obtained contained a highly active growth factor that had the ability to stimulate growth in dilution of 1/1,000,000. This activator was butyl insoluble.

The effect of these activators was studied on the growth of the colon bacillus. They were observed to possess a great acceleration of carbohydrate consumption in synthetic mediums. The effect on the growth curve was marked by an acceleration of the rate of growth, an increase in the population of the colon bacillus in a 1 per cent peptone medium after the microörganisms had reached their maximum population.

The colon bacillus was shown to possess the faculty to produce its own activator in a synthetic medium. A method is described for the isolation of the colon bacillus activator.

The ability of the colon bacillus to utilize amino acids and amino acid-like substances was also investigated. A considerable variation in the rate of utilization of the various amino acids was noted. In the case of cysteine it was shown that the SH group of this amino acid was responsible for the stimulation of growth. The amino acids that had a marked effect on the growth of the colon bacillus are as follows: Cysteine, glutamic acid, aspartic acid, asparagine, tryptophane, tyrosine, histidine and proline. High concentrations of cysteine and tyrosine were observed to retard the rate of growth of the microörganisms.

A comparison between the effect of the most influential amino acids and that of the activator on the rate of growth of the colon bacillus was also investigated.

STUDIES ON THE EXTRACTION OF A PRECIPITABLE SUBSTANCE FROM THE GENUS BRUCELLA

DOROTHY O. REITER

CHICAGO

The genus Brucella, or Alcaligenes, is composed of three commonly recognized varieties or species, the melitensis, the abortus, and the suis. These varieties, although closely related morphologically, biochemically, and serologically, differ somewhat in glucose, nitrogen, and sulfur metabolism, sensitivity to dyes, and pathogenicity.

McAlpine and Slanetz[1] studied the metabolic activity of representative cultures and found that abortus strains of bovine origin could be separated from abortus strains of porcine and human origin and from melitensis strains on the basis of their nitrogen and glucose metabolism. Huddleson[2] separated the genus into three distinct groups or species according to the time and rate of H_2S production. McAlpine and Slanetz[3] have shown that CO_2 stimulates the growth of the bovine strains, but partially inhibits the growth of the other varieties.

Differences have been observed among the strains when grown on the various dye mediums; the dye plate method of Huddleson[2] or the semi-solid method of Meyer and Zobell.[4] By their growth differences on these mediums, strains can be classified into three varieties, the melitensis, the abortus, and the suis.

Slight differences have been observed in the pathogenicity of the various strains for monkeys. Fleischner, Vecki, Shaw, and Meyer[5] found melitensis strains more pathogenic than abortus strains. Huddleson and Hallman[6] observed that suis strains were the most invasive and like Fleischner and his collaborators reported that melitensis strains were more pathogenic than those of the abortus variety.

Various serological studies have been made of the members of this genus. By direct agglutination no appreciable differences are observed between the varieties but, by agglutination absorption the genus can be divided into two varieties, the melitensis and the abortus; agglutination absorption does not differentiate the bovine and porcine varieties. Reciprocal agglutination absorption studies show the close relationship of the strains. Evans[7] found that

Received for publication, May 21, 1935.

From the Department of Hygiene and Bacteriology, The University of Chicago.

1. J. Infect. Dis. **42:** 66 and 73, 1928.
2. Undulant Fever Symposium, New York, American Public Health Association, 1929, p. 18.
3. J. Infect. Dis. **43:** 232, 1928.
4. J. Infect. Dis. **51:** 72, 1932.
5. J. Infect. Dis. **29:** 663, 1921.
6. J. Infect. Dis. **45:** 293, 1929.
7. Studies on Brucella (Alkaligenes) Melitensis, Hyg. Lab. Bull. 143, 1925.

strains of the abortus variety absorbed 87.5 per cent of the agglutinins from serum of the melitensis A variety and that the reciprocal relationship was the same. Futamura's[8] absorption tests likewise show the close relationship between the abortus and melitensis varieties.

Few attempts have been made to study the chemical nature of the varieties of the genus Brucella. Favilli and Biancalani[9] obtained polysaccharides of the immunological behavior of incomplete antigens from melitensis and paramelitensis strains, but failed to isolate a polysaccharide from the abortus strain. Their failure to isolate a polysaccharide from the abortus variety is interesting in view of the close morphological, biochemical, and serological relationship of the members of this genus.

Because of the close relationship between the varieties of the genus Brucella, a study was made of the alcohol insoluble antigenic substance of representative melitensis, abortus, and suis strains. The strains were obtained from the National Institute of Health through the courtesy of Dr. Geo. W. McCoy. Strains 456 and 428 have been used by the National Institute of Health as type strains of the abortus and melitensis varieties. Strain 41–1, porcine abortus, was more recently isolated.[10]

The strains were tested for their reaction on dye mediums, using Meyer's semi-solid method. Table 1 summarizes the results.

TABLE 1.—*Bacteriostatic Action of Dyes*

Dye	Strain		
	A456	S41–1	M428
Fuchsin	+	0	+++
Pyronine	+++	0	+++
Thionine	0	+++	+++
Methyl violet	0	0	+

+ = growth.
0 = no growth.

The results of the direct agglutination tests using living antigens, organisms grown on glycerol liver infusion agar for forty-eight hours at 37 C., are summarized in table 2.

TABLE 2.—*Direct Agglutination Tests*

Strain	Dilution of serum						
	80	160	320	640	1280	2560	Control
			Serum A456				
A456	++++	++++	++++	++++	+	0	0
S41–1	++++	++++	++++	++++	+	0	0
M428	++++	++++	++++	++	0	0	0
			Serum S41–1				
A456	++++	++++	++++	++++	+++	0	0
S41–1	++++	++++	++++	++++	+++	0	0
M428	++++	++++	++++	+++	+	0	0
			Serum M428				
A456	++++	++++	++++	++	±	0	0
S41–1	++++	++++	++++	+++	±	0	0
M428	++++	++++	++++	+++	0	0	0

8. J. Japanese Soc. Vet. Sc. **3:** 127, 1924.

9. Sperimentale, Arch. di biol. **86:** 357, 1932.

10. These strains are designated respectively as A456 (abortus type), M428 (Melitensis), and S41–1 (suis).

Table 2 shows that strain M428 did not agglutinate to so high a titer as the other strains with the heterologous serums, and that it did not stimulate quite so rapid an immuue response in animals. The animals all had been immunized in the same way.

This change in antigenicity is interesting, since the results of agglutination studies performed two years previously showed no difference in the height of the titer when this strain was tested with heterologous serums.

By agglutination absorption, strains A456 and S41–1 partially absorbed the agglutinins from serum M428 and completely exhausted A456 and S41–1 serums of agglutinins. Strain M428 likewise partially removed the agglutinins from serums A456 and S41–1 and completely exhausted serum M428 of agglutinins.

All the strains formed homogeneous suspensions in saline and did not spontaneously agglutinate.

MORPHOLOGICAL CHARACTERISTICS OF THE STRAINS

Due to the fact that two of the strains, A456 and M428, were older laboratory cultures, a study was made of the colony morphology of the organisms. Henry,[11] Gwatkin,[12] McAlpine, Plastridge and Brigham,[13] and Plastridge and McAlpine[14] have shown that variants occur in the brucella group which differ from the ordinary form in colony morphology, biochemical activity, glucose utilization, and serology.

The strains were grown in veal infusion broth and glycerol liver infusion broth, streaked on the corresponding agar mediums and the colonies examined with the colony microscope.

In veal infusion broth the strains caused a slight clouding of the medium with no surface ring or pellicle and slight or no sediment in forty-eight hours at 37 C. After incubation for two weeks at 37 C. the strains produced a slight ring and sediment.

In glycerol liver infusion broth the strains likewise caused an even clouding of the medium with slight or no sediment. After two weeks' incubation strains A456 and S41–1 produced a pellicle and a heavier viscid sediment. Strain M428 produced a ring and a slight sediment. In spite of the pellicle and sediment, the broth remained turbid.

Strains A456 and S41–1 on veal infusion agar and glycerol liver infusion agar produced colonies of practically uniform size, smooth, and glistening. Strain M428, however, produced colonies of two sizes, large and small. The smaller colonies were clearer and more transparent and could readily be observed only with a colony microscope after seventy-two hours' growth.

Transfers made from the larger colonies to veal infusion broth showed a slight clouding in twenty-four hours. Transfers made from the smaller colonies seldom showed an appreciable clouding before forty-eight hours. Transfers from such broth cultures to veal infusion agar or glycerol liver infusion

11. Proc. Soc. Exper. Biol. & Med. **26:** 101, 1928.
12. Canad. Pub. Health J. **23:** 485, 1933.
13. J. Infect. Dis. **45:** 485, 1929.
14. J. Infect. Dis. **46:** 315, 1930.

agar showed no marked differences in colony size after forty-eight hours' incubation. However, when transfers were made to veal infusion agar or glycerol liver infusion agar slants, incubated forty-eight hours, kept in the ice box for a short time and replated, two colony types were again discernible. The colony types did not seem to be stable forms, but rather seemed to revert from one to the other upon subsequent transfer. The larger and smaller colonies were tested bacteriostatically, but no differences were observed in their reactions on the dye mediums. The strain was not spontanaously agglutinable, was serologically active, and was therefore used for extraction purposes. Several more recently isolated strains of the different varieties were likewise grown in broth and streaked on veal infusion agar and glycerol liver infusion agar. Colonies of two sizes were observed. McAlpine, Plastridge and Brigham[13] likewise observed large and small colonies on liver infusion agar. Henry[11] reported the occurrence of two colony types, the opaque and the transparent, on plates made from twenty-three stock cultures.

EXTRACTION OF PRECIPITABLE SUBSTANCE

The method used for extracting a precipitable substance from the varieties of the genus Brucella was similar to that used by Furth and Landsteiner[15] in obtaining a precipitable substance from the bacilli of the salmonella group and consisted of alcohol and saline extraction, followed by precipitation of the saline soluble constituents with an excess of 95 per cent alcohol. Favilli and Biancalani,[9] in obtaining the polysaccharides from the brucella group, also used alcohol and saline extraction, followed by precipitation of the saline soluble constituents with alcohol. Their material from the paramelitensis strain was purified by the addition of trichloracetic acid followed by precipitation with absolute alcohol from an alkaline solution. The polysaccharide from the melitensis strain was purified by precipitation with uranium acetate followed by precipitation with alcohol.

METHOD OF EXTRACTION USED IN THIS WORK

The organisms were grown on glycerol liver infusion agar prepared, with slight modifications, according to the method of Huddleson, Hasley, and Torrey.[16] In order to simplify the preparation of the medium, the albumin precipitation was omitted, the broth was filtered only through tightly packed glass wool, and five per cent glycerol and Merck's finely powdered agar were added. The medium was relatively clear and gave an abundant growth of the organisms.

Petri dishes were inoculated with the growth from forty-eight hour glycerol liver infusion agar slants. Approximately eighty to one hundred plates were inoculated with each strain. After incubation at 37 C. for seventy-two to eighty-four hours the bacterial mass was obtained by emulsifying the growth in physiological salt solution. The bacteria were washed with saline and centrifuged, and 300–400 cc. of 95 per cent alcohol was added to the residue and placed in the ice box for twelve to eighteen hours.

15. J. Exper. Med. **49:** 727, 1929.
16. J. Infect. Dis. **40:** 352, 1927.

The centrifuged bacterial mass was boiled with 250–300 cc. of absolute alcohol under a reflux for one hour and filtered hot through a hot water filter. The extracts from all the strains filtered readily, and the filtrates usually remained clear even after standing at room temperature or at ice box temperature for several days.

The bacterial residue was extracted with 300–400 cc. of 75 per cent alcohol for two hours on a water bath and filtered hot through a hot water filter. The material usually filtered slowly, although differences were observed with the various strains: for example, strains A456 and S41–1 filtered readily and yielded a clear filtrate, whereas M428 filtered slowly and yielded an opalescent filtrate.

The bacterial residue which remained after absolute alcohol and 75 per cent alcohol extraction was boiled with 400–500 cc. of 0.9 per cent sodium chloride for two hours, centrifuged, and the slightly opalescent supernatant was evaporated by boiling to about three-fourths of its volume. The material when cold was precipitated with normal hydrochloric acid and centrifuged. The acid was added drop by drop until further addition no longer brought down a precipitate. The white flocculent precipitate yielded a strongly positive biuret and xanthoproteic reaction and precipitated homologous and heterologous immune serums in low dilutions, 1:50, 1:100 up to 1:500. No differences were observed in the height of the titer or in the amount of the precipitate.

To the clear supernatant, obtained after the protein precipitate had been removed by centrifugalization, N/10 HCl and N/10 NaOH were added drop by drop in order to make sure that the optimum precipitation point had not been passed. Any precipitate that formed was removed by centrifuging. The solution was alkalinized by the addition of 1/10 the volume of normal NaOH and precipitated with four volumes of absolute alcohol. Precipitation was complete in twenty-four to forty-eight hours. The material, after being washed several times with 95 per cent alcohol, was dried with absolute alcohol and ether.

CHEMICAL CHARACTERISTICS OF THE ALCOHOL PRECIPITABLE SUBSTANCE

The dried precipitable substance from all the strains was a white powder soluble in water. The substances gave a negative xanthoproteic reaction and were not precipitated by any of the substances used to precipitate proteins, such as picric acid, tannic acid, or trichloracetic acid. The substances gave a negative biuret test when 2 cc. of a 10 per cent NaOH solution was mixed with 2 cc. of a concentrated solution of the precipitable substance and 0.1 per cent $CuSO_4$ solution was added. When different concentrations of the reagents were used different results were obtained. For example, when 1 cc. of a saturated solution of NaOH was added to 4 cc. of a concentrated solution of the precipitable substance, mixed, and 2 drops of diluted Fehling's solution A was added, $2\frac{1}{2}$ cc. of Fehling's solution diluted with 10 cc. of distilled water, the precipitable substances from the strains A456 and S41–1 gave a slightly positive test while the extract from strain M428 gave a negative test. The material when dissolved in water did not reduce Fehling's solution. After hydrolysis with N/3 HCl for five hours extracts from the three varieties strongly reduced Fehling's solution.

Repeated attempts to further purify the material by precipitation with trichloracetic acid and picric acid from acid and alkaline solutions failed. Alcohol precipitation from acid and neutral solutions also was unsuccessful.

IMMUNE REACTIONS OF THE PRECIPITABLE SUBSTANCE

Rabbits were immunized with organisms grown in liver infusion broth and on liver infusion agar slants for forty-eight hours. The growth from the broth cultures was centrifuged, washed with saline, and adjusted to a density of 2 on McFarland's nephelometer. The growth from the agar slants was emulsified in saline, centrifuged, and the sediment adjusted to a density of 2. The antigens were heated at 60 C. for forty minutes and tested for sterility in liver infusion broth and on glycerol liver infusion agar.

Rabbits were immunized by injecting 2 cc. of the heated vaccines intravenously. They were bled from the heart on the sixth day after the injection, reinjected on the following day, and again bled from the heart twelve to fourteen days later.

Broth and agar antigens were used in order to study their effect on the precipitation reaction. The broth antigens were used in order to eliminate cross reactions due to anti-agar immune substances. In 1931, Sordelli and Mayer[17] showed that serums prepared by immunizing animals with agar cultures of B. anthracis or Bact. typhosum contained precipitins for agar. Zozaya and Medina[18] confirmed these findings and indicated that false cross agglutination and precipitation might occur when agar cultures were used for immunization and for the preparation of test suspensions or extracts.

PRECIPITATION TEST

The antigen used in the precipitation test was a saline solution of the dried precipitable substance. A weighed amount of the material was dissolved in saline and quantitative dilutions were prepared. In the test, 0.2 cc. of the saline solution of the antigen was mixed with 0.2 cc. of immune serum, incubated for two hours at 37 C. in a water bath, and placed in the ice box for twelve to eighteen hours. Readings were taken after ice box incubation with artificial light against a dark background.

The results of the precipitation tests are summarized in table 3.

The alcohol insoluble substances extracted from the abortus, the suis, and the melitensis varieties of the genus Brucella precipitated homologous and heterologous immune serums. Considered from the standpoint of precipitability of abortus and suis immune serums, the strains fall into three varieties. Arranged in the order of antigenic activity they are: the abortus, precipitable in dilutions of 1:50,000, the suis, precipitable in dilutions of 1:10,000 to 1:25,000, and the melitensis, precipitable in dilutions of 1:1000 to 1:5000.

17. Compt. rend. Soc. de biol. **107:** 736, 1931; **108:** 675, 1931.
18. J. Exper. Med. **57:** 41, 1933.

TABLE 3.—*Precipitation Tests*

Serum	Precipitable substance	Dilution						
		500	1000	2500	5000	10,000	25,000	50,000
A456 (broth)	A456	++++	++++	++++	++++	++++	+++	+
	S41–1	++++	++++	++++	+++	+	0	0
	M428	+++	++	+	0	0	0	0
S41–1 (broth)	A456	++++	++++	++++	++++	++++	++	+
	S41–1	++++	++++	++++	++++	++	+	0
	M428	++++	+++	++	+	0	0	0
M428 (broth)	A456	++++	++	+	0	0	0	0
	S41–1	++++	+	±	0	0	0	0
	M428	++++	+++	+	±	0	0	0
A456 (agar)	A456	+++	++++	++++	++++	++++	++	+
	S41–1	+++	++++	++++	++++	+++	+	0
	M428	++++	++++	+++	+	0	0	0
S41–1 (agar)	A456	++++	++++	++++	++++	++++	+++	++
	S41–1	++++	++++	++++	++++	+++	+	0
	M428	+++	+	0	0	0	0	0
M428 (agar)	A456	+++	+	0	0	0	0	0
	S41–1	+++	+	0	0	0	0	0
	M428	++++	+++	++	+	0	0	0

In Br. melitensis var. melitensis antiserum no such differences are observed. In general the precipitating titer is low for all strains and is slightly higher with the homologous than with the heterologous precipitable substance.

The abortus variety not only precipitates its own serum in high dilutions, but also precipitates heterologous suis serum in higher dilutions than the suis precipitable substance. The abortus extract is active in the same dilution, 1:50,000, in both abortus and suis antiserums. The suis extract is likewise active, with one exception, to approximately the same titer, 1:25,000, in both abortus and suis antiserums.

Serums from two other strains, 481 and 89, were also used in precipitation tests. The characteristics of these strains may be briefly considered. Strain 481 was classified by Evans[7] as the only representative of the serological group to which it belonged. She observed that it was the only strain isolated in this country which precipitated spontaneously in saline. Because of its spontaneous agglutination it was difficult to carry out the simple agglutination tests, and its relationship to the other groups was established only by testing its property of absorbing the agglutinins from the various serums. The strain when used in these studies spontaneously agglutinated in saline, and no satisfactory bacterial suspension was obtained even by reducing the salt content to 0.2 to 0.4 per cent. Nine-day liver infusion broth cultures showed pellicle formation, a viscid sediment, and clearness of the broth. On the usual dye mediums growth was obtained only in thionin, indicating the strain to be of the porcine variety.

Strain 89 was classified by Francis,[19] in 1931, as of the melitensis variety. When used in the present studies, the strain was not agglutinated by A456, M428, or S41–1 antiserums although it still gave the dye reactions of the melitensis variety. It caused an even clouding of liver infusion broth, was

19. Pub. Health Rep. **46:** 2416, 1931.

readily emulsified in saline, and produced unusually small colonies on glycerol liver infusion agar.

The agglutinating titers of serums 481 and 89 are shown in tables 4 and 5. Living antigens were used and the tests were incubated at 56 C. for four hours and then placed in the ice box overnight.

Tables 4 and 5 show that strains A456, M428, and S41–1 either were not agglutinated or were agglutinated to only a low titer by the serums from strains 481 and 89. Strain 89 was likewise agglutinated in only a comparatively low titer.

TABLE 4.—*Serum 481*

Antigen	Dilution of serum						
	20	40	80	160	320	640	Control
A456	±	0	0	0	0	0	0
M428	++++	+	±	0	0	0	0
S41–1	++	+	0	0	0	0	0
89	++++	++++	++++	+++	+	0	0

TABLE 5.—*Serum 89*

Antigen	Dilution of serum						
	20	40	80	160	320	640	Control
A456	±	0	0	0	0	0	0
M428	++++	++	±	0	0	0	0
S41–1	++++	++	±	0	0	0	0
89	++++	++++	++	+	0	0	0

Table 6 shows the results of precipitation tests obtained with serums 481 and 89 and the precipitable substance from strains A456, S41–1, and M428.

TABLE 6

Serum	Precipitable substance	Dilution							
		500	1000	2500	5000	10,000	25,000	50,000	75,000
481	A456	++++	++++	++++	++++	++	++	0	0
	S41–1	++++	++++	++++	+++	++	+	0	0
	M428	++++	++	+	0	0	0	0	0
89	A456	+++	++++	++++	++++	++++	++++	++	0
	A41–1	++++	++++	++++	++++	+++	+	0	0
	M428	++++	++++	++++	++++	++	0	0	0

The precipitation tests indicate that strains 481 and 89 produced an immune response in rabbits which could be demonstrated when an alcohol precipitable substance was used as an antigen, but which was not readily demonstrable when the whole bacteria were used as antigens. It seems that the precipitable substance is a more sensitive antigen than the bacteria.

SPECIFICITY OF THE PRECIPITABLE SUBSTANCE

Reference to table 3 indicates that practically no differences are observed in the precipitating titer of a serum or in the extent of the cross precipitation reactions when serums obtained by injecting organisms grown in broth or on agar are used. It seems that the cross reactions are due to a substance extracted from the bacteria rather than to the agar on which the bacteria were grown.

In order to learn something of the strain specificity of the precipitating substances, immune serums were absorbed with the extracts from strains A456, S41–1, and M428. In the first series of absorptions 1 cc. of immune serum was mixed with 1 cc. of a saline solution of the precipitable substance, incubated four hours at 37 C., and placed in the ice box overnight. The precipitate was removed by centrifuging and the serums diluted and used in the agglutination test.

The agglutinating titer of the absorbed serums was used as an index of the extent of absorption, because it is difficult to accurately read the precipitating titer when diluted serum is used. The results of the absorption tests are given in table 7.

TABLE 7.—*Absorption of Immune Serum with Precipitable Substances*

Serum	Absorbed with	Dilution	Agglutination test						
			Dilution						
			Antigen	20	40	80	160	320	Control
A456	A456	1:500	A456	++++	++++	++++	++	0	0
			S41–1	++++	++++	+++	+	0	0
			M428	++++	+++	+	0	0	0
	S41–1	1:500	A456	++++	++++	+++	+	0	0
			S41–1	++++	++++	+++	++	0	0
			M428	++++	++++	++	0	0	0
	M428	1:250	A456	++++	++++	++++	+++	±	0
			S41–1	++++	++++	++++	+++	±	0
			M428	++++	++++	+++	+	0	0
S41–1	A456	1:500	A456	++++	++++	+++	++	±	0
			S41–1	++++	++++	+++	++	±	0
			M428	++++	+++	+	0	0	0
	S41–1	1:500	A456	++++	++++	+++	+	0	0
			S41–1	++++	++++	+++	+	0	0
			M428	+++	++	+	0	0	0
	M428	1:250	A456	++++	++++	++++	++++	++	0
			S41–1	++++	++++	++++	++++	++	0
			M428	++++	++++	++++	+++	+	0
M428	A456	1:250	A456	+++	+	0	0	0	0
			S41–1	+++	+	0	0	0	0
			M428	+++	+++	±	0	0	0
	S41–1	1:250	A456	+++	+	0	0	0	0
			S41–1	+++	+	0	0	0	0
			M428	++++	+++	±	0	0	0
	M428	1:250	A456	+++	+	0	0	0	0
			S41–1	+++	±	0	0	0	0
			M428	++++	+++	±	0	0	0

The unabsorbed serums had an agglutinating titer of approximately 1:1280 (table 2). After absorption with the precipitable substances, the agglutinating titers were reduced; the extent of the reduction depending upon the substance used. For example, the extracts from strains A456 and S41–1 in 1:500 dilutions removed more antibodies from the corresponding serums than the extract from strain M428 in a 1:250 dilution. The agglutinating titer of the absorbed serum M428 was lower than that of the other serums; however, unabsorbed M428 serum also had a slightly lower titer than the other serums. Furthermore, more of the antibodies may have been removed because a lower dilution of the precipitable substance of strains A456 and S41–1 was used for absorbing the serum.

In order to determine whether the agglutinating titer could be further reduced by absorption with precipitable substance, serum was mixed with an equal amount of the precipitable substance (as in the previous tests), incubated at 37 C. for four hours, centrifuged, and 1 cc. of the substance was added to the supernatant. The serum was incubated for two hours at 37 C., placed in the ice box overnight, centrifuged, and used for the agglutination test.

No differences were observed in the agglutination results, whether the serums were absorbed once or twice with the precipitable substances.

In order to determine whether the reduction in the agglutinating titers was due to a non-specific change in the serum constituents, S. schottmülleri and S. aertrycke serums were absorbed with the precipitable substances from brucella strains. No reduction in the agglutinating titer was observed when the absorbed serums were tested with the homologous organisms.

Brucella antiserums were also treated with the chemical precipitate produced by the addition of sodium hydroxide to absolute alcohol. No reduction in the agglutinating titer was observed.

These experiments indicate that the reduction of the agglutinating titer of brucella antiserums is due to some substance specific for the genus, but not specific for the different varieties of the genus.

IN VIVO ANTIGENIC ACTIVITY OF THE PRECIPITABLE SUBSTANCE

Rabbits were injected intravenously with 2 cc. of a 1:200 dilution of the precipitable substances. Approximately 30 mg. of the extracts from strains A456, S41–1, and M428 were injected. The rabbits were bled six days after the last injection, and the serum was tested for precipitating and agglutinating antibodies. The results are summarized in tables 8 and 9.

TABLE 8.—*Precipitating Titer of Serum due to Injection of Precipitable Substance*

Immunized with	Antigen	Dilution			
		100	200	500	1000
A456	A456	++++	+++	+	0
	S41–1	++++	++++	++	0
	M428	++++	+++	+	0
S41–1	A456	+++	+	0	0
	S41–1	++++	++	0	0
	M428	+++	+	0	0
M428	A456	+++	+	0	0
	S41–1	+++	++++	+	0
	M428	++++	+++	+	0

Favilli and Biancalani[9] attempted to immunize rabbits with the purified material extracted from melitensis and paramelitensis strains. The serum of their animals did not show a precipitating titer when tested with the polysaccharides. They did not report agglutination or anaphylactic experiments.

The stimulation of antibodies in rabbits following the injection of precipitable substance may be due to the presence of a small residue of protein material. In order to determine whether the immune response was due to the presence of protein material, guinea pigs were injected intravenously with 15 mg. of the precipitable substances dissolved in saline. Ten days later they were injected intravenously with 50 mg. of the same material.

The guinea pig injected with the extract from strain A456 showed a typical anaphylactic reaction, but did not die. The animal that received extract M428 showed only a slight reaction, difficulty in breathing, and roughness of the fur. In the case of the guinea pig sensitized with the S41–1 extract, an attempt was made to determine whether one-half of the shock dose (25 mg.) would cause an anaphylactic reaction. Only a slight reaction was obtained, roughness of the fur, urination, and slight difficulty in breathing. No further symptoms were observed after a second injection of 25 mg. about fifteen minutes later.

TABLE 9.—*Agglutinating Titer of Serum Due to Injection of Precipitable Substance*

Immunized with	Antigen	Dilution						
		10	20	40	80	160	320	Control
A456	A456	++++	++++	++++	++++	++++	+++	0
	S41–1	++++	++++	++++	++++	++++	+++	0
	M428	++++	++++	++++	++++	++++	++	0
S41–1	A456	++++	++++	++	±	0	0	0
	S41–1	++++	++++	+	±	0	0	0
	M428	++++	++++	+	0	0	0	0
M428	A456	++++	++++	++++	++	+	0	0
	S41–1	++++	++++	++++	++	+	0	0
	M428	++++	++++	++++	++	+	±	0

Another explanation may be suggested to account for the immune response in animals. Zinsser[20] found that when alkaline extracts of pulverized bacteria of several varieties were precipitated with acid in the cold, boiled with acid, alkalinized to a p_H 7, and again filtered, a small amount of an alcohol-precipitable material remained which reacted negatively to the biuret, Hopkins-Cole, Millon, and sulfosalicylic acid protein tests. Such filtrates, however, gave precipitation turbidity with ten volumes of absolute alcohol which varied in intensity in different preparations. He suggested that the alcohol-precipitable material was merely incidental, carrying down the antigenic material with it, since antigenic potency did not parallel alcohol precipitation. His material was not antigenic in animals. There is a possibility that the alcohol-precipitable material may be antigenic in the absence of protein material, if a sufficiently large molecule of the alcohol precipitate is obtained. Zozaya[21] has shown that polysaccharides can be rendered antigenic by haptogenic absorption upon a colloid carrier. He used collodion, aluminum hydroxide, casein, and bacterial cells as colloids, and polysaccharides from B. anthracis, the meningococcus, Streptococcus viridans (Bargen), B. proteus, S. morgani, B. dysenteriae, both the Shiga and Hiss type, and the pneumococci.

---

20. J. Exper. Med. **37:** 275, 1923.
21. J. Exper. Med. **55:** 325, 1932.

DISCUSSION

While this investigation was in progress a paper appeared by Favilli and Biancalani[9] on the extraction of hydrocarbons from organisms of the brucella group. By using alcohol and saline extraction followed by alcohol precipitation, they obtained antigenic substances of the nature of haptenes from a melitensis and a paramelitensis strain, but not from an abortus strain. They suggested that their failure to isolate a carbohydrate from the abortus variety was due to the fact that in this strain the carbohydrate is more intimately linked with the bacterial protein.

In the work reported here preparations of a carbohydrate nature were extracted from the three varieties of the genus, the melitensis, the abortus, and the suis. Unlike the results obtained by the Italian workers, a carbohydrate substance was as readily extracted from the abortus variety as from the other two.

These preparations, like those of Favilli and Biancalani,[9] precipitated both homologous and heterologous brucella antiserums. The preparation from the abortus strain was the most active, precipitating abortus and suis antiserums in a dilution of 1:50,000. The suis extract precipitated in dilutions of 1:10,000 to 1:25,000. The melitensis extract precipitated melitensis antiserum in a dilution of 1:5000, abortus antiserum in dilutions of 1:2500 to 1:5000, and suis antiserum in dilutions of 1:1000 to 1:5000. The melitensis carbohydrate extracted by the Italian workers precipitated melitensis antiserum in a dilution of 1:800 and abortus antiserum in a dilution of 1:12,800. They also found, as I did, that melitensis serum was precipitated in relatively low dilutions by extracts of homologous and heterologous strains.

The polysaccharids extracted by Favilli and Biancalani[9] were of the nature of haptenes. The preparations obtained in this investigation stimulated the production of precipitating and agglutinating antibodies. Definitely positive precipitation tests, however, were obtained only when low dilutions of the precipitable substances were used (1:100 to 1:200). The agglutinating titers also were low, except in the case of the rabbit immunized with extract A456. This extract also was the only preparation which caused typical anaphylaxis in a guinea pig. The preparations from the other strains caused only a mild reaction characterized by slight difficulty in breathing. The antigenic response in animals may be due to the presence of a slight protein residue or may be due to the fact that the extracts were absorbed on a sufficient amount of an alcohol precipitable substance to render them antigenic. Zinsser[20] found that alcohol precipitable substances obtained from various bacteria were not antigenic in animals. His material, however, was precipitated at p_H 7. It is possible that by increasing the alkali content of a solution a precipitate of larger molecular size is obtained which may be feebly antigenic.

The results of the precipitation tests using the substances extracted in this work indicate a closer relationship between the abortus and the suis varieties than between these and the melitensis variety. By agglutination absorption tests differences have likewise been observed between the melitensis and the abortus varieties, but not between the bovine and the suis varieties.

There is a possibility that the differences between the three varieties of the genus Brucella may be due to their residence in different animal hosts. Theobald Smith[22] believed "that the porcine variety has been developed from cattle in recent times in the Middle West as a result of the very close association of the two species in the feed lots and the adaptation of the bovine variety to the pig under certain unknown conditions." Differences in the serological reactions of the organisms of the brucella group may also be caused by prolonged growth on artificial mediums. Plastridge and McAlpine[14] have shown that the mucoid variant is not agglutinated by antiserum prepared against the ordinary strains of the brucella organisms, but mucoid antiserum agglutinates both the mucoid variant and the ordinary strains, indicating that the mucoid variant possesses a double antigen complex, whereas only one complex is present in the normal form.

The method of chemical fractionation has been used in studying many groups of bacteria, yeasts, and fungi. Furth and Landsteiner[15] prepared specific precipitable substances from the main serological types of the typhoid-paratyphoid group and found that the specificity of the precipitin reactions of these substances paralleled in a general way the so-called small flaking agglutination. In some instances, as in the case of the pneumococci, highly type specific carbohydrates were obtained. In other instances, as in the case of the C substance of the pneumococci, group characteristics were found. Occasionally preparations from different species of organisms show chemical similarities, as in the case of the Friedländer's bacillus, the type II pneumococcus, and one variety of yeast.

In the brucella group, a group practically indistinguishable morphologically, serologically, biochemically, and pathogenically, the carbohydrate substance isolated from the three strains was specific for the species, but not for the varieties.

The results of the precipitation absorption tests seem to indicate that the differences between the preparations may be quantitative rather than qualitative, since the preparations from all the strains were able to reduce the agglutinating titers of the serums to about the same extent. If the alcohol precipitable material may be considered incidental carrying down the specific material with it, then differences in the amount of absorption might account for the differences in the activity of the preparations from the three varieties.

SUMMARY

Specific precipitable substances of polysaccharide nature were prepared from the three varieties of the genus Brucella by saline extraction, followed by precipitation with alcohol. These substances were feebly antigenic in rabbits, but failed to give any of the usual chemical tests for proteins with

22. J. Exper. Med. **43:** 207, 1926.

the exception that under certain conditions the substance from strains A456 and S41–1 gave a doubtfully positive biuret test. The specific substance from the abortus strain caused a typical anaphylactic reaction in a guinea pig when 15 mg. was used as a sensitizing dose. The specific substance from the melitensis and the porcine strains failed to give a typical reaction. The preparations from the three varieties precipitated brucella antiserums, but did not precipitate heterologous serums from the salmonella group. Serums absorbed with the precipitable substances from the three varieties showed a considerable reduction in the agglutinating titer of both homologous and heterologous brucella antiserums, indicating that the differences observed in the specific precipitable substances from the three strains may be quantitative rather than qualitative.

SALIVARY GLAND DISEASE OF MICE

JUANITA THOMPSON

NEW YORK

The salivary glands from fifty apparently healthy adult mice were examined during the winter of 1932 at Toronto, Canada. Microscopically, all showed pathological changes consisting of focal accumulations of mononuclear cells. In 60 per cent of the glands, large inclusion-bearing cells were observed.[1] Since the lesions appeared analogous to those produced by certain viruses, it was decided to ascertain whether a virus disease existed in mice from this colony.

During the present year (1934–5) the opportunity was afforded to continue the investigation in New York. It was essential to import mice from the Toronto colony to find out whether after an interval of two years the salivary glands of the offspring presented a similar microscopic picture. Positive findings were definitely established.

METHOD

A preliminary microscopic survey of the salivary glands of adult mice obtained from a colony in New York City showed no inflammatory foci or inclusions. Therefore, it was decided that mice of this stock were suitable for the experimental work. Preliminary studies were designed to serve as a histological control. For this purpose, ten days prior to inoculation, one-half of the submaxillary gland from approximately two hundred mice was removed. Since these glands showed no pathological changes, this procedure was discontinued. Two weeks following injection, the experimental mice were killed by ether. Using aseptic precautions, the salivary glands were removed; a portion was saved for microscopic study and the remainder emulsified for serial passage.

A sterile technic used in preparing the emulsions was consistently followed. The tissue was placed in a mortar with sand and in the process of grinding 5.0 cc. of distilled water per gland was added gradually. This mixture was centrifuged at slow speed for a few minutes. The supernatant fluid was decanted and aerobic and anaerobic cultures made in order to rule out the presence of bacteria.

RESULTS

By the injection of an emulsion of affected glands it has been found possible to produce a chronic inflammatory reaction with inclusion bodies. Lo-

---

Received for publication, May 23, 1935.

From the Laboratory of Experimental Neurology, Department of Neurology, New York University College of Medicine.

This work was aided by a grant from the Rockefeller Foundation.

1. Thompson, J.: Am. J. Path. **10:** 676, 1934.

calization occurred only in the salivary glands irrespective of the site of inoculation (whether intraglandular, subcutaneous, intraperitoneal, intratesticular or intracerebral). Transmission of tissue other than submaxillary gland from an affected animal produced no reaction in the submaxillary gland of the new host.

Histologically, the inclusion-bearing cells were confined to the acinar tissue of both the serous and mucous portions of the submaxillary glands. Occasionally the duct cells and more rarely the alveolar cells of the parotid contained inclusions. The affected cells were usually found to be remote from the associated inflammatory areas. The number of inclusion-containing cells and the degree of the inflammatory reaction did not appear to have any definite relationship.

The altered cells were greatly hypertrophied. Their contour was irregular and seldom clearly defined. The nuclei showed considerable variability. Some were entirely filled by a bland mass, the acidophilic center gradually becoming basophilic toward the periphery. Since no unstained zone surrounded the inclusions it was thought that only partial margination of the chromatin had taken place. Nucleoli were infrequently recognized. Other nuclei differed in having a relatively large unstained halo surrounding the inclusion. In these, the chromatin appeared to have almost entirely marginated. Only a few filamentous chromatin remnants bridged the intervening gap between the inclusion and the nuclear membrane. The inclusion body was acidophilic and consisted of aggregated minute spherules. The nucleoli usually adherent to the nuclear membrane were clearly defined. The cytoplasm of the affected cells was basophilic and varied in character. In some cells it appeared finely granular; in others, relatively large more or less spheroidal granules were scattered throughout. Frequently fusion of two or more altered cells, each with its separate inclusion, occurred.

Many degenerative variants from the preceding typical picture were observed. Gradations were found ranging from the typical to fragmented cytoplasmic masses devoid of nuclear body and consisting merely of a conglomeration of irregularly stained basophilic granules.

In serial passage to the fifteenth generation, there has been consistently found a small percentage of glands in each group showing only chronic inflammatory foci. Despite the apparent absence of inclusions, it is probable that a very small number may have been overlooked even on serial section. However, in the above connection, one should consider the possibility of the disintegration of a small number of primary inclusions in the course of the disease.

The effect of intracerebral injection of the so-called "mouse salivary virus" was studied. Both adult and immature mice were used. Emulsions of glands prepared from the 4th, 8th and 12th serial passage were employed. In order to follow the histological response, some animals of each group were killed at periods from six to thirty days.

In the present study, none of the mice injected intracerebrally showed any notable clinical manifestations. All remained apparently well until sacrificed.

Histologically, 12 of 50 experimental mice killed between the sixth and twelfth day showed a slight localized meningitis characterized by a mononuclear exudate. In many of the cells, intranuclear inclusions were found. In the majority of these, the brain showed no significant changes. In four of the mice, inflammatory foci of mononuclear cells, some containing inclusions, were irregularly scattered throughout the cerebral tissue. In two of these, inclusions were present within the nuclei of some of the endothelial cells lining the choroid plexus. The number of positive findings bore no relation to either the serial passage from which the emulsion was made nor to the age of the mice. The remaining mice showed nothing of note.

In all the mice, the inoculation of 0.03 cc. was sufficiently potent to produce characteristic submaxillary changes.

An attempt was made to investigate the host range. It was thought that this particular "mouse salivary virus" might be adaptable to other species since the original strain of mice from which it was derived had been reared in close association with a colony of rats and guinea pigs which have previously been found to harbor submaxillary inclusions.[2] However, injections either intracerebrally or in the submaxillary region in rats, rabbits, and young guinea pigs produced no significant alterations. Intracerebral injections in cats gave equivocal results. It is of interest to note that 10 per cent of apparently healthy adult New York cats showed focal areas of chronic inflammatory cells in the submaxillary tissue. No inclusions were found. The findings in a small series of inoculated cats were difficult to interpret in that a larger percentage of the animals showed a reaction similar to that found in "normal" cats. In this connection, it might be interpolated that in monkeys mononuclear aggregations frequently occur in this region.

DISCUSSION

During the past few years investigators have repeatedly drawn attention to the incidental finding of inclusions in various tissues of apparently healthy animals. A knowledge of any intracellular phenomena which may occur spontaneously in common laboratory animals is of especial importance to those interested in virus research.

Experimental evidence would appear to indicate that the causative factors giving rise to an inflammatory reaction together with inclusions in the cells of the salivary glands of rodents (e.g., guinea pig;[3,2] hamster;[4] rat;[4,2,1] mole;[5] and mouse[4,1] are of low pathogenicity. The conditions essential for the transfer between the different species has not been discovered to date. Nevertheless, it is thought that the etiological agents in the different species of animals are closely related if not identical. Since, in humans, lesions similar to those demonstrated in animals have been found concomitant with

---

2. Thompson, J.: J. Infect. Dis. **50:** 162, 1932.
3. Cole, R. and Kuttner, A. G.: J. Exper. Med. **44:** 855, 1926.
4. Kuttner, A. G., and Wang, S.: J. Exper. Med. **60:** 773, 1934.
5. Rector, E. J., and Rector, L. E.: Am. J. Path. **10:** 629, 1934.

severe disorders,[4] the possible pathogenic rôle of this so-called "group of viruses" remains doubtful.

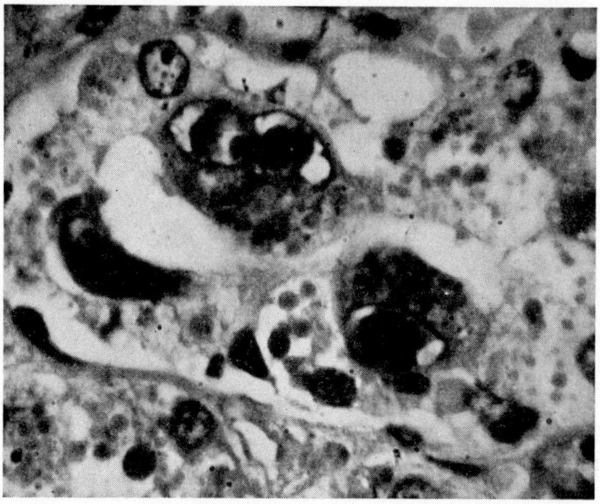

Fig. 1.—Inclusion bodies in the cells of the submaxillary gland.

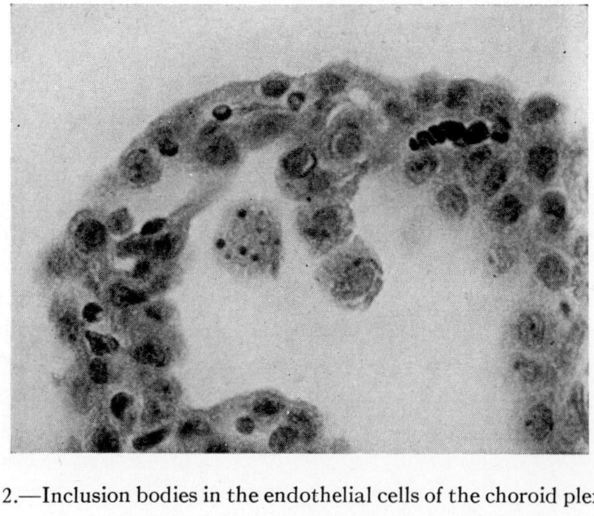

Fig. 2.—Inclusion bodies in the endothelial cells of the choroid plexus.

CONCLUSIONS

From experimental studies it is concluded that a focal mononuclear reaction together with inclusion-bearing cells in the salivary glands of apparently healthy mice indicates a virus disease.

The evidence to support this view is:

(a) Using the presence of an inflammatory reaction together with inclusions as an index, the condition was found to be transmissible to normal mice in series by the inoculation of bacteriologically sterile emulsions of affected glands.

(b) Localization occurred only in the salivary glands following intraglandular, subcutaneous, intraperitoneal, intratesticular or intracerebral injection.

(c) When the intracerebral route was used, a localized encephalomeningitis developed in some of the mice.

Histologically, the inclusion bodies in the cells of the salivary glands of mice resemble those of the guinea pig, hamster, rat and mole.

The salivary gland disease of mice after becoming established in a colony is transmitted for generations as is the case in submaxillary gland disease of the guinea pig.[3]

The condition has not been successfully transmitted to other common laboratory animals.

THE DESTRUCTION OF TUBERCLE BACILLI WITHIN PHAGOCYTES IN VITRO

B. J. CLAWSON

MINNEAPOLIS

Observations of lesions in experimental tuberculosis and the fact that tuberculosis in people may heal indicate that the tubercle bacilli are reduced in number or disappear in lesions in animals and individuals. The mechanism by which the reduction or destruction of the organisms is brought about is not entirely agreed upon.

Römer and Joseph[1] decided that increased resistance to tuberculosis in animals was due to an inhibitory action by the tissues rather than to lysis of the organisms. The finding of living virulent organisms by Opie and Aronson[2] in and around old pulmonary lesions supported this idea. Evidences of lysis of the tubercle bacilli were observed in the peritoneal cavity of immunized guinea pigs by Deycke and Much,[3] Much and Leschke[4] and Kraus and Nofer.[5] These conclusions were based upon the observations of a rapid disappearance of tubercle bacilli from the peritoneal fluid and the appearance of nonstaining forms and granules resembling remnants of bacteria. Manwaring and Bronfenbrenner[6] called attention to the fact that a rapid decrease of tubercle bacilli in the peritoneal fluid may not be due to destruction of organisms but to absorption of the organisms by the peritoneal lymphatics or to adhering of the bacteria to the peritoneal surfaces. These authors contended that the evidence cited in support of the belief that lysis of tubercle bacilli takes place is not adequate to establish the conclusions beyond doubt. In the repeated experiments later carried on by Manwaring and Bronfenbrenner on lysis of tubercle bacilli, they decided that the bacilli rapidly disappeared from the peritoneal fluid of tuberculous animals but persisted in normal animals. The intraperitoneal lysis was due, according to these experimenters, to specific changes in the fixed peritoneal cells of the tuberculous animals.

Lurie[7] by culturing various organs from animals previously injected with tubercle bacilli observed a rapid disappearance of bacilli in immunized animals while in normal animals injected in a similar manner the bacilli actually increased.

Received for publication, June 3, 1935.

From the Department of Pathology, University of Minnesota.

1. Beitr. z. Klin. d. Tuberk. **17:** 287, 1910.
2. Arch. Path. **4:** 1, 1927.
3. Beitr. z. Klin. d. Tuberk. **15:** 277, 1910.
4. Beitr. z. Klin. d. Tuberk. **20:** 405, 1911.
5. Deutsche med. Wchnschr. **38:** 1227, 1912.
6. J. Exper. Med. **18:** 601, 1913.
7. J. Exper. Med. **50:** 747, 1929.

The purpose of the experiments reported in this paper is to see if tubercle bacilli can be reduced significantly outside of the body in the presence of living mononuclear leucocytes and normal or immune serum. The relation of the degree of lysis to the concentration of antibodies (agglutinins) in the serums and to the allergic state in the animals from which serums or leucocytes were obtained was also carefully studied.

Material and methods.—The tubercle bacillus used in the experiments, both for immunizing the animals and for the experiments in lysis was the Calmette-Guérin bacillus (BCG). This organism was used because of less possible danger to the worker and because immune serum could be developed in animals without producing tuberculosis. It was assumed that more virulent strains of tubercle bacilli would be lysed to some extent at least in a similar manner.

Following the method described by Hughes[8] the mononuclear leucocytes were obtained in an almost pure suspension. One hundred cc. of paraffin oil was injected into the peritoneal cavity of a rabbit. Four days later the rabbit was killed and the oil and the cell content of the peritoneal cavity was washed out with 200 cc. of citrated salt solution. All salt solution used in the experiments contained 0.1 per cent of gelatin to give a viscosity approximately that of serum.

The heavy suspension of leucocytes obtained from the peritoneal cavity was separated from the oil by allowing the mixture to stand for a few minutes in a tall cylinder. The oil soon collected at the top of the cylinder. The cells were removed with a large pipette and washed twice in salt solution by centrifuging at a moderate speed for 3 minutes. If the centrifuge was run at full speed the leucocytes became packed so that it was difficult to get them into a smooth suspension.

To 0.1 cc. of the suspension of leucocytes were added equal amounts of bacterial suspension and immune serum. One drop of this mixture from a standard capillary pipette was spread evenly over a measured surface (6.25 sq. cm.) on a glass slide. The suspension of leucocytes was diluted and gaged by its turbidity so that 25 oil immersion fields from the mixture on the slide contained approximately 350 leucocytes.

The suspension of tubercle bacilli was prepared by grinding the organisms in a mortar in salt solution. The suspension was then centrifuged for a few minutes to throw down all visible clumps. The fine suspension was pipetted off and diluted so that in 25 oil immersion fields of the mixture, as described above, there were about 1500 bacilli. It was impossible, at different tests, to have the same number of leucocytes or bacilli in the suspensions but, with each suspension, from 20 to 30 serums were tested. This reduced the possibilities of errors decidedly. It was found, however, by experimenting, that suspensions of both leucocytes and bacilli could be duplicated fairly closely by observing the degree of turbidity.

The immune serums were obtained from rabbits which had been vaccinated with BCG so as to obtain high antibody titers in the serums of some

8. J. Immunol. **25:** 102, 1933.

animals and low titers in others. The methods of immunizing the animals are described in other publications.[9] The lowest titers were obtained by vaccinating the rabbits subcutaneously with heat killed BCG, and the highest titers by injecting 4 mg. of living BCG subcutaneously in one area and after 3 weeks following this with 4 intravenous injections of 1 mg. each of heat killed BCG at weekly intervals. The serums in the tests were diluted 1–25. This dilution when mixed with equal volumes of suspensions of leucocytes and bacilli gave a final dilution of 1–75. It was found from repeated tests that best comparative results were obtained when this dilution of serum was used. Two to 4 normal control serums (1–75 dilution) were used in each test.

Equal amounts (0.1 cc.) of the leucocyte suspension, bacterial suspension and diluted serum were added to a vial 6 cm. long and 1.5 cm. in diameter. From 20 to 30 vials were tested at one time. The vials were stoppered tightly with corks which had been dipped in melted paraffin. The vials were then rotated on a mixing wheel (as described by Robertson and Sia[10] and Sutliff and Rhoades[11]) at 37 C. for one hour. Repeated tests showed 1 hour to be the best time of incubation for obtaining comparative results.

At the end of the hour of incubation and mixing the vials were removed and a drop from the same standard capillary pipette from each vial was evenly spread on a measured area (6.25 sq. c.) on respective slides. The pipette was washed out between suspensions with salt solution. The smears on the slides were dried quickly under an electric fan and fixed with methyl alcohol. They were then stained by the acid fast stain and counterstained with methylene blue so that both acid fast and non acid fast organisms could be shown. The number of leucocytes and the number of bacilli outside or inside leucocytes were counted in 25 evenly distributed oil immersion fields on each slide and the percentage of disappearance of organisms calculated. The numbers of bacilli visible were determined in the following combinations:

1. Bacilli+gelatin salt solution;
2. Bacilli+normal or immune serum;
3. Bacilli+normal mononuclear leucocytes;
4. Bacilli+normal mononuclear leucocytes+normal serum;
5. Bacilli+normal mononuclear leucocytes+immune serum;
6. Bacilli+normal mononuclear leucocytes+various concentrations of immune serum.
7. Bacilli+mononuclear leucocytes from animals which were both immune and allergic to the strain of tubercle bacillus used in the experiments.

Counts were made in all these combinations from the suspensions before and after incubation and mixing.

Results of the experiments.—Repeated counts of the number of bacilli in a gelatin salt suspension showed no appreciable difference in the numbers on

9. J. Infect. Dis. **56:** 297, 1935; Arch. Path., **19:** 673, 1935.
10. J. Exper. Med. **46:** 239, 1927.
11. J. Clin. Investigation **9:** 43, 1930.

the slides made from the mixtures before and after incubation. The same was found when normal or immune serum without leucocytes was incubated with the bacilli. When tubercle bacilli and normal mononuclear leucocytes were mixed and incubated an occasional bacillus was found to be phagocytosed, but the total number of bacilli visible in or outside of leucocytes was always practically the same as in the suspension of bacilli which had not been incubated.

When bacilli were mixed with normal mononuclear leucocytes and normal serum and incubated with mixing for one hour a degree of phagocytosis took place but the total number of bacilli seen either outside or within the leucocytes always approximated the number in the suspension before incubation. This combination (bacilli+normal mononuclear leucocytes+normal serum) was used as a standard for comparing the degrees of lysis in the further studies.

TABLE 1.—*Lysis of Tubercle Bacilli (BCG) When Mixed with Normal Mononuclear Leucocytes and Normal or Immune Serums (Dilution 1–75) and Incubated at 37 C. with Constant Mixing for One Hour*

Kinds of serums	No.	Percentage of lysis
Normal	8	0
Immune	32	68

When tubercle bacilli were mixed with normal leucocytes and immune serums, different results were obtained. In table 1 is seen a comparison of the degrees of lysis when the only variable factor was the serum. The serums from 8 normal animals and from 32 animals which had previously been immunized were tested and compared in respect to the amount of lysis produced. In the tests in which the normal serums were used the number of bacilli visible after incubation was approximately the same as was found in the same dilution of organisms before incubation. The average percentage of lysis was zero. The amount of lysis brought about by the 32 immune serums in the presence of mononuclear leucocytes averaged 68 per cent.

To determine whether an increase in the concentration of antibodies in the serums brought about a greater degree of lysis an experiment was performed which is recorded in table 2. Animals were selected which showed varying dilutions of antibodies as indicated by agglutinins. The agglutination titers of these 32 immune animals ranged from less than 1–50 to 1–6400. As the agglutination titers rose from 1–50 to 1–6400 the percentage of lysis

TABLE 2.—*Degree of Lysis of Tubercle Bacilli (BCG) with Various Concentrations of Antibodies (Agglutinins) in the Serums*

No.	Kinds of serums	Agglutination titers	Percentage of lysis
4	Normal	0	0
9	Immune	1–50 or less	29
4	Immune	1–100	55
6	Immune	1–200	60
2	Immune	1–400	80
4	Immune	1–800	85
2	Immune	1–1600	92
2	Immune	1–3200	92
3	Immune	1–6400	95

rose from 29 per cent to 95 per cent. The serums of the 4 normal animals caused no lysis of the bacilli. It appeared evident that a high titered serum in the presence of normal mononuclear leucocytes was capable of bringing about a significantly greater degree of lysis than a normal or low titered serum.

The question arose whether washed mononuclear leucocytes would cause a greater degree of lysis, if they were taken from animals which were immune and also allergic. Rich and Lewis[12] and Aronson[13] found by tissue cultures that cells from tuberculous allergic animals washed free from serum were still hypersensitive to tuberculin. To answer this question in regard to the mononuclear leucocytes in the peritoneal cavity, leucocytes for the test were collected from an animal which had previously been injected subcutaneously with living BCG. The serum of the animal had an agglutination titer of 1–100 and tuberculin skin test was positive (++) (table 3).

TABLE 3.—*Lysis of Tubercle Bacilli (BCG) when Mixed with Leucocytes from an Animal both Immune and Allergic to Tubercle Bacilli and with Normal or Immune Serums*

No.	Kinds of serums	Percentage of lysis
6	Normal	0
38	Immune	72
1	Immune homologous	75

With the leucocytes from this animal the serums of 6 normal animals brought about no lysis. The serums of 38 immune animals caused an average of 72 per cent of lysis. The serum from the rabbit from which the leucocytes were taken plus the homologous leucocytes gave an average of 75 per cent of lysis or practically the same amount as that which occurred with the other immune serums. It appeared evident that these leucocytes as tested in this experiment had no advantage over the normal mononuclear leucocytes in producing the lysis of tubercle bacilli.

Experiments were also performed to find whether the serums from immune animals which were allergic had an advantage or disadvantage in inducing lysis over the serums from animals which were found to be immune but gave a negative skin tuberculin test. The relation of allergy to resistance is discussed in other papers.

Rabbits were vaccinated so as to produce allergy in some and no allergy in others. Ten animals were selected from each group (table 4). The animals

TABLE 4.—*Degree of Lysis of Tubercle Bacilli (BCG) with Serums from Allergic and Non-allergic Animals*

No.	Degree of allergy	Percentage of lysis
10	0	70
10	++ to +++	80

in the first group showed grades of allergy from ++ to +++. The serums from these animals in the presence of mononuclear leucocytes caused 80 per

12. Bull. Johns Hopkins Hosp. **50:** 115, 1932.
13. J. Exper. Med. **54:** 387, 1931.

cent lysis of the tubercle bacilli. The serums from the 10 non-allergic animals under similar conditions resulted in 70 per cent of lysis which was practically the same as with the serums from the allergic animals. The lysis was slightly greater in the allergic animals but the titers of the immune serums were also greater in this group. In producing allergy in the animals it was, as a rule, necessary to use living organisms which tended to give a more concentrated immune serum than when heat killed organisms were used. The property in the serum to bring about lysis of tubercle bacilli through mononuclear leucocytes appeared to bear no necessary correlation to the phenomenon of allergy.

DISCUSSION

In these experiments a method is described for measuring the degree of lysis of tubercle bacilli in vitro. The degree of lysis was estimated from the degree of failure of the bacilli to take the acid fast stain or to be stained by ordinary methods.

It was found that lysis of tubercle bacilli would not take place except when leucocytes were present. It was obvious from the presence of the bacilli in the leucocytic cells in various stages of disintegration that lysis took place intracellularly.

Measurable amounts of lysis did not occur in the presence of normal serum and leucocytes in one hour. To bring about lysis in this time it was necessary to have the bacilli in contact with leucocytes and immune serum. The degree of lysis increased as the concentration of the antibody content of the serums increased.

The mononuclear leucocytes from animals immune and allergic to tubercle bacilli showed no advantage over normal mononuclear leucocytes in producing lysis of tubercle bacilli. The allergic state in the animals from which immune serums were taken had no apparent influence upon the process of lysis.

CONCLUSIONS

Tubercle bacilli undergo lysis in vitro after being phagocytosed by normal mononuclear leucocytes in the presence of immune serum.

The lysis is greatly accelerated in the presence of immune serum and the degree of lysis tends to correlate the concentration of antibodies in the immune serum.

The mononuclear leucocytes of immune and allergic animals when washed free from serum appear to be no more sensitive in bringing about lysis than normal leucocytes.

The degree of lytic action of the serum appears to bear no necessary relation to the allergic state in the animals from which the serums were taken.

Lysis of tubercle bacilli, phagocytosed by mononuclear leucocytes, is a probable method of destroying the organisms in the tuberculous infected body.

RURAL TYPHOID FEVER

BÉLA JOHAN

BUDAPEST

One of the most important aims of urban sanitation was to free cities of typhoid fever. The studies directed towards discovering the cause of typhoid fever epidemics in centers of population are well known, and have clearly shown a causal relationship between the disease and water, milk, or food stuffs in general. The net result of control work based on these studies is that typhoid fever morbidity and mortality rates in the large cities of civilized countries show an important decrease as compared with data of the preceding century.

Much less has been done to free villages of typhoid fever. The number of studies concerned with the disease in the rural field has been much smaller. Furthermore, the careful investigations of the typhoid fever epidemics of cities have given only very restricted enlightenment as to the causes of rural typhoid fever.

The aim of the study here reported was to discover the causes of rural typhoid fever and the conditions under which it occurs, and to determine the factors responsible for the frequency of the disease, in order that these may be controlled. The paper summarizes part of the results of three years of epidemiological research work conducted at the suggestion of the International Conference on Rural Health, initiated by the Health Section of the League of Nations.

At the outset, two questions must be raised:

(1) Do international and national statistics indicate that typhoid fever is more prevalent today in villages than in cities?

(2) Is rural typhoid fever a special problem?

If the causes of rural typhoid fever are identical with those of city epidemics, identical methods of control can be used in both instances. If the contrary is true, then a special plan of operation must be prepared for the fight against rural typhoid fever.

It is hardly possible to obtain the necessary data for answering the first question on a large scale, but some enlightenment is furnished if we compare the typhoid fever mortality rates of various countries with the same rates in their respective capital towns. Such data were collected from the Monthly Epidemiological Reports of the League of Nations. Unfortunately, however, these data were not gathered according to identical systems. The statistics for the different capital cities do not furnish a true picture of the situation, because some of them include figures for typhoid fever patients transported from the rural field to the city hospitals and deceased there.

Received for publication, June 3, 1935.

From The State Hygienic Institute of Hungary.

Table 1 shows that typhoid fever mortality in the capital cities of certain countries (Bulgaria, Czechoslovakia, Greece, Hungary, Spain) is lower, in some instances considerably so, than the typhoid fever mortality rate of the whole country. In the other countries studied, both rates are more or less the same, or the urban rate is higher than that for the country as a whole. As a rule, with the exception of Portugal, the countries in the latter group

TABLE 1.—*Typhoid Fever Mortality Rate per 100,000 Population (Averages for the Years 1929–33)*

Country	Typhoid Fever Mortality	Capital City	Typhoid Fever Mortality
England	0.64	London	0.70
Austria	1.93	Vienna	2.03
Bulgaria	7.00	Sofia	6.70
Czechoslovakia	6.87	Prague	3.83
Denmark	0.62	Copenhagen	1.70
Greece	22.42	Athens	19.53
Jugoslovaia	3.65	Belgrade	7.26
Hungary	16.19	Budapest	8.20
Germany	1.18	Berlin	0.86
Norway	0.74	Oslo	1.46
Portugal	18.24	Lisbon	18.30
Rumania	3.32	Bucarest	5.50
Spain	15.88	Madrid	8.07

are those where typhoid fever is not very prevalent. The higher mortality rate in the capital cities might be the result of including in the reckoning rural patients referred to the city hospitals and deceased there.

Let us consider the position of this problem in Hungary. Here morbidity statistics concerning typhoid fever are fairly reliable, and we may compare those for Budapest with those for other parts of the country.

TABLE 2.—*Typhoid Fever Morbidity Rate in Hungary per 100,000 Population*

	1931	1932	1933
Entire country	99.6	257.6	87.4
Counties, excluding cities	103.4	281.0	88.9
Cities, including Budapest	83.9	159.9	76.8
Cities, excluding Budapest	148.9	283.3	114.1
Budapest alone	40.5	77.7	52.2

According to the data in table 2 typhoid fever morbidity is much lower in Budapest than in the counties excluding the cities with statutory powers, which are the largest cities. The county data, however, include returns from both villages and county towns. The lower typhoid fever rate of the cities, as compared with that of the counties is connected with the low rate of Budapest, because if this is omitted, then the rate of cities is higher, in all three years, than the corresponding rate of the counties. A further analysis of these data would be necessary to establish how far the high morbidity rate of these cities is connected with the typhoid fever morbidity conditions of their suburban (farming districts) territories. The fact that as a rule notification in the cities with statutory powers is better than in the counties, may contribute to the higher rate. But the table also shows that a city like Budapest, provided with all modern sanitary conveniences, has a comparatively favorable typhoid fever rate. The position of other cities is often unfavorably influenced by the fact that a considerable part of their territory is not urban in character, but decidedly rural. Thus, from the point of view of epidemiological research our cities are not uniformly urban, but include both urban and rural territories. This explains why they stand, as far as typhoid fever is concerned, on the same level as the counties with their incorporated villages and towns. Indeed the situation has the appearance of being worse in cities, because there public health service is better than in the villages, and notification brings more cases to the knowledge of the authorities.

Undoubtedly, there is a difference from year to year between the morbidity rates of the large cities and other territories of the country. Therefore the typhoid problem in the large cities and in the smaller agglomerations is not identical. "Other territories" not being homogeneous, it is obvious that the character of rural typhoid will be revealed only if we study in detail the typhoid fever picture of a rural district.

The district of Mezökövesd was selected and studied in 1931, 1932, and 1933 for this purpose. The number of inhabitants in the 29 villages of the district was 71,963 in 1932, calculated from the data of the census of 1930. The largest commune had a population of 20,806 in 1930, the smallest a population of 658. Twelve communes had populations between 1,000 and 2,000.

The average number of persons per dwelling house, which usually had two living rooms and a kitchen, was 4.8. In about 24 per cent of the dwelling houses there were no privies, and where privies existed they were very often in a neglected state. Of the public wells, 37 per cent were safe from the health point of view. The majority of the people were engaged in agricultural work. In the years 1931–33, 13.8 per cent of the population was employed as seasonal agricultural laborers, working in different parts of the country and being absent for about six months from their homes.

The district is highly infected with typhoid as shown by the morbidity rates of 180,730, and 147 per 100,000 for the years 1931, 1932, and 1933, respectively, whereas in Budapest the rates for the corresponding years were 40, 77, and 52 per 100,000. The case fatality rates for the district were 8.5, 11.6, and 11.3 respectively.

In the year 1932 only 8.9 per cent of the cases occurring in the district were referred to hospital, the other patients, 91.1 per cent, remained in their homes during the entire course of the disease. Careful analysis of the cases showed that at least 43 per cent were the result of contact infections occurring either within one dwelling or among visitors, especially relatives, of the patients. Careful local observations showed that simultaneous infections are very rare (Dr. Ralovich). In Budapest in those years 5.9 to 10.8 per cent of all typhoid fever cases were due to contact infections. In Budapest 90 to 95 per cent of typhoid fever patients are admitted to hospital.

It has been said that an important number of typhoid fever cases in the rural field are contracted through direct contact with a patient suffering from this disease. The question now arises as to what are the sources of infection of the isolated cases, and of the first cases in group infections.

Rural typhoid fever, like urban typhoid fever, has two epidemiologically different types of appearance. One type, aseasonal typhoid fever epidemy, may occur at various times of the year and is independent of the season. The other type, seasonal typhoid fever epidemy, occurs in the so-called typhoid fever season and is dependent on the season. In Hungary the typhoid fever season begins towards the end of July or early in August and lasts till the end of November or the middle of December.

Research concerning the causes of the aseasonal typhoid fever epidemy, is assisted by the fact that the disease is mostly restricted to a circumscribed territory and causes there the illness of a large number of people. Epidemics caused by foodstuffs and contaminated water belong to this group. These may occur not only in the typhoid fever season but during any month of the

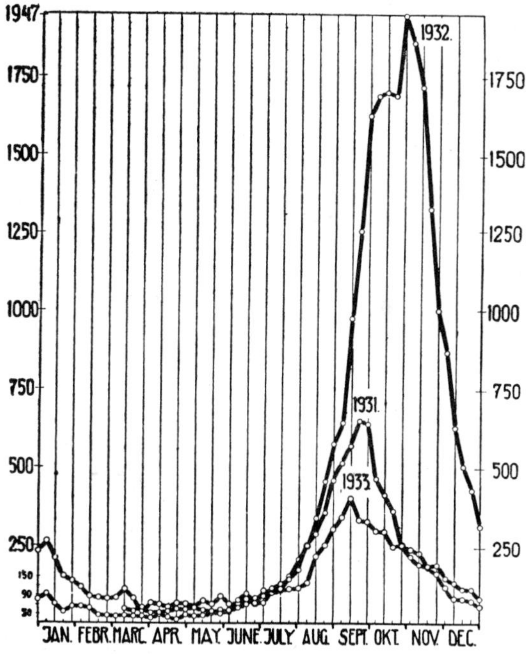

Fig. 1.—Curves showing typhoid fever in Hungary in the years 1931–33.

year. Typhoid fever epidemics observed in boarding schools, caserns, etc., may be considered under this heading. In such epidemics a carrier of typhoid fever bacilli or a patient suffering from a mild form of the disease generally plays an important part; through the medium of foodstuffs or water he communicates the excreted typhoid fever bacilli to a large group of healthy individuals, some of whom become subsequently ill with typhoid fever. Etiological research concerning this type of epidemy is very frequently successful. General sanitation of the water supplies of cities and villages considerably reduces such epidemics. Epidemics of this type were frequent in the past in the countries where much milk was consumed in a raw state; however with the introduction of careful pasteurization their number was reduced.

In rural areas of Hungary water-borne typhoid fever is not an important problem. Water supplies in the villages are seldom centralized, and a contaminated well is a source of infection only to the persons using it. Some typical water-borne epidemics in rural regions have been studied in Hungary, but these are not numerous and are not responsible for the high typhoid incidence in the villages. Furthermore large groups of the rural population are seldom exposed to the danger of infection through foodstuffs owing to the decentralization of food supply as well as to the widely practiced rural autarchy. In this respect there is undoubtedly a difference between the typhoid fever risk of the urban and the rural population.

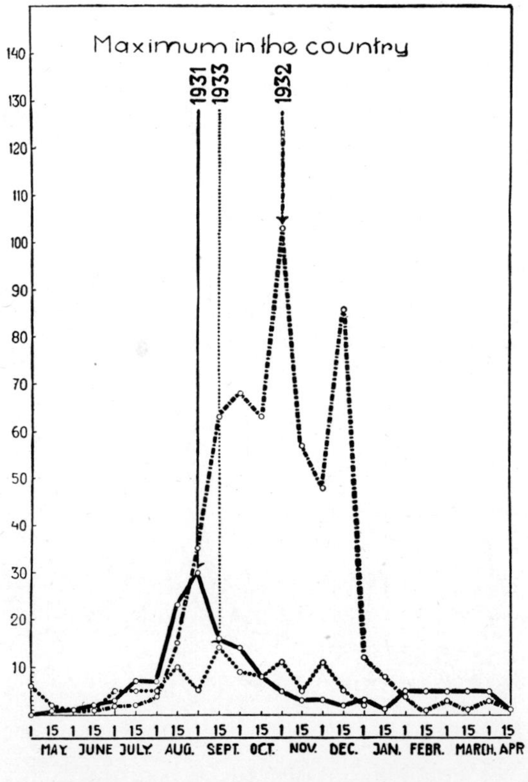

Fig. 2.—Curves showing typhoid fever morbidity of the district Mezökövesd in 1931–33. The date when the national curve reached the maximum in the same years is given.

The causes of the outbreak of the so-called seasonal typhoid fever epidemics are much harder to determine. There is a certain period of the year in the temperate climate, when the number of typhoid fever cases increases. In Hungary the increase begins each year at exactly the same time, namely the month of July, and rises abruptly during the second half of August, reaching the maximum between the middle of September and October; after this there is a sudden decrease in the number of cases. This is so characteristic that American authors designated as "normal" the epidemiological curve remaining after the elimination of the above mentioned aseasonal typhoid fever epidemics. Rosenau used the term "residual typhoid curve" and Sedgwick "prosodemic typhoid curve" to express the idea.

The questions arise as to whether this increase of typhoid fever observed in the late summer and the autumn is a regular phenomenon of rural typhoid fever, and what relation the rural typhoid fever curve bears to the typhoid fever curve of cities and of the whole country.

For the purpose of studying this question, the typhoid fever curve of the district of Mezökövesd for the years 1931, 1932, and 1933 is presented. On the same diagram the time of the peak of the national typhoid curve is also shown (diagram 2). It can be established that in Mezökövesd District the increase begins in July, as it does in the country as a whole (see diagram 1), and the curve becomes steeper in August.

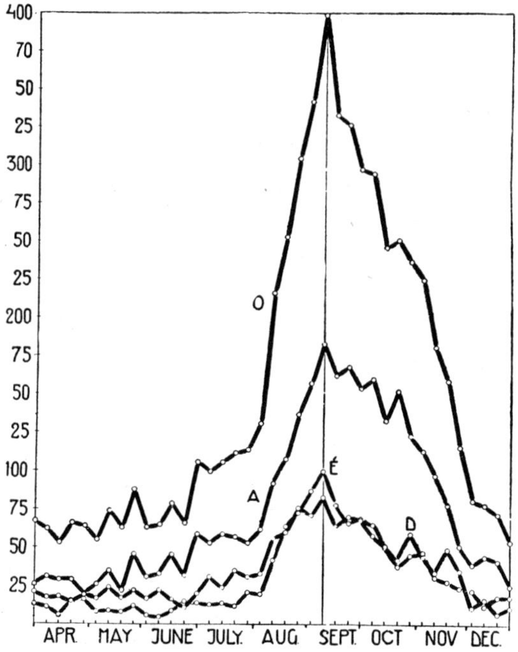

Fig. 3.—Typhoid morbidity curve of Hungary as a whole (O) and of the different parts of the country (A, E, D) in 1933.

The typhoid fever curve of the district of Mezökövesd reached its high point in 1931–33 at the same time as the national curve. It may be mentioned that the typhoid fever curve of Budapest also shows a marked increase in the autumn. The time of the peak of the typhoid fever curve of the cities with statutory power, which are the largest cities in Hungary, corresponded in 1933, for instance, exactly with that of the peak of the typhoid fever curve of both the country and the district of Mezökövesd. Dr. Petrilla has proved that the curves of typhoid fever incidence in different parts of the country in the same year reach their high point during the same week (diagram 3).

For many years in Hungary, the time at which the typhoid fever curve begins to climb steeply has been the same. With regard to the time of the culmination of the curve there are differences from year to year. The maximum was reached in 1931 early in September, in 1932 towards the end of October, in 1933 during the middle of September. In general, the later the culmination of the typhoid fever curve, the higher the number of typhoid fever cases.

Based on the above related facts, it is safe to speak of a "normal" typhoid fever curve if this same shows an increase during the late summer and early autumn months. The question arises as to what may be the reason—especially in the villages—for the autumn increase.

The question is an old and interesting problem of the epidemiology of typhoid fever. The cause of the rise of the typhoid fever curve is certainly not local because, as has been demonstrated, it appears comparatively simultaneously in the whole country, in different parts of the country, in the capital city as well as in the studied district. Therefore, only a generally represented cause can be considered. An increased excretion of bacilli by carriers, which might occur for some reason in that period of the year, might have some part in this. Also the greater susceptibility at this time of the persons exposed to the infection might play a rôle. Some changes—up to now unknown—occurring about the same period in the condition of water and of foodstuffs or in the living conditions of flies might contribute to the spread of the disease.

As early as 1931, the thought presented itself that carriers might perhaps excrete larger quantities of bacilli in summer, during the time when much fruit is consumed, than late in the autumn, in the winter, or in the spring. The so-called intermittent carriers were thought of, and the question arose whether the negative cultures presented by these persons from time to time did not tend to appear during the winter and spring months, when the smaller number of typhoid fever cases might be a consequence of the restricted excretion of bacilli. To obtain light on this matter, a carrier study was undertaken. During the first year of the study, in the winter of 1931 as a matter of fact, only a very small number of carriers were found. Later the reason for this was discovered, namely, that specimens of feces had not been sent in for examination immediately, but several days after they had been obtained.

Another circumstance which must be considered in carrier work is the possibility that the person under observation may submit fecal specimens from some other individual. Such a subterfuge is natural on the part of persons like waiters, dairy workers, etc., who would not be permitted to follow their occupations if they were found to be carriers of bacilli. Two methods are used to preclude this possibility: The doctor may apply suppositories to the person under examination, and as these produce a movement in about 8–10 minutes, he may wait and take the sample himself; or he may administer a dose of fine vegetable seeds in a capsule and instruct the patient to bring a specimen of the next day's stool for examination. In laboratory examination it is easy to detect the seeds and to establish whether the specimen was obtained from the patient who was given the seeds and whose feces should be examined for typhoid fever bacilli. In case several members of the same family are to be examined, different seeds must be administered to each and notes taken as to which person received which seed. Thus the laboratory can easily determine whether any exchange has been practiced. This method was worked out by Dr. B. Zboray in our Institute. He recommended a 0.5 to 1.0 gram doses of the following seeds:

Anethum graveolens	Ruta graveolens
Gypsophylla scorsoneriae folia	Salvia officinalis
Lavandula vera	Salvia sclarea
Nigella damascena	Sinapis alba
Plantago psyllium	

Taking all these precautions, it was found that the number of the so-called "intermittent" carriers cannot be very high. Dr. Lovrekovitch examined in this Institute over a period of nearly three years about a thousand specimens of feces secured from eleven carriers living in rural districts, and as a rule he obtained regularly a long series of positive results with the same patient (diagram 4). This also indicates the reliability of the technique used in the laboratory. Negative findings were also made, but the majority of these were obtained during the summer. The heat probably diminished the positives among the specimen sent by mail. If our supposition had been right, the highest number of positive results should have been obtained in summer. However, these researches demonstrated that there is not a sufficiently regular and pronounced difference between the seasons of the year from the point of view of excretion of bacilli by the carriers to explain the seasonal rise of the typhoid fever curve.

Dr. Petrilla of our Institute has indicated lately that there is a decided correlation—at least in the past three years—between the changes of the daily average temperature and the fluctuation of the typhoid fever curve. According to his observations, whenever the daily average temperature rose about 20 C., this was followed approximately 4 weeks later by an ascending tendency of the typhoid fever curve. The sinking under this level of the daily average temperature was followed, also approximately 4 weeks later, by a descending tendency of the typhoid fever curve. If this observation is confirmed by data in subsequent years, then one step will have been made towards the solution of the problem of the so-called seasonal typhoid fever. However, even then the problem remains unsolved as to how the higher temperature causes an increase in the number of typhoid fever cases. It is not probable that the higher temperature acts directly on the human organism by lowering its power of resistance. If such direct action occurred, the rise of the typhoid curve would follow more promptly the rise of temperature.

Certain observations make one suspect the rôle of flies. If there is an important correlation between the lack of adequate hygienic pit privies and rural typhoid fever, and typhoid fever is more frequent in rural areas, even then the existence of a factor must be supposed which carries the infection from the excreta of the bacillus-carrier found in inadequate privies to the susceptible individual, especially during the late summer and early autumn days. It has been established that carriers excrete bacilli during the entire

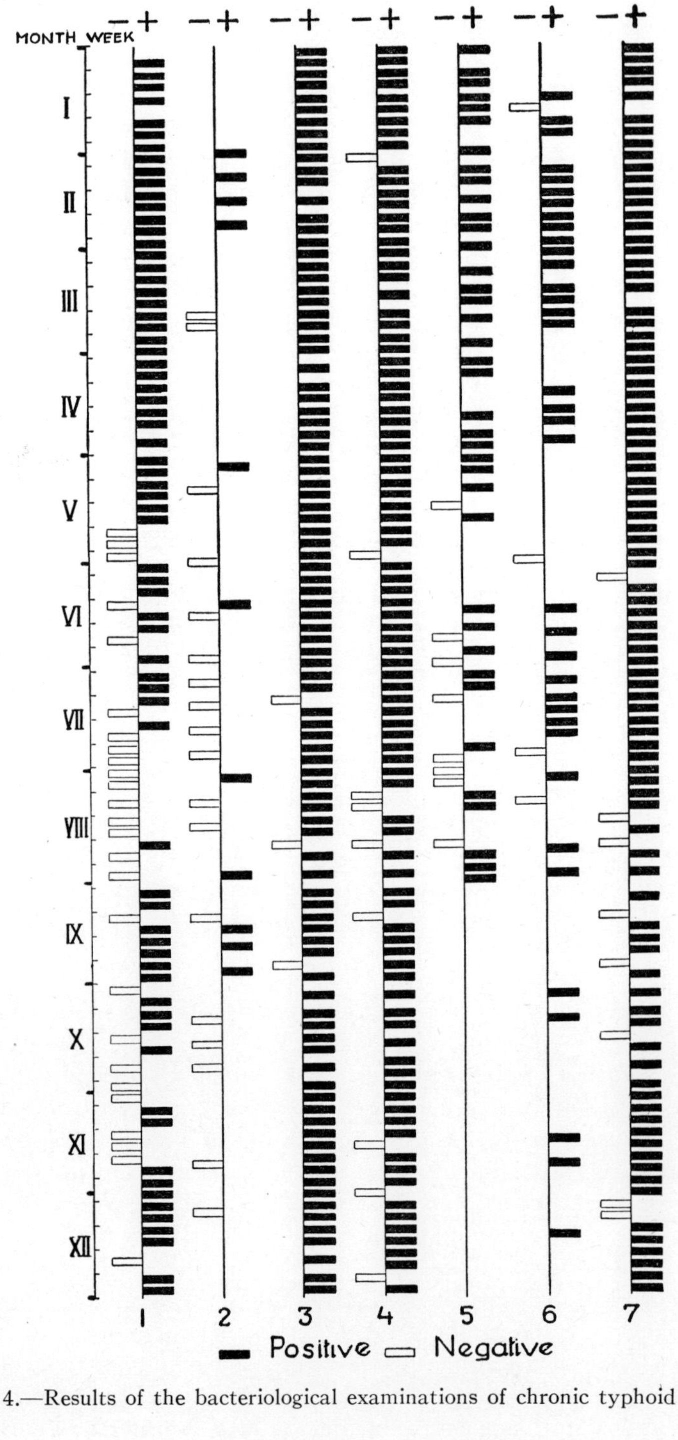

Fig. 4.—Results of the bacteriological examinations of chronic typhoid carriers.

year. The pit privies are used uniformly by the population throughout the year, and the state of these privies does not deteriorate during the period of time preceding the outbreak of the epidemics. Excluding the probability of a greater susceptibility of the population to infection in this period, we must suppose that they are more exposed to infection during this time of the year than at other periods. Because of the predilection of flies for decaying, decomposed material, and the fact that these insects are constant carriers of polluting material, they have been suspected for a long time of playing a part in the spread of typhoid fever. It must be mentioned, however, that during the autumn of 1933 more than 1,000 flies caught in the houses of rural typhoid fever patients were examined without a culture of typhoid fever bacilli being obtained from any of them.

The part played by water in the outbreak of the aseasonal typhoid fever epidemics is well known. However, we do not think that water has an important part in causing seasonal typhoid fever epidemics. It would be difficult to explain why infected wells should cause typhoid fever epidemics only or largely in August or September. As it happens, at the time of the upward tendency of the typhoid fever curve observed early in the autumn, isolated cases of the disease occur in communities where the entire population is served by the same water supply; and this in itself militates against the theory of seasonal infection caused by water. Another argument against water as a source of seasonal infection is the fact that simultaneous infections in the same house are rare. Furthermore in this country typhoid fever is frequent in many communes provided with a sufficient number of deep wells giving safe drinking water. The following thesis therefore cannot, at least generally, be sustained: contaminated wells may cause typhoid fever; an important proportion of rural wells in Hungary are polluted; in consequence the cause of rural typhoid fever must be sought in the contaminated wells. In the first place, polluted water is not always synonymous with contaminated wells. Typhoid fever epidemics caused by contaminated water have special epidemiological characteristics and therefore only when these are established may a typhoid fever epidemic be labelled as water borne.

In outbreaks of aseasonal typhoid fever epidemics, caused by contaminated foodstuffs, water, etc., or contact infections, the carriers of bacilli play an important part. Even in seasonal typhoid fever epidemics, their part is important, as they conserve bacilli during the epidemic-free periods. However, the existence of carriers of bacilli does not explain the characteristic summer-autumn outbreak of typhoid fever. Laboratory examinations proved that in the excretion of bacilli by carriers there is no such seasonal fluctuation as would explain the seasonal changes of the typhoid fever curve. The bacillus carrier is living in a community of people all the year round and is excreting bacilli about evenly in all seasons. Therefore, besides carriers of bacilli, the permanent sources of infection, some other factor must be playing a part in the increase in the number of infections during the so-called typhoid fever season. Some agent must be thought of, which carries the excreted typhoid bacilli to the susceptible individual especially in this period.

During the period 1931–1933, over 5,000 feces and urine specimens from the district of Mezökövesd were examined. A large part of the examinations were performed with the aim of discovering carriers of bacilli. The number of chronic carriers found was 27. Researches on the premises could prove that in 10.6 per cent of all typhoid fever cases, a carrier of bacilli was the primary cause of the disease.

SUMMARY

The results of epidemiological studies and laboratory examinations concerning the importance, forms of appearance, and causes of rural typhoid fever establish certain facts. The majority of rural typhoid fever patients are not admitted to hospital, which factor plays a very important rôle in the spread of the disease in Hungary. There is ample opportunity in the village for members of the patient's family and relatives visiting him to contract the disease through direct contact. In rural areas simultaneous infections are rare, contact infections frequent. In cities simultaneous infections caused by foodstuffs and in certain instances by water are more common, and contact infections comparatively rare. Besides typhoid fever patients, carriers of bacilli are the sources of infection.

Rural typhoid fever may be considered under aseasonal and seasonal epidemics. In outbreaks of the first mentioned type, contaminated wells and eventually foodstuffs may have a part. Seasonal typhoid fever epidemics appear simultaneously in the whole country, and the epidemiological curve reaches its high point in all localities about the same time, sometimes even during the same week. The correlation between the average daily temperature, over 20 C., and the fluctuation of the typhoid fever curve observed by Dr. Petrilla is very striking. However, this relationship is probably not direct but presupposes at this period a larger number or a greater activity of the infection carrying factor—perhaps the fly.

The part—at least the direct part—played by insanitary rural wells in the seasonal typhoid fever epidemics, is probably not very large. The neglected state, or the complete lack, of rural pit privies is much more important.

The carriers of bacilli conserve the sources of infection, but this fact in itself does not explain the late summer-autumn epidemics. According to examinations the excretion of the bacilli by the carriers does not show such seasonal fluctuations as would explain the typical seasonal changes of the epidemiological curve of typhoid fever.

Thus, rural typhoid fever is different, at least as far as origin and spread are concerned, from typhoid fever of large cities. Therefore, rural typhoid fever must be studied separately. In the fight against this disease, experiences obtained during urban campaigns against typhoid fever must be utilized, but in addition the special characteristics of rural typhoid fever must be considered and such procedures worked out as conform to the character of this disease.

STUDIES ON INFLAMMATION. XI.

INVASIVENESS AND VIRULENCE IN RELATION TO RESISTANCE

VALY MENKIN

BOSTON

The earlier studies of the writer[1] have demonstrated that various materials, including dyes, ferric chloride, a foreign protein, and bacteria, injected into an area of acute inflammation, are retained in situ, so that they fail to disseminate to the tributary lymphatics as readily as under normal circumstances. The mechanism of this fixation of foreign substances was found to be referable to an obstructuve barrier in the form of coagulated plasma and thrombosed lymphatics in acutely inflamed tissue.[2] These observations suggested further study with some common pyogenic microorganisms in an endeavor to obtain an insight into the nature of invasiveness. The localizing property of the staphylococcus was ascribed to the prompt formation of an obstructive barrier, as described above.[3] Within one hour after intracutaneous inoculation of this organism, a vital dye, trypan blue, injected into the infected focus, failed to reach the tributary lymphatic vessels and nodes. The fixation of this dye was correlated with the finding of fibrinous plugs in the lymphatics of the inflamed area. Varying amounts of fibrin deposits were also observed. In the case of type I pneumococcus, the "Walling-off" process was manifested a trifle later, i.e., about 6 to 9 hours following the inoculation of the microorganisms. The results obtained with hemolytic streptococci were particularly interesting in this connection. The lymphatic lumina remained unoccluded for a period of almost 2 days. Throughout this time, trypan blue freely diffused from the site of bacterial inoculation into the draining lymphatic channels. Thereafter the inflammatory reaction had progressed to such a point that completely occluded lymphatics with dense leucocytic thrombi were to be noted, as well as a heavy cellular infiltration. Only then would the vital dye injected into the inflamed focus fail to reach either the afferent and efferent tributary lymphatic vessels or the lymph node. These findings offered a satisfactory explanation for the spreading capacity of the streptococcus in contrast to the localizing properties of the staphylococcus. The conclusion reached was that the rapidity and the intensity with which a bacterial or chemical inflammatory irritant circumscribed itself, by inducing a mechanical barrier, doubtless was an important factor in determining its invasive capacity. These results on the differential

Received for publication, June 6, 1935.

From the Department of Pathology, Harvard University Medical School.

This study was aided by grants from the DeLamar Mobile Research Fund and from the William W. Wellington Memorial Research Fund.

1. J. Exper. Med. **50:** 171, 1929; Arch. Path. **12:** 802, 1931.
2. Menkin, V.: J. Exper. Med. **53:** 171, 1931; **56:** 157, 1932.
3. Menkin, V.: J. Exper. Med. **57:** 977, 1933.

behavior of staphylococcus and streptococcus have recently been confirmed by Dennis and Berberian.[4]

The invasive property of a microorganism has often been taken as a criterion of its virulence and vice versa.[5] Some bacteriologists have, however, recognized that, properly speaking, virulence and invasiveness are different properties[6] and that there is no justification therefore for employing the two terms synonymously.

The terms virulence, invasiveness, and resistance, as used by the writer in the present communication, may be defined as follows:

Virulence represents the capacity of a pathogenic microorganism to produce generalized deleterious effects when inoculated in a given host. The maximum effect of the damage is obtained with the death of the animal. The rate at which this end-point is reached serves as an index of the resistance of the host to a given dose of the infecting microorganism.

Invasiveness, on the other hand, represents the capacity of a microorganism to disseminate to the circulating blood from its point of cutaneous inoculation. The extent of invasiveness is evidently largely regulated by the intensity of the local inflammatory reaction induced in the host by the pathogenic microorganism.

As above defined therefore, virulence refers to the ability of the microorganism per se to induce in the host generalized damage; whereas invasiveness is associated with the degree of localized inflammatory reaction developed in the host owing to the presence of the pathogenic microorganism.

The experimental observations to be reported in the present communication indicate that the invasiveness of a virulent microorganism (type III pneumococcus) from the site of its cutaneous inoculation may be delayed by a superimposed injection of an inflammatory irritant that causes prompt "walling-off." This procedure may retard the dissemination of the virulent microorganisms, and even in some cases, apparently, allow sufficient time for the local inflammatory reaction to dispose of them in large part. In this way massive blood stream invasion and death may be delayed and in a few cases even aborted. Nevertheless the data to be presented do not indicate that the virulence of the pathogenic microorganism has been in any way altered by delaying its invasiveness.

EXPERIMENTAL

White rabbits were inoculated intracutaneously with varying quantities of a virulent strain of type III pneumococcus grown on blood broth.[7] The site of inoculation was always in the skin of one of the forelegs. The amounts inoculated ranged from 0.1 cc. to 0.5 cc. The cultures were about 18 to 24 hours old. For each experimental rabbit a control was inoculated with the same amount of culture. The injection of pneumococci in the experimental rabbit was immedi-

---

4. J. Exper. Med. **60:** 581, 1934.

5. Zinsser, H.: Resistance to Infectious Diseases, New York, Macmillan Company, 4th edition, 1931.

6. Topley, W. W. C.: An Outline of Immunity, Baltimore, William Wood & Company, 1933.

7. SV strain obtained through the courtesy of Dr. J. Enders.

ately followed by the inoculation, in the same cutaneous site, of 1.5 cc. of a virulent strain of Staphylococcus aureus (grown on broth). In the control animal an injection of 1.5 cc. of sterile broth was superimposed upon the inoculation of pneumococci. To control the possible effect of the two microorganisms on one another, in a few rabbits a mixture of aleuronat (5 per cent) and starch (3 per cent) and 0.5 per cent saline was substituted for the staphylococci. In such experiments the control animal was injected with 0.5 per cent saline following the inoculation with pneumococci. In one case 0.5 cc. turpentine was employed as the circumscribing irritant. Both control and experimental rabbits were kept as a rule in the same cage, and the survival time was observed. A thorough postmortem was performed in many of the cases, and blood from the heart was cultured on blood agar.

The results on the survival time of experimental and control animals are summarized in table 1. In every instance the experimental animal survived for a longer interval of time than did its respective control. None of the latter lived over 5 days. Since each experimental rabbit was inoculated with an identical volume of the same culture as its control, and practically at the

TABLE 1.—*Effect of a Superimposed Inflammatory Irritant on the Survival Time of Rabbits Infected with Virulent Pneumococci*

Control Animals				Experimental Animals			
Rabbit no.	Quantity of pneumococcus culture inoculated	Quantity of broth or saline injected	Survival time	Rabbit no.	Quantity of pneumococcus culture inoculated	Quantity of staphylococcus culture or chemical irritant injected	Survival time
	cc.	cc.	Days		cc.	cc.	Days
10–68	0.1	1.5 broth	3	10–69	0.1	1.5 Staph.	9
11–08	0.2	1.0 broth	1	11–21*	0.2	1.0 Staph.	4
10–54	0.2	3.0 saline	1	10–53	0.2	3.0 Aleuronat	3
10–94	0.2	5.0 saline	3	11–29	0.2	5.0 Aleuronat	5
10–66	0.25	3.0 saline	4	10–64	0.25	3.0 Aleuronat	5
11–24	0.3	0.5 H_2O	2	11–28	0.3	0.5 Turpentine	11
10–78	0.3	1.5 broth	5	10–77*	0.3	1.5 Staph.	64 Alive and well
11–12	0.4	1.5 broth	2	11–13*	0.4	1.5 Staph.	3
11–99	0.5	1.5 broth	2	12–00	0.5	1.5 Staph.	3
11–02	0.5	1.5 broth	3	11–01	0.5	1.5 Staph.	4
11–97	0.5	1.5 broth	4	10–86	0.5	1.5 Staph.	9
10–61	0.5	1.5 broth	3	11–98	0.5	1.5 Staph.	34 Alive and well (Killed subsequently)

* With the exception of these rabbits, all animals were inoculated with the same strain of Staphylococcus aureus.

same time, the results obtained in regard to longevity are entirely comparable. The greater survival time of the experimental rabbits as compared with the controls was marked in many instances irrespective of the type of irritant. Two rabbits (11–98 and 10–77), inoculated with pneumococcus and staphylococcus, survived inoculation of the virulent strain of pneumococcus. After a month and two months respectively, both these animals were still alive and well. One of them (11–98) was sacrificed on the 34th day. The other (rabbit 10–77) showed definite increase in weight and was well, to all intents and purposes, two months after its inoculation. All other animals succumbed to massive pneumococcal invasion of the blood stream, as indicated by blood culture.

The observations show that the superimposition of an inflammatory irritant, e.g. Staphylococcus aureus, aleuronat, or turpentine, delayed the full manifestation of infection with virulent type III pneumococcus, as evidenced by a significant increase in survival time. In two instances, the animals even survived the infection. It is conceivable that in these two (rabbit 11–98 and 10–77), the apparently greater effectiveness of Staphylococcus aureus as a superimposed irritant over the protective effects of aleuronat or turpentine may have been due to the proliferation of that microorganism at the site of inoculation, resulting in an unusually marked local reaction.

Section of the tissue at the site of cutaneous inoculation revealed, in both control and experimental rabbits, dense cellular infiltration consisting principally of mononuclear phagocytes extending into a thickened subcutaneous tissue, with considerable extravasation of red cells. Many lymphatics and small blood vessels were found occluded by fibrinous thrombi. Mural thrombi were not infrequently seen in the capillaries of such regions. Gram-Wiegert stained sections revealed in many cases pneumococci; sometimes these were observed outside of the cells; and at other times they were seen within the fibrinous meshwork occluding the lumina of lymphatics. In a number of instances large masses of microorganisms were also found in the vascular lumina, thus confirming histologically the positive blood culture findings. At death the microscopic appearances in both experimental and control rabbits were almost indistinguishable, the density of cellular infiltration being perhaps a trifle more striking in the experimental animals.

Are the favorable results obtained by the superimposition of an inflammatory irritant at the site of pneumococcal inoculation referable to alterations in the virulence or in the invasiveness of the microorganisms? On the other hand, might they not be due to differences in degree of leukocytic infiltration, or finally, perhaps to neutralizing principles seeping through the walls of the damaged capillaries?

In an endeavor to answer these questions, a series of experiments was set up.

It has previously been pointed out that when a vital dye is introduced into a skin area at various intervals of time after bacterial inoculation of this site, the degree of walling-off of the infected focus may be determined by the extent to which the dye can drain into the regional lymphatics.[3]

In a series of tests two white rabbits were inoculated intracutaneously in the skin of the foreleg with 0.5 cc. of a blood broth culture of the same strain of type III pneumococcus as used in the foregoing experiments. Immediately following this inoculation, 1.5 cc. of a broth culture of Staphylococcus aureus was injected into the same site in one of the rabbits, while the other animal, serving as control, received a superimposed equal volume of sterile broth. At varying intervals thereafter, ranging from about 2 to 19 hours, 2.5 cc. of 1 per cent trypan blue in saline were injected with a fine needle (gauge 24 or 25) into the inflamed area. The same amount of dye was introduced into the other foreleg as a control. The lymph from the efferent vessel draining the axillary lymphatic node was collected, as described in a previous paper.[8] The subclavian vein was exposed in the axillary region. Alongside and somewhat below the vein an efferent lymphatic vessel was seen to emerge from one of the axillary lymph nodes. The lymph was drawn by puncturing this vessel with a capillary pipette. Immediately after sacrificing the animals, both the lymph and the lymphatic nodes were studied for the presence of the dye. By means of a platinum loop, blood obtained from the ventricle was cultured on blood agar plates for the presence of pneumococci. The local area of inflammation was removed and fixed in 10 per cent formaldehyde for microscopic sectioning. Many of these preparations were stained by

8. Menkin, V. J. Exper. Med. **50:** 171, 1929.

Gram-Weigert in order to study the distribution of the microorganisms at the site of their inoculation.

The results of these experiments are shown in table 2. It is clear that at least for the first seven hours following the intracutaneous inoculation of pneumococci superimposed with broth, trypan blue freely diffuses from the inflamed area to the regional lymphatic nodes (see control rabbits, table 2). When longer intervals have elapsed between the injection of the irritant and that of the dye, there is definite evidence that the dye is retained at the site

TABLE 2.—*Retention of Trypan Blue at the Site of Inflammation Induced by the Inoculation of Virulent Pneumococci and Staphylococci*

Rabbit no.	Interval between injection of irritant and that of dye	Total duration of inflammation prior to examination of the lymph	Presence of dye on inflamed side		Presence of dye on normal side		Presence of pneumococci in Blood stream
			Lymph of efferent lymphatic	Lymph node	Lymph of efferent lymphatic	Lymph node	
	hrs.: mins.	hrs.: mins.					
10–81 (exp.)*	2:19	4:58	0	Faint Trace	+	+ to ++	0
10–80 (control)*	2:11	5:05	+	++	Trace	+	0
11–11 (exp.)	3:30	5:45	0	0	+	+	0
11–96 (control)	3:35	6:03	+++	Trace	++	+ to ++	+
10–55 (exp.)	3:00	5:50		+		++	0
10–48 (control)	2:47	6:10	++	++	+	+	+
11–26 (exp.)	7:55	9:35	0	0	++	++	0
11–23 (control)	7:40	9:34	Faint trace	Trace	+	Trace	+
11–36 (control)**	7:17	9:17	+	++	+	+	+
11–25 (exp.)**	13:15	15:45	Faint trace	0	+++	++	+
11–34 (exp.)	13:15	16:05	0	0	+	++	0
11–39 (control)	13:10	16:10	Trace	Trace	+	+	+
10–57 (exp.)	19:02	21:59	0	0	Trace to +	+	+ (2 colonies)
10–63 (control)	18:55	22:08	0	0	+ to ++	+	+ (12 colonies)

* Exp. refers to rabbits inoculated with pneumococci and staphylococci in broth. Control refers to animals inoculated with pneumococci and broth.

** Performed on separate days and with different cultures of pneumococci and staphylococci.

of inflammation. This is well illustrated 19 hours after the inoculation of pneumococci and broth (see control rabbit 10–63, table 2). On the other hand, examination of the results obtained in experimental rabbits inoculated intracutaneously with pneumococci immediately followed by administration of Staphylococcus aureus reveals the inability of the dye to permeate freely to the regional lymphatics, a failure evident at a very early stage. In the experimental rabbits, in contrast to the controls, definite evidence was obtained that 2 to 3 hours after bacterial inoculation, the area of inflammation had become circumscribed, as indicated by the failure of the dye to reach the regional lymphatics.

Histological studies correlate the passage of dye in the control rabbits with the presence of patent lymphatics (see fig. 1, rabbit 10–80, table 2). In the later stages of the inflammatory reaction in the control animals, the failure of the dye to diffuse outward is associated with fibrinous occlusion of the lymphatic vessels and with the presence of coagulated plasma in the inflamed area. The superimposition of staphylococci hastens the blockage of lymphatic drainage owing to the injurious effects of this microorganism on small vessels. This was indicated both by the inability of the dye to diffuse away from the site of inflammation and also by the presence in such areas of deposits of fibrin in the extra-capillary spaces and of partial or complete occlusion of the lymphatic lumina by fibrinous thrombi (see figs. 2, 3, and 4, rabbits 10–81, 10–55, and 11–26, table 2).

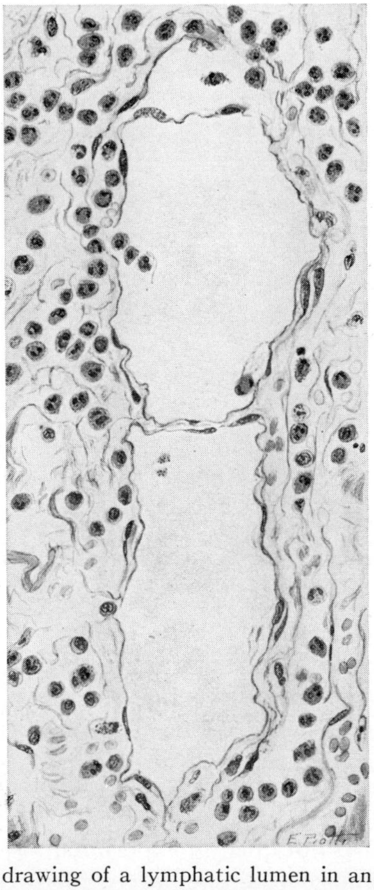

Fig. 1.—Camera lucida drawing of a lymphatic lumen in an inflamed area of about five hours duration induced by the intracutaneous inoculation of pneumococci type III followed by sterile broth. The lumen is unoccluded and trypan blue drained freely to the regional lymph node. × 540 (control rabbit 10–80, table 2).

The delay in the invasiveness of pneumococci in the above experiment is doubtless due to the presence of an intense irritant, Staphylococcus aureus, which, as has been demonstrated previously,[3] induces an early walling-off of the inflamed area. This is likewise indicated by the blood culture findings (table 2). The reader's attention is called to the fact that in the control animals, pneumococci can be recovered in the blood stream about 6 hours following their cutaneous inoculation (see control rabbit 10–48, table 2). In the experimental rabbits pneumococci were recovered in one case only, after about 16 hours had elapsed subsequent to the cutaneous inoculation of the microorganisms. In the experimental animals, studies of Gram-Weigert sections frequently revealed in the local areas of inoculation great numbers of pneumococci and clumps of staphylococci. The pneumococci for the most part were situated extracellularly. It is interesting to note in this connection that Ward and Lyons[9] regard virulence as the resistance of a microorganism to phagocytosis. These observations apparently support the view that ani-

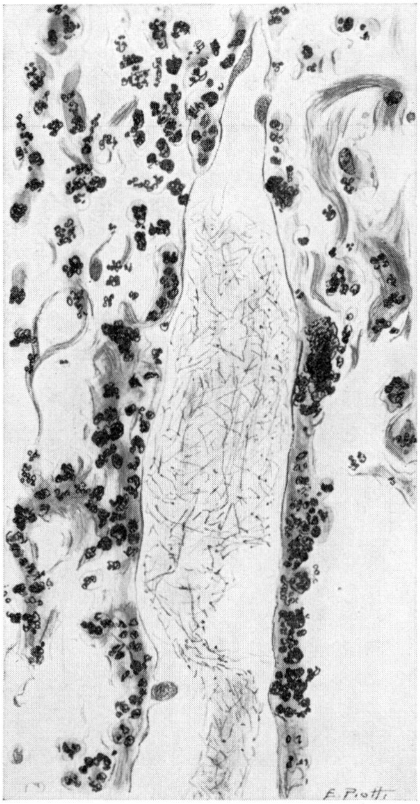

Fig. 2.—Camera lucida drawing of a lymphatic lumen in an inflamed area of about five hours duration induced by the inoculation of pneumococcus type III followed immediately by Staphylococcus aureus injection. The lymphatic lumen is occluded in large part by a delicate fibrinous reticulum. Trypan blue drained only in minute traces to the regional lymph node. × 760 (experimental rabbit 10–81, table 2).

mals infected almost simultaneously with pneumococci and staphylococci probably owe the increase in their survival time to the delay in invasiveness of the virulent pneumococci, occasioned by the early formation of an obstructive barrier to free lymphatic drainage.

The possibility remains that the increased survival time obtained by the superimposition of an acute inflammatory irritant in a pneumococcus infected area may be referable to differing degrees of leucocytic response. An added cellular infiltration, in addition perhaps to an increase in plasma seepage, may be largely responsible for the effects evoked. The fact that at death the local cellular reaction at the site of inoculation both in control

9. J. Exper. Med. **61:** 515, 1935.

and experimental animals, is not materially different as well as the fact that a very great number of the pneumococci are situated extracellularly, would suggest that the leukocytes as a factor are perhaps not of primary significance in explaining the results.

Solution of this question was sought, however, by means of direct tests. An attempt was made to prevent lymphatic blockage while maintaining at the same time the dense cellular infiltration induced by the superimposition

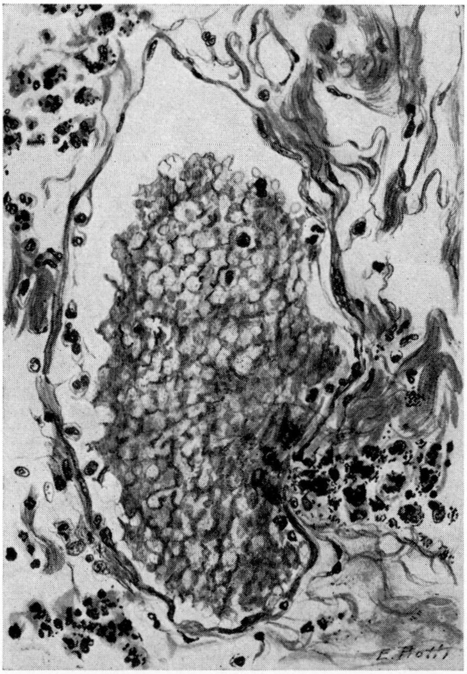

Fig. 3.—Camera lucida drawing of a lymphatic lumen in an inflamed area of about six hours duration induced by inoculation of type III pneumococcus followed immediately by Staphylococcus aureus injection. The lymphatic lumen is occluded in large part by a thrombus composed of a coarse fibrinous meshwork. The dye injected into the inflamed area reached the regional lymphatic node in distinctly smaller amounts than appeared in the control axillary lymphatic node. ×540 (experimental rabbit 10–55, table 2).

of Staphylococcus aureus. This was accomplished by injecting concentrated urea solution at the site of inoculation. It may be recalled that previous studies have clearly demonstrated that this substance dissolves fibrin in vivo, and this allows the free escape in the tributary lymphatics of various foreign substances injected into acutely inflamed areas.[10] At the same time concentrated urea not only fails to inhibit the seepage of fluid through the capillary endothelium but it apparently enhances the passage in the tissues of dyes and plasma. There is always a moderately dense cellular infiltration following the injection of urea. Hence as far as objective observations allow, the sole effect of concentrated urea in an inflamed area is to prevent lymphatic blockage by its dissolving effect on fibrin.

10. Menkin, V.: J. Exper. Med. **56:** 157, 1932.

A series of white rabbits was inoculated in the skin with 0.5 cc. to 0.8 cc. of a culture of pneumococcus type III. This was immediately followed by the inoculation in the same area of 1 cc. of 50 per cent urea solution. Experimental animals received in addition a superimposed injection of 1.5 cc. of Staphylococcus aureus culture, while an identical amount of sterile broth was administered to the control animals. The animals were then allowed to die of their infection.

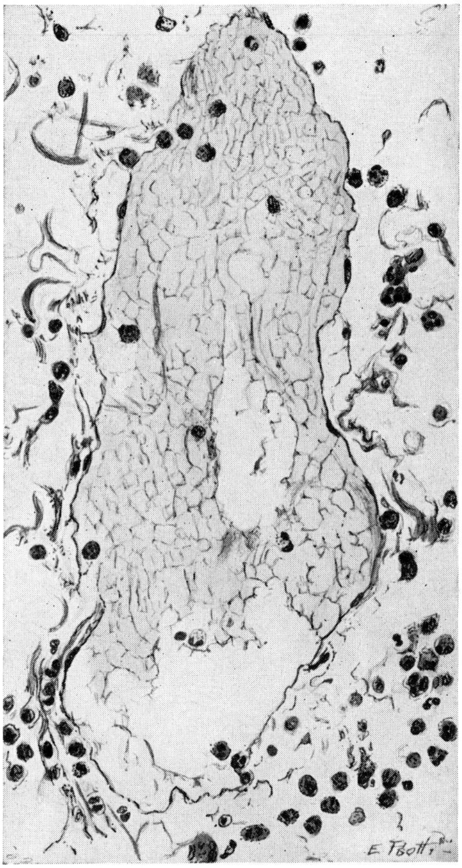

Fig. 4.—Camera lucida drawing of a lymphatic lumen in an inflamed area of over nine hours duration induced by type III pneumococcus followed by Staphylococcus aureus inoculation. The lumen is plugged by a fibrinous reticulum. Trypan blue injected into the area of inflammation failed to reach the regional lymph node. ×400 (experimental rabbit 11–26, table 2).

Contrary to the consistent results on the increase in the survival time inoculated with only pneumococci and staphylococci (table 1), the present series of experiments in which in addition concentrated urea was added, revealed no such favorable effects. In fact in several cases the experimental rabbits succumbed a day or two earlier than the controls inoculated with urea and broth in addition to pneumococci. Microscopic study of the inflamed area in an experimental animal killed 6 hours after both bacterial inoculations and injection of urea revealed dense leukocytic infiltration, extravasation of red cells, and some congestion of capillaries. This picture differed in only one important respect from that in animals similarly treated save that they had received no urea. Instead of finding areas containing much coagulated plasma, and with lymphatics with lumina obstructed by fibrinous plugs, there was no coagulated plasma in the urea treated rabbits and the lymphatics were distended and perfectly patent, containing no fibrin or at most a few isolated strands. Evidently the addition of concentrated urea, by preventing the formation of fibrin in the area of the inflammation, prevented the staphylococci from retarding the spread of pneumococci.[11] This occurred in spite of the heavy leukocytic infiltration and vascular reaction induced by the superimposition of Staphylococcus aureus. The failure to obtain an increase in the survival time in this set of experiments is evidently referable to unobstructed lymphatic drainage due to the fibrinolytic effect of urea.

There is no indication that the virulence or toxic property of the pneumococcus as such is in any way altered by the superimposed inoculation of another irritant. When pneumococci that had been recovered from the blood of an experimental animal were subsequently injected into the skin of a normal rabbit, the latter died within 2 days, thus indicating that the virulence had in no way been modified by the original experimental procedure. In another experiment pneumococci were recovered directly from the site of skin inoculation of an experimental rabbit about 2 days after the beginning of the experiment. These organisms when injected into a normal animal induced massive infection followed by death several days later. The organisms recovered from the blood of such an animal revealed capsulated pneumococci. In vitro studies showed no effect on the viability of pneumococci by the presence in the same culture medium of staphylococci. Furthermore the use of inert irritants, such as aleuronat or turpentine, would rule out a specific effect of the staphylococci on the pneumococci.

DISCUSSION

The observations reported in this communication demonstrate that the rapidity with which a virulent microorganism is able to produce its full systemic effect may be in large part a function of its disseminating capacity. Virulent pneumococci fail to disseminate readily from an inoculated area if one superimposes a bacterial or chemical irritant which, by its injurious action, induces prompt "walling-off" of the inoculated site. For a considerable interval of time after inoculation, pneumococci cannot be found in the circulation of experimental animals, whereas they are present in the blood stream of control rabbits. The delay in the passage of bacteria in experimental animals is referable to an early blockage of normal lymphatic drainage, as indicated both by the inability of a dye to diffuse to the regional lymphatics and also by the histological findings. The delay in the invasion of virulent pneumococci by the superimposed injection of an irritant is associated with an increase in the survival time of such infected rabbits. Two out of twelve experimental animals did not succumb at all. There is no indication

11. To rule out the possible effect of urea per se on the viability in vivo of staphylococci, platinum loopfuls obtained from skin inoculated previously with urea and this microorganism were cultured on blood agar plates. Prolific growth of numerous colonies of Staphylococcus aureus was obtained.

that the virulence of the pneumococcus is altered in any way by the superimposed inoculation of another irritant. The early formation of an effective barrier, by circumscribing a large proportion of the virulent pneumococci at the point of their inoculation, may allow sufficient time for leukocytes, opsonizing bodies, and possibly other defensive factors, to assemble in this area.

The foregoing studies demonstrate that the local inflammatory reaction, by restricting invasion, is an important factor in immunity. The resistance of the host infected with a virulent microorganism is the resultant of a number of factors, including among others the invasiveness and the virulence of the bacteria. By experimentally modifying the factor of invasiveness, as was done in the present series of experiments, the importance of this variable can be estimated in studying resistance. It is worth pointing out in this connection that resistance to a virulent microorganism is not to be taken as a measure of the invasive capacity of the latter, as has been done by various writers. Clark[12] has shown that "preparing" a pleural cavity by preliminary introduction of an inflammatory irritant does not protect rabbits inoculated subsequently into that cavity with virulent pneumococci, type I. This does not indicate, as has apparently been assumed by some writers,[13] that the acute inflammatory reaction has failed to prevent the spread of virulent pneumococci. Fixation is not to be measured by the resultant of a number of factors which collectively may perhaps be appropriately termed resistance. As shown by the writer,[14] invasiveness or dissemination is measured as a quantitative factor and therefore even if but a few extremely virulent microorganisms can escape into the circulation through the mechanical barrier induced in an area of inflammation, their virulence may prove of sufficient magnitude to overcome the resistance of the animal.

CONCLUSIONS

The inoculation of a culture of Straphylococcus aureus, or aleuronat, or turpentine, into a skin area into which virulent type III pneumococci have been injected is accompanied by an increase in the survival time of rabbits.

The increase in resistance thus manifested is due to a delay in the spread of the pneumococci from the site of their inoculation, and this is referable in turn to early mechanical obstruction by thrombosed lymphatics and coagulated plasma in the inflamed area. The presence of such a barrier in the experimental animals has been correlated both with the inability of a dye to diffuse readily into the regional lymphatics from the site of inflammation, and by studies on the presence of pneumococci from the blood stream.

The observations indicate that the rapidity of invasion of a microorganism, as modified by the local inflammatory reaction, is a significant factor in determining the resistance or immunity of the host, but induced alterations in the rate of dissemination may leave the virulence of the bacteria essentially unaffected.

---

12. Arch. Path. **8:** 464, 1929.
13. Rich, A. R., and McKee, C. M.: Bull. Johns Hopkins Hosp. **54:** 277, 1934.
14. J. Exper. Med. **53:** 647, 1931.

EFFECT OF DISSOCIATION OF STREPTOCOCCI ON THEIR FIBRINOLYTIC AND ANTICLOTTING ACTIVITY

RUTH TUNNICLIFF

CHICAGO

STREPTOCOCCUS HEMOLYTICUS

Tillett and Garner[1] made the interesting observation that broth cultures of beta hemolytic streptococci of human origin rapidly dissolve the normal human fibrin clot and that the dissolving action is dependent upon an extracellular substance. With the exception of some strains of Staphylococcus aureus, fibrinolysis appears to be peculiar to the hemolytic streptococcus and it has not been demonstrated with other bacteria including Streptococcus viridans, pneumococcus and most strains of hemolytic streptococci of animal origin.

Hadfield, Magee and Perry[2] found a greater variation in the dissolving power of their strains of hemolytic streptococci than described by others. They observed that the strains of hemolytic streptococci which were virulent for mice and formed colonies corresponding to the colonies called smooth in this country, were the strongest fibrinolytic strains. As their strains became less virulent they became less fibrinolytic.

For my tests streptococci were grown 20 hours in meat extract 1 per cent dextrose broth, p_H 7.0. If they would not grow in this medium one drop of defibrinated sheep blood was added to 5 cc. of dextrose broth.

In general the method of Tillett and Garner was followed. As it is more convenient to use small amounts of blood, it is collected from the finger or ear into bent capillary pipets containing 2 per cent sodium citrate in salt solution. Two-tenths per cent potassium oxalate give the same results. Two parts of blood are drawn into a pipet containing one part of the anticoagulant and diluted at once with eight parts of physiological salt solution and centrifuged. The plasma is used within one hour after the blood has been collected, although it may be kept 24 hours in the ice box before using. Four parts of the diluted plasma are mixed with two parts of broth culture and one part of 0.25 per cent $CaCl_2$ in small test tubes. The mixtures are incubated at 36–37 C. The control containing plasma, uninoculated broth and $CaCl_2$ clots in from 5–15 minutes. When broth cultures of hemolytic streptococci dissolve the plasma clot, it occurs in from 15 minutes to 24 hours after its coagulation.

Nineteen strains of hemolytic streptococci, from scarlet fever (8), erysipelas (6, including the pigmented yellow dissociant), septic sore throat (2),

Received for publication, June 15, 1935.

From the John McCormick Institute for Infectious Diseases.

1. J. Exper. Med. **58:** 485, 1933.
2. Lancet **1:** 834, 1934.

malignant endocarditis (1), septicemia (1), and sore throat (1) were examined for their dissolving activity on normal human plasma clot. All of these strains dissolved the clot. I find that the strongest fibrinolytic activity is associated with the virulent strains which show capsules[3] and produce smooth colonies.[4] This property is gradually lost as the cocci form more granular colonies and finally become dull, rough and flat with irregular lacy edges and change from round diplococcus forms into the large round or flattened cocci in twisted chains or into bacillary and filamentous forms, characteristic of the rough type of streptococci. Hemolytic streptococci generally lose their dissolving power before they are completely stabilized as rough. As the rough forms revert to the smooth, morphologically and colonially, the cocci again acquire the power to dissolve the fibrin clot.

Reich[5] observed that on passing a strain of S. hemolytic, lytic for human fibrin through 22 rabbits it was transformed into a strain which did not dissolve the clot. It was reverted to the original lytic type by the seventh subculture on routine culture medium. He made no record of any morphological or colonial changes during this transformation so one cannot correlate these observations with the S→R→S dissociation, to which they seem to correspond.

According to Morales-Otero and Pomales-Lebron[6] the N. Y. No. 5 scarlet fever strain is the only strain of thirty human hemolytic streptococcus strains examined by them which does not dissolve the normal human fibrin clot. My culture of this strain, which now turns chocolate agar green and forms flat, granular colonies (RS) composed of large irregular cocci in long chains, does not dissolve the normal fibrin clot. After transferring it three times in blood dextrose broth it dissolves the clot in 24 hours and after the seventh transfer it dissolves it in 45 minutes. It now forms smooth conical colonies, most of which do not turn chocolate agar green. These are characteristics of S. scarlatinae.

STREPTOCOCCUS VIRIDANS

My observations are in accord with those of Dennis and Berberian[7] that strains of Streptococcus viridans do not dissolve the fibrin clot but may

---

3. Capsules on virulent S. hemolytic streptococci may be demonstrated as previously described (Tunnicliff, R.: J. Infect. **49:** 357, 1931) or after fixing with methyl alcohol, dilute the Giemsa stain with an equal amount of 10 per cent acetic acid instead of with distilled water and then stain 5–10 minutes. The capsule stains a pinkish tan, the cocci blue. To demonstrate capsules the streptococcus is grown in 1 per cent dextrose broth, p_H 7, containing 1 per cent defibrinated sheep blood. In this medium S type of hemolytic streptococci begins to show capsular material as soon as growth starts, as described by Seastone (J. Bact. **28:** 481, 1934), if the culture is a stabilized S type, otherwise not until after 24–72 hours incubation, depending on the stage of dissociation. Capsules may be still demonstrated on dead cocci in 2 week old cultures. Capsules are not found on cocci in R streptococcus cultures. Seastone was unable to demonstrate capsules in cultures after 6–8 hours' growth, using a medium similar to mine.
4. J. Infect. Dis. **49:** 357, 1931.
5. Proc. Soc. Exper. Biol. & Med. **32:** 639, 1935.
6. Proc. Soc. Exper. Biol. & Med. **32:** 111, 1935.
7. J. Exper. Med. **60:** 581, 1934.

inhibit its formation. I examined five strains from subacute and malignant endocarditis, two from measles and one from sore throat. One anhemolytic strain from endocarditis now turns blood agar green. One strain of an anhemolytic streptococcus from endocarditis behaves like the greening cocci. As in the case of the hemolytic streptococcus, virulence of the green producing streptococcus is generally associated with the smooth type. As the cocci of smooth strains change into the rough type they lose their virulence and show the same morphological and colonial variations as seen in rough cultures of hemolytic streptococci.[8] When they revert to the smooth form of colony they also revert morphologically. I find that the anticlotting property of the viridans group is associated with the smooth virulent type. If the cocci change into the rough form they lose this property, but acquire it if they revert to the smooth type.

Although the greening colonies may appear smooth for several days, if the broth culture does not prevent clotting of the plasma, rough projections with their bacillary forms will be seen at the edge of the colony, generally within a week.

The greening diplococci from measles (D. morbillorum) prevent clotting of normal plasma so long as they form depressed colonies. When they lose this characteristic although the colony appears smooth for several days, the cocci no longer inhibit clotting of normal plasma, and at the end of a week rough projections with bacillary forms may be found.

To determine whether one is examining a smooth or rough streptococcus broth culture, it is advisable to make a subculture onto blood agar and examine the colonies with a culture microscope for signs of roughness.

Dennis and Berberian observed in one strain of S. hemolyticus from erysipelas both the fibrinolytic and the "antifibrinogenic" or anticlotting action, the lytic usually masking the inhibitory action, which was brought out by dilution of the filtrate. They thought Tillett and Garner missed the inhibitory factor in S. viridans cultures because their medium containing less glucose was unfavorable for demonstrating anticlotting activity. It seems more likely that one medium favored dissociation more than the other. Anticlotting occurs with my smooth greening and anhemolytic cultures whether containing 0.5 or 1.0 per cent glucose. One of my erysipelas strains also shows both the lytic and the inhibitory actions, depending on the character of the culture. So long as it shows fairly smooth hemolytic colonies it dissolves the fibrin clot, but as it gets rougher it becomes less hemolytic and slightly green and now inhibits clotting. When it reverts to the smooth hemolytic form it again dissolves the clot.

In a previous article[9] on the dissociation of hemolytic streptococci from erysipelas, I described a pigmented yellowish hemolytic, a S. viridans and an anhemolytic streptococci among the dissociants. Since then I have dissociated from one of these hemolytic strains a R type which produces green

8. Cooley, L. E.: J. Infect. Dis. **50:** 358, 1932; Tunnicliff, R.: J. Infect. Dis. **52:** 39, 1933; Tunnicliff, R., and Woolsey, C. I.: J. Infect. Dis. **56:** 116, 1935.

9. J. Infect. Dis. **48:** 511, 1931.

colonies without hemolysis on blood agar. These observations together with the inhibitory action of the RS greenish dissociant of a hemolytic streptococcus indicate a close relation between the hemolytic and the greening and anhemolytic streptococci.

Two strains of hemolytic streptococci recently isolated from scarlet fever, one from the blood, dissolved the normal fibrin clot in 15 minutes but suddenly, in one case after subculturing in blood dextrose broth they completely inhibited clot formation. Both had lost their power to lake blood and formed smooth conical greening colonies on blood agar.

In this connection it is of interest that Howell and Werner[10] isolated only anhemolytic streptococci on a number of blood agar plates from the throats of patients with typical scarlet fever and that the three strains, tested by the opsonic method with the serum of a horse immunized with hemolytic streptococci from scarlet fever appeared to belong immunologically to the group of hemolytic streptococcus specific for scarlet fever. Lately Pilot and Stocker[11] have described a hemolytic streptococcus from scarlet fever dissociating into a viridans type whose toxin is identical with that of the hemolytic strain from which it originates.

RESISTANCE TO FIBRINOLYTIC AND ANTICLOTTING FACTORS BY PLASMA OF PATIENTS RECOVERING FROM INFECTIONS WITH HEMOLYTIC AND GREENING STREPTOCOCCI

It has been demonstrated (Tillett, Edwards and Garner[12]; Meyer, Keefer and Holmes, Jr.[13]; Hadfield, Magee and Perry[2]) that the plasma clot of patients recovering from hemolytic streptococcus infections may become more resistant to fibrinolysis than plasma clot from normal persons and patients with infections caused by other microorganisms.

I thought it would be worth while to study whether the plasma of persons with infections associated with greening streptococci might become resistant to their anticlotting property, with improvement in symptoms or recovery. The plasma of patients with subacute endocarditis (S. viridans) and measles with which greening diplococci (D. morbillorum) are closely associated, was therefore studied. The plasma was obtained from patients of Doctor Archibald L. Hoyne, Doctor Frank B. Kelly, Doctor Frank V. Theis and Doctor Eugene F. Traut. The plasma showed no resistance to the anticlotting property of two S. viridans strains from malignant endocarditis. One of these was originally anhemolytic. Any resistance to the anticlotting property was demonstrated with S anhemolytic and greening endocarditis strains and a freshly isolated greening strain from measles, all preventing clotting of normal plasma. As with the fibrinolytic activity of hemolytic strains there appears to be no specificity in the anticlotting action of green and anhemolytic streptococci.

---

10. J. Infect. Dis. **43:** 525, 1928.
11. Proc. Soc. Exper. Biol. & Med. **31:** 181, 1933.
12. J. Clin. Investigation **13:** 47, 1934.
13. J. Clin. Investigation **14:** 119, 1935.

The plasma of two patients with subacute endocarditis from whose blood cultures of S. viridans had been isolated, was studied. The two R strains isolated twice from each patient, did not prevent the clotting of normal human plasma but the S form in the second culture of one did. After one of these R strains had been changed to an S form by subculturing in blood dextrose broth, it prevented clotting. The plasma of one of these patients examined only once a short time before death, did not show any resistance to the anticlotting action of the anhemolytic strain. The plasma of the other patient was examined six times at weekly intervals and when signs of improvement were noted the plasma developed partial resistance to the anticlotting property of the anhemolytic endocarditis strain, and complete resistance to that of the homologous smooth S. viridans strain and of the greening strain from measles. Neither patient showed resistance to the lytic action of S. hemolyticus.

The plasma of a person immunized with S. viridans for transfusion, with an opsonic index of 27.0 for this strain, did not resist the anticlotting property of the anhemolytic strain, but showed partial resistance to that of the greening coccus from measles.

Of the plasma of five patients examined after recovery from measles, two, one at the end of one and the other at the end of three weeks after the onset, showed no resistance to the anticlotting property of the greening diplococcus from measles; one at the end of two weeks showed partial resistance and two, two and three weeks respectively after the onset of measles, developed complete resistance. The plasma of one of these patients examined at weekly intervals for four weeks, beginning three weeks after the attack, developed also partial resistance to the anticlotting action of the anhemolytic streptococcus during the fourth week but lost it one week later. The plasma continued to be resistant to the anticlotting action of the greening diplococcus from measles throughout the experiment. No resistance to the anhemolytic strain was observed with the plasma of the other patients, perhaps because they were not examined late enough after the attack.

The plasma clots of only one of the five measles patients showed resistance to the lytic action of S. hemolyticus. This patient had recovered from an attack of scarlet fever just before getting measles.

Two patients recovering from hemolytic streptococcus infections, one with endocarditis following scarlet fever, developed resistance to the lytic action of S. hemolyticus and partial resistance to the anticlotting action of the anhemolytic streptococcus. One of these patients with a hemolytic streptococcus pharyngitis also developed resistance to the anticlotting action of the greening diplococcus from measles. After the hemolytic streptococci disappeared from the throat, the plasma lost its resistance to both the lytic action of the hemolytic streptococcus and the anticlotting action of the anhemolytic streptococcus, but three weeks later it still resisted the inhibitory action of the greening coccus.

The plasma clot of two patients with endocarditis following sore throat and arthritis, from whose blood no streptococci were isolated, with improvement, developed resistance to the lytic action of the hemolytic streptococcus.

The plasma of one showed resistance to the inhibitory action of the anhemolytic streptococcus, the other to the greening. The plasma of one of these patients examined four times, lost its resistance to both the lytic and anticlotting action during a relapse.

These few observations suggest that during recovery from a hemolytic streptococcus infection the plasma may develop resistance to not only the fibrinolytic activity of the hemolytic streptococcus but also some resistance to the anticlotting property of anhemolytic and greening cocci. The plasma of a patient showing improvement in subacute bacterial endocarditis (S. viridans) and of persons following an attack of measles may develop resistance to the anticlotting action of anhemolytic and greening cocci, but not for the lytic property of S. hemolyticus unless recovering from an infection with this organism.

SUMMARY

The fibrinolytic action of hemolytic streptococci appears to be associated with the virulent smooth type. This power is lost as the organism becomes rough, and is regained as it reverts to the smooth form.

Smooth and rough cultures of Streptococcus viridans and of anhemolytic streptococci do not show any power to dissolve the normal fibrin clot, but smooth cultures completely prevent its forming. If the smooth form changes to the rough type it loses its anticlotting action and regains it if it reverts to the smooth form.

The plasma clot of patients recovering from hemolytic streptococcus infections appears to resist the lytic action of the hemolytic streptococcus, and the plasma appears to resist the anticlotting property of greening and anhemolytic streptococcus strains. The plasma of patients after an attack of measles or in a remission from S. viridans subacute endocarditis may develop resistance to the anticlotting action of greening and anhemolytic cocci, but the clot does not resist the lytic action of the hemolytic streptococcus unless the patient is also recovering from an infection with this organism.

PROPERTIES OF HOMOGENIZED HERPES VIRUS

C. W. BUGGS
AND
R. G. GREEN
MINNEAPOLIS

In this laboratory we have had occasion to make an extensive series of intracerebral inoculations with herpes virus, the H. F. strain of which was obtained from Doctor Simon Flexner. At the outset of our experiments we followed the usual procedure of triturating the virus brains either with or without sterile sand for the preparation of suspensions. In our hands such virus suspensions, aged not more than two weeks, produced death in rabbits on the third or fourth day following the intracerebral injection of 0.3 cc. of one per cent virus in normal saline.

Employing homogenized brain virus (as prepared by Green et al.[1]) of the same age, in the same dosage, and by the same route, it was found that rabbits regularly succumbed to herpes encephalitis within thirty hours after inoculation. The increase in the potency or activity of herpes virus after homogenization is explained on the basis that the virus within the infected brain tissue is intracellular, and that a high degree of dispersion of the cellular elements releases the virus in maximum quantity.

HOMOGENIZATION OF VIRUS BRAINS

Our usual procedure is to obtain the brains from rabbits immediately after they have succumbed to an experimental infection. In a few cases the necropsies were delayed for as long as twelve hours. The brains are removed sterilely and either homogenized at once or placed in sterile 50 per cent glycerol. Fresh or glycerolated brain tissue is triturated for a few minutes in a sterile mortar, and made into a 10 per cent suspension with 50 per cent sterile glycerol of p_H 7.4. The suspension is then slowly passed through an homogenizer three or more times, the resulting product being a highly homogeneous suspension of finely divided tissue elements.

The homogenizer was the model L Hurrell Homogenizer. It is of the smooth-surface type of dispersion apparatus and depends only upon hydraulic shearing forces for its effect. It consists essentially of a smooth, revolving surface, the rotor, which revolves in a smooth-surfaced stator ring. The adsorption of films of fluid upon each of the working surfaces causes tremendous shearing stresses in the rest of the liquid between them. Under these stresses the material held in suspension is dispersed into particles of the order of magnitude of one micron. Smears of such an homogenized

---

Received for publication, June 21, 1935.
From Department of Bacteriology and Immunology, University of Minnesota.
1. Am. J. Hyg. **19:** 343, 1934.

preparation have been fixed and stained, but only rarely is one able to demonstrate intact neurons.

ACTIVITY OF HOMOGENIZED VIRUS BRAINS

Fresh, homogenized H. F. herpes encephalitis virus is exceedingly active during the first two weeks of refrigeration. When injected intracerebrally into rabbits in doses of 0.3 cc. of a one per cent suspension an infection is produced which is fatal within 30 hours after inoculation. It was also found that virus brains could be glycerolated for at least two weeks before homogenization without any noticeable loss in virulence. The group of animals described below represents a set of typical results.

Five rabbits were inoculated intracerebrally with 0.3 cc. of a one per cent virus suspension. The virus brain had been glycerolated for two weeks before homogenization. All the animals inoculated died well within the 30-hour, limit, one each after intervals of 10, 11, 16, 17, and 24 hours. Sections of the brains showed the characteristic necrotic neurons, mononuclear infiltrations, perivascular infiltrations with similar cells, and microscopic hemorrhages which are typical of herpes encephalitis. Inclusion bodies were demonstrated in two of the brains.

Symptoms in two animals developed with explosive violence. From three to five hours before death the animals became greatly excitable, running about the cages in a wild manner, and salivating profusely. Loss of equilibrium set in rapidly, and within two hours both rabbits were unable to stand without support. Opisthotonos was marked and frequent.

After standing at 5 C. for two or more weeks, homogenized H. F. virus loses its ability to produce death in rabbits within 30 hours. However, the virus does reach a degree of virulence at which it remains for a considerable length of time. When tested at intervals of 28 days over a period of 7 months, one preparation of homogenized virus was found to produce death consistently on the third day. In a few instances rabbits have survived until the fourth day, when a dose of 0.3 cc. of a one per cent suspension was employed; but in no case has one survived until the fifth day. We have never had an animal recover once an infection had started, no matter how small the dose.

In table 1 are recorded the results of inoculating rabbits with diminishing doses of glycerolated homogenized virus (aged several months), and with cerebrospinal fluid obtained from such infected animals. Beginning with a 10 per cent suspension of virus, dilutions were made up with normal rabbit serum (some with normal saline) so that 1 cc. of preparation contained from 5.0 mg. to 0.001 mg. of brain tissue. When definite symptoms of encephalitis developed in rabbits injected with these various dilutions, cerebrospinal fluid was drawn by cisterna puncture and injected intracerebrally into normal rabbits.

These results show that homogenized H. F. herpes virus is extremely potent, amounts as small as one ten-millionth of a gram of infected brain tissue producing death within five or six days. Infection was produced in each case in which cerebrospinal fluid from herpetic rabbits was inoculated into normal rabbits.

COMPARISON OF THE ACTIVITIES OF TRITURATED AND HOMOGENIZED VIRUS

Fresh, herpetic brains were weighed and triturated in a sterile mortar for 10 minutes. The brain substance was then made into a 10 per cent suspension with 50 per cent glycerol. A portion of this emulsion was designated triturated brain virus. A similar portion of the suspension was further triturated with a small amount of sterile sand and centrifuged at low speed for a few minutes, after which the supernatant fluid was removed by pipetting. This portion was designated virus triturated with sand. The remaining suspension was homogenized and constituted the homogenized virus.

TABLE 1.—*Infection of Rabbits with Small Doses of Homogenized H. F. Herpes Encephalitis Virus, and with Cerebrospinal Fluid Obtained from such Infected Rabbits. Virus aged in Glycerol*

No. of Rabbit	Material Injected	Total Dosage in ccs.	Virus Dosage in mgs.	Time of Death
161	Normal serum and virus	0.5	2.5	3 days 14 hours
162	Normal serum and virus	0.5	2.5	3 days 19 hours
165	Normal serum and virus	0.5	0.5	4 days 12 hours
169	Spinal fluid from 165	0.5		4 days 2 hours
170	Spinal fluid from 165	0.5		4 days 15 hours
171	Spinal fluid from 170	0.1		6 days 14 hours
172	Normal serum and virus	0.5	0.5	3 days 9 hours
173	Normal serum and virus	0.5	0.5	4 days 3 hours
176	Normal serum and virus	0.5	0.05	3 days 10 hours
177	Normal serum and virus	0.1	0.01	4 days 6 hours
178	Spinal fluid from 172	0.5		5 days 14 hours
179	Spinal fluid from 172	0.5		5 days
186	Spinal fluid from 176	0.5		5 days 8 hours
187	Spinal fluid from 177	0.5		5 days 11 hours
180	Normal serum and virus	0.5	0.005	4 days 3 hours
181	Normal serum and virus	0.1	0.001	4 days 5 hours
182	Normal serum and virus	0.1	0.001	4 days 18 hours
183	Saline and virus	0.5	0.005	4 days 7 hours
184	Saline and virus	0.1	0.001	4 days 15 hours
185	Saline and virus	0.1	0.001	3 days 2 hours
188	Saline and virus	0.5	0.0005	5 days 11 hours
189	Saline and virus	0.1	0.0001	6 days

Six rabbits of about the same weight were inoculated intracerebrally, in sets of two, with the three virus preparations. The results, as tabulated in table 2, indicate that a direct relationship exists between the degree of dispersion of the brain tissue and the activity of the virus contained therein. Activity increases with an increase in the destruction of the cellular elements of the tissue. The necessary conclusion is that the virus of herpes encephalitis is found mainly within the cellular elements of the brain tissue.

TABLE 2.—*Comparative Results of the Activity of Virus Brain in Different Degrees of Dispersion. 1 Per Cent Suspensions*

No. of Rabbit	Dosage	Time of Death
	Triturated Virus	
57	0.3 cc.	69 hours
58	0.3 cc.	63 hours
	Virus Triturated with Sand	
59	0.3 cc.	50 hours
60	0.3 cc.	42 hours
	Homogenized Virus	
61	0.3 cc.	18 hours
62	0.3 cc.	21 hours

It has been shown by Goodpasture[2] and Goodpasture and Teague[3] that the virus of herpes propagates itself along the axis-cylinders of peripheral nerves in traversing the distance from the cornea, or some other extracranial focus, to the central nervous system, and does not make its entrance by way of the perineural spaces. Thus, it is a relatively simple process for the virus to penetrate the nerve cells in its immediate vicinity when it is implanted directly in the brain substance, and to infect the majority of them rapidly by way of the axial filaments of the neurons and the processes of the glial cells.

Table 3 summarizes the time intervals between inoculation and death for a number of rabbits as obtained by Flexner and Amoss,[4] using triturated virus, and by us, employing homogenized virus.

TABLE 3.

Results Obtained by Flexner and Amoss on the Activity of Triturated H. F. Herpes Encephalitis Virus. Animals given Various Dosages of Virus

Rabbits Used	Treatment of Virus	Time of Death
1	Triturated Fresh Virus	4th day
1	Triturated Fresh Virus	2nd day
1	Triturated Fresh Virus	6th day
1	Triturated Fresh Virus	6th day
1	Triturated Fresh Virus	4th day
1	Triturated Fresh Virus	5th day
1*	Triturated Glycerolated Virus, Paper Filtered	3rd day
1*	Triturated Glycerolated Virus, Paper Filtered	3rd day
1*	Triturated Glycerolated Virus, Paper Filtered	3rd day
?	Berkefeld Filtrate of Glycerolated Virus. Three Separate Experiments. Virus Triturated.	All animals Survived
1	Berkefeld Filtrate of Fresh, Triturated Virus	Succumbed
1	Berkefeld Filtrate of Fresh, Triturated Virus.	Succumbed

The Activity of Homogenized H. F. Herpes Encephalitis Virus. Animals Injected with 0.25 cc. of a 5 Per Cent Suspension or Product Therefrom

Rabbits Used	Treatment of Virus	Time of Death
1	Homogenized Fresh Virus	12 hours
1	Homogenized Fresh Virus	12 hours
1	Homogenized Fresh Virus	12 hours
1	Homogenized Fresh Virus	14 hours
1	Homogenized Fresh Virus	24 hours
1	Homogenized Fresh Virus	24 hours
1	Homogenized Fresh Virus, Paper Filtered	20 hours
1	Homogenized Fresh Virus, Paper Filtered	17 hours
1 1	Homogenized Fresh Virus, Paper Filtered	12 hours
1	Homogenized Fresh Virus, Paper Filtered	24 hours
1	Berkefeld Filtrate of Homogenized, Glycerolated Virus	90 hours
1	Berkefeld Filtrate of Homogenized, Glycerolated Virus	96 hours
1	Berkefeld Filtrate of Homogenized, Glycerolated Virus	102 hours
1	Berkefeld Filtrate of Homogenized, Glycerolated Virus	115 hours
1	Berkefeld Filtrate of Fresh, Homogenized Virus	33 hours
1	Berkefeld Filtrate of Fresh, Homogenized Virus	29 hours

* These animals were inoculated with 0.01, 0.05, and 0.1 cc. respectively of a 5 per cent virus suspension.

The smallest volume of suspension employed by Flexner and Amoss in these tests has been calculated on the weight basis. Their suspension was 5 per cent. Their smallest volume, 0.01 cc., is equivalent to 0.5 mg. of brain tissue, and produced death on the third day following intracerebral inoculation. Employing homogenized virus brain (aged not more than 5 weeks) and a similar dosage, we have succeeded in producing death before the end of the second day. With virus glycerolated for over seven months, and in a dosage of 0.001 mg., we have produced death in from three to four days following inoculation.

2. Am. J. Path. **1:** 11, 1925.
3. J. M. Research **44:** 139, 1923.
4. J. Exper. Med. **41:** 233, 1925.

Table 3 shows that in all cases homogenized virus is more active than virus preparations prepared by simple trituration. It also shows the absolute inactivity of Berkefeld filtrates of virus brain, as employed by Flexner and Amoss, which has been glycerolated for any length of time. In all our cases, rabbits receiving glycerolated virus which had been passed through a Berkefeld V candle died of typical herpetic encephalitis on the third day following intracerebral inoculation.

FILTRATION OF HOMOGENIZED VIRUS

A Berkefeld filtrate of virus is a desirable preparation to work with, but we encounter a serious obstacle in obtaining a suitable quantity of active filtrate. The pores of the filter become clogged, even when a 1 per cent suspension is used, before a suitable quantity of the product is obtained. It is often found that such filtrates are only slightly active as the major portion of the virus remains in the tissue when simple trituration is practiced. The following method was found to be simple and efficient in producing a filtrate of high potency in large quantities.

A 10 per cent homogenized glycerolated brain suspension was employed. The virus was first filtered through sterile paper pulp which was loosely packed into a small Büchner funnel. By applying suction it was possible to obtain 200 cc. of a slightly turbid liquid in a few minutes. The filtrate was next put through sterile paper pulp which was very tightly packed to a depth of one-half inch. The resulting filtrate was almost water-clear, and required only about 10 minutes for passage through the pulp.

This last product was passed through a Berkefeld V candle. Ninety cubic centimeters of filtrate were collected in a few minutes, and was immediately tested for its activity by intracerebral inoculation into rabbits. Controls were run with unfiltered virus, as well as with the filtrate obtained from passage through the tightly packed paper pulp. The results obtained are summarized in table 4.

TABLE 4.—*The Activity of Filtered, Glycerolated Herpes Encephalitis Virus*

No. of Rabbit	Dosage	Time of Death
	Berkefeld Filtrate	
103	0.3 cc.	100 hours
104	0.3 cc.	121 hours
105	0.3 cc.	105 hours
	Paper Pulp Filtrate	
106	0.3 cc.	74 hours
107	0.3 cc.	88 hours
108	0.3 cc.	91 hours
	Unfiltered Virus	
109	0.3 cc.	77 hours
110	0.3 cc.	74 hours
111	0.3 cc.	86 hours

It is evident from the figures obtained from paper pulp filtrate and unfiltered virus that filtering through pulp removes a negligible amount of active virus. There is no significant difference between the time of death in the two groups. On the other hand, Berkefeld filtrate is slightly less potent than unfiltered virus, though not as much as one would ordinarily expect.

This filtration experiment was performed a second time. However, instead of employing glycerolated brains, fresh 10 per cent virus suspension was used. Three rabbits inoculated with the Berkefeld filtrate died at the end of 43, 45, and 50 hours, respectively. Three rabbits injected with unfiltered virus died before the end of the second day.

There is probably no significant difference between the action of the Berkefeld filtrate and the unfiltered virus. However, comparing these results with those obtained in the previous experiment (table 4), it is seen that fresh virus, either filtered or unfiltered, is more active than glycerolated virus. It should be noted that the dosages of fresh virus employed were 0.02, 0.05, and 0.1 cc. for both groups of rabbits.

INACTIVATION OF HERPES VIRUS BY ETHER

Levaditi and Harvier[5] found the virus of herpes to be ether-resistant, We attempted to take advantage of this information and develop a method of separation of virus from brain lipoids by a process of ether flotation. By taking a constant volume of 10 per cent virus suspension and adding purified ether to it in increments of 1 cc., it was determined that 40 cc. of the suspension required 10 cc. of ether to bring about the production of two distinct layers. The upper floating layer consisted of the brain lipoids adsorbed to ether droplets.

After thoroughly shaking such a virus-ether mixture for a few minutes in a separatory funnel and allowing 15 minutes for separation into two layers, the bottom, watery layer was drawn off into a second separatory funnel where cotton-filtered air was bubbled through it in order to evaporate more quickly what ether was present. As the ether was removed, the fluid was drawn from this second funnel into a sterile flask. This treatment gives the clear, watery product of the filtered virus, free from all discernible particles of brain tissue.

Three rabbits were employed in each of two separate experiments designed to test the activity of such ether-treated virus suspensions. In no case were we successful in producing an infection by the intracerebral injection of such preparations. Five control rabbits succumbed within 20 hours after the inoculation of virus not treated with ether.

We are unable to account for the positive results obtained by Levaditi and Harvier, except on the assumption that the brain material they employed was only coarsely triturated, and that enough virus was contained in the intact cells not penetrated by the ether to produce an infection on their subsequent disintegration.

SUMMARY

Homogenized H. F. herpes encephalitis virus is extremely potent, producing death in rabbits within 5 days when inoculated intracerebrally in

5. Compt. rend. Soc. de biol. **83:** 1140, 1920.

doses of one ten-millionth of a gram of infected brain tissue. It produces death in rabbits regularly on the third day after intracerebral injection of 0.3 cc. of a one per cent aged suspension. When employed in the fresh state, homogenized herpes virus is fatal to rabbits in from 12 to 30 hours following intracerebral inoculation.

Evidence is advanced, from differences in the activity of homogenized and triturated brain tissue, to support the viewpoint that herpes encephalitis virus is found mainly within the cellular elements of the central nervous system.

Homogenized H. F. herpes virus is not ether-resistant, and a method of ether flotation cannot be employed for the separation of the fatty brain tissue from the virus.

A rapid method is given for the preparation of highly potent Berkefeld filtrates of herpes virus.

COMPARATIVE OBSERVATIONS ON STREPTOCOCCI FROM HUMAN GASTRO-INTESTINAL ULCERATIONS AND FROM BOVINE MASTITIS

JOHN C. TORREY

AND

ELIZABETH MONTU

NEW YORK

In several publications Saunders[1,2,3] has described a streptococcal type which he has found constantly associated with ulcerative processes in the gastro-duodenal region and also with gastric carcinoma. He also reported that this organism was identical with three streptococcal strains isolated from bovine mastitis milk.[2,3] In a recent paper the writers[4] described the cultural and agglutinative relationships among intestinal streptococci (enterococci) isolated from ulcerative colitis, comparing these strains with the Saunders type and with the reported characteristics of the Bargen diplostreptococcus. It was concluded that the Saunders organism should be classified as an enterococcus. When the foregoing study was nearing completion, Dr. J. A. Bargen was kind enough to send us five recently isolated strains of his organism, and also Dr. E. W. Saunders placed at our disposal more representatives of his type. This has permitted a direct comparison of authentic Bargen strains with our isolations, with the Saunders type and with bovine mastitis streptococci, which were either type strains or isolated directly from milk specimens.

The identity claimed by Saunders for his streptococcal type and that commonly causing bovine mastitis, would seem to call for further inquiry as it has been generally held that the Streptococcus mastitidis of bovine origin is not pathogenic or infective for humans. If it were otherwise, mastitis being so frequent in dairy herds, exposure to infection would be almost constant in communities where unpasteurized milk is still commonly used. In this paper, evidence both cultural and serological is presented which indicates that the typical Streptococcus mastitidis is not related to the Saunders organism. It is also shown that authentic strains of the Bargen diplostreptococcus may or may not show serological relationships to the Saunders streptococcus or to each other.

Received for publication, June 22, 1935.

From the Department of Public Health and Preventive Medicine, Cornell University Medical College.

1. Arch. Int. Med. **45:** 347, 1930; Ann. Surg. **92:** 222, 1930.
2. Ann. Surg. **95:** 327, 1932.
3. Saunders, E. W.; Holsinger, H. B., and Cooper, M. A.: Am. J. M. Sc. **187:** 246, 1934.
4. J. Infect. Dis. **55:** 340, 1934.

TABLE 1

Strain	Disease	Source	Hemolysis (Blood Agar)	Fermentations							Gelatin	H₂S Production	Methylene Blue Milk	SodHippurate Hydrolysis	MacConkey Agar Medium	Heat Resistance 30 Minutes	
				Lactose	Sucrose	Salicin	Mannitol	Raffinose	Inulin	Esculin Bile medium						60 C	63 C
L. S. (Bargen)	Ulcerative colitis	Lesion	0	+	+	0	0	+	0	0	0	+	R*	+	+	+	+
W. M. (Bargen)	Ulcerative colitis	Lesion	0	+	+	0	0	+	0	0	0	+			+	+	+
O. J. T. (Bargen)	Ulcerative colitis	Lesion	0	+	+	0	0	+	0	0	0	+			+	+	+
H. D. (Bargen)	Ulcerative colitis	Lesion	0	+	+	0	0	+	0	0	0	+	R	+	+	0	0
J. B. (Bargen)	Ulcerative colitis	Lesion	0	+	+	+	+	+	0	+	0	+++	R	+	+	+	0
3	Ulcerative colitis	Stool	0	+	+	+	±	0	0	0	0	+			+	0	0
13	Ulcerative colitis	Lesion	++	+	0	+	±	0	0	+	0	+++	R	+	+	+	0
24	Ulcerative colitis	Stool	++	+	0	+	±	0	0	+	0	+++	R	+	+	+	0
32	Ulcerative colitis	Lesion	0	+	0	+	±	0	0	+	0	+++				+	0
5	Ulcerative colitis	Stool	0	+	+	+	±	0	0	+	+	+++	R	+	+	+	0
66 (Saunders)	Gastric ulcer carcinoma	Lesion	+	+	+	+	+	0	0	+	0	+++	R	+	+	+	0
83 (Saunders)	Gastric ulcer	Lesion	+	+	+	+	+	0	0	+	0	+++	R	+	+	+	0
138 (Saunders)	Gastric ulcer	Lesion	+	+	+	+	0	0	0	0	0	+++	0	+	0	0	0
142 (Saunders)	Gastric ulcer	Lesion	0	+	0	0	0	0	0	0	0	+	R	0	+	0	0
125 (Saunders)	Gastric ulcer carcinoma	Tissue	0	+	+	+	+	0	0	+	0	+++	R	0	+	+	0
127 (Saunders)	Gastric ulcer carcinoma	Tissue	0	+	+	+	+	0	0	+	0	+++	R	0	+	+	0
131 (Saunders)	Gastric ulcer carcinoma	Tissue	0	+	+	+	+	0	0	0	0	+++	R	+	+	+	0
140 (Saunders)	Gastric ulcer carcinoma	Tissue	+	+	+	+	0	0	0	0	0	0	0	+	0	0	0
143 (Saunders)	Gastric ulcer carcinoma	Tissue	0	+	+	+	0	+	+	+	0	0	0	0	+	0	0
128 (Saunders)	Breast carcinoma	Tissue	0	+	+	+	+	0	0	+	0	+	R	+	+	+	+
4784 (A)	Bovine mastitis	Milk	+	+	+	0	0	0	0	0	0	0	0	+	+	0	0
4787 (A)	Bovine mastitis	Milk	0	+	+	0	0	0	0	+	0	++	0	+	0	0	0
110 (A)	Bovine mastitis	Milk	0	+	+	+	0	0	0	0	0	+	0	+	+	0	0
123 (A)	Bovine mastitis	Milk	0	+	+	+	0	0	0	0	0	+++	0	+	+	0	0
3G (A)?	Bovine mastitis	Milk	0	+	+	0	0	0	0	0	0	+++	R	+	0	0	0
4G (A)	Bovine mastitis	Milk	0	+	+	0	0	0	0	0	0	+++	0	+	0	0	0
1A (A)	Bovine mastitis	Milk	0	+	0	+	0	0	0	0	0	++			+	0	0
1B	Bovine mastitis	Milk	0	+	+	+	+	+	+	+	0	+++	R	+	+	+	0
90 (B)	Bovine mastitis	Milk	0	+	+	+	±	0	0	+	0	+++	R	+	+	+	0
91 (B)	Bovine mastitis	Milk	0	+	+	+	±	0	0	+	0	+++	R	+	+	+	0
AB-13 (Cecil)	Rheumatoid arthritis	Blood	++	+	+	+	0	0	0	0	0	++	0	+	0	0	0
RB-5 (Cecil)	Rheumatic fever	Blood	0	+	+	+	+	+	0	+	0	+++	R	+	+	+	0

* Methylene blue reduced.

HISTORY OF CULTURES

The following data was kindly supplied by Dr. J. A. Bargen in regard to the five strains received from him. Strain O. J. T. from a man, 38 years old, and experiencing a mild relapse of ulcerative colitis after 8 years freedom from the trouble. Strain L. S., man, age 28, 3 months bloody diarrhea, ulcerative process involving only rectum and sigmoid. Strain W. M., woman, age 56, year's history of rectal bleeding, only rectum involved. Strain J. B. isolated directly from rectal ulcers of a man, age 37, with history of 20 months trouble; typical proctoscopic picture with intensity of one plus (on basis of four). Disease involved only rectum and sigmoid. Strain H. D., woman, age 40, disease of several years duration. The organism was isolated in 1931. Given the serum treatment. Between May 1932 and January 1933, several mild exacerbations of symptoms and again early in 1934 when the strain was isolated.

Strains 3, 5, 13, 24 and 37, were among those described in a previous article[4] and all from ulcerative colitis cases.

Of the 10 Saunders strains, No. 66 is a type strain isolated directly from gastric ulcer carcinoma and described in his papers.[2,3] Strains 83, 128, 138 and 142, are later isolations from gastric ulcers, and 125, 127, 131, 140 and 143, from gastric ulcer carcinoma tissues.

Of the bovine mastitis strains, 4784 and 4787 were received from the American Type Culture Collection with a history having come originally from the Rockefeller Institute of Medical Research, Princeton, N.J. Strains 110 and 123 were received from Dr. G. J. Hucker, Geneva, N.Y., the former having originally come from the above Rockefeller Institute and the latter from the Veterinar-Hygienisches Institut der Universitat, Leipsig, Germany, as Streptococcus agalactiae, No. 1. Strains 3G, 4G, 1A, 1B, were isolated from samples of bovine mastitis milk received through the courtesy of Dr. J. A. Sweet. Strains 90 and 91 were from a similar source and received from Dr. E. W. Saunders. Strains AB-13 and RB-5 were received from Dr. E. E. Nichols and were isolated from the blood of cases of rheumatoid arthritis and rheumatic fever respectively as reported by Cecil, Nichols and Stainsby.[5]

CULTURAL CHARACTERISTICS

In table I are detailed cultural data in regard to these strains.

The fermentation tests were conducted with sterilized semi-solid meat extract peptone agar, with bromcresol purple indicator, to which the various highly purified test carbohydrates were added in $\frac{1}{2}$ or 1 per cent amounts, tubed and sterilized by exposure for 10 minutes for three consecutive days in the Arnold. The esculin bile medium is that of Harrison and Van der Lack.[6] Tests were also made with esculin without bile salts. The medium for detection of H_2S production is the sodium thio-sulphate, lead acetate combination recommended by Tilley[7] and prepared according to the formula of Kahn.[8] In tests for hydrolysis of sodium hippurate the pepsin peptone medium of Ayer and Rupp[9] was employed and for reduction of methylene blue sterile skim milk containing one part of the dye to 5000 parts milk was employed as recommended by Avery.[10] The aqueous solution of methylene was sterilized separately and then added to the sterile milk and then allowed to stand several days before seeding as recommended by Plastridge et al.[11] Readings were made after 1, 3 and 7 days incubation. Unfortunately, five strains were lost before these last two tests were carried out. The heat resistance tests were made according to the method described in a previous publication.[4]

Bargen and Logan,[12] in 1925, described their diplostreptococcus of ulcerative colitis (20 strains) as mannitol and inulin negative but positive for salicin and raffinose when first isolated.

---

5. Arch. Int. Med. **43:** 571, 1929; J. Exper. Med. **50:** 617, 1929.
6. Centralbl. f. Bakt. (Abt. 2) **22:** 547, 1909.
7. J. Bact. **8:** 115, 1923.
8. J. Bact. **10:** 439, 1925.
9. J. Infect. Dis. **30:** 388, 1922.
10. J. Exper. Med. **50:** 463, 1929.
11. Storrs Agric. Exper. Sta. Bull. 195, March 1934.
12. Arch. Int. Med. **36:** 818, 1925.

TABLE 2.—*Agglutination Titers of Streptococci from Human Gastro-Intestinal Ulcerations and from Bovine Mastitis*

Strain	Disease	Immune Serums										
		H. D. (Bargen)	J. B. (Bargen)	24	5	83 (Saunders)	142 (Saunders)	128 (Saunders)	140 (Saunders)	110	4784	1 A
L. S. (Bargen)	Ulcerative colitis	0*	0	200	800	3200	0	0	0	0	0	0
W. M. (Bargen)	Ulcerative colitis	0	0	800	200	3200	0	0	0	0	0	0
O. J. T. (Bargen)	Ulcerative colitis	0	0	3200	200	0	800	0	0	0	0	0
H. D. (Bargen)	Ulcerative colitis	3200	1600	100	0	0	0	0	0	0	0	0
J. B. (Bargen)	Ulcerative colitis	3200	3200	0	0	0	0	200	0	0	0	0
3	Ulcerative colitis	0	0	0	12800	100	0	0	0	0	0	0
5	Ulcerative colitis	0	0	0	12800	100	0	100	0	0	0	0
13	Ulcerative colitis	0	0	800	0	0	0	0	0	0	0	0
24	Ulcerative colitis	0	0	3200	0	0	200	0	0	0	0	0
32	Ulcerative colitis	0	0	3200	0	0	400	0	0	0	0	0
66 (Saunders)	Gastric ulcer carcinoma	0	0	400	0	800	0	800	0	0	0	100
83 (Saunders)	Gastric ulcer	0	0	200	400	12800	0	800	0	0	0	0
138 (Saunders)	Gastric ulcer	0	0	0	12800	200	0	0	0	0	0	0
142 (Saunders)	Gastric ulcer	0	0	0	0	0	6400	800	400	0	0	0
125 (Saunders)	Gastric ulcer carcinoma	0	0	800	0	3200	0	400	0	0	0	0
127 (Saunders)	Gastric ulcer carcinoma	0	0	0	400	800	0	800	0	0	0	0
131 (Saunders)	Gastric ulcer carcinoma	0	0	0	200	800	0	800	0	0	0	100
140 (Saunders)	Gastric ulcer carcinoma	0	1600	0	200	0	200	0	3200	200	100	400
143 (Saunders)	Gastric ulcer carcinoma	0	0	0	0	0	0	0	0	0	0	0
128 (Saunders)	Breast carcinoma	0	0	0	800	800	0	1600	0	0	0	0
4784 Group A	Bovine mastitis	0	0	0	0	0	0	0	0	6400	6400	0
4787 Group A	Bovine mastitis	0	0	0	0	0	0	0	0	0	0	12800
110 (Hucker) Group A	Bovine mastitis	0	0	0	0	0	0	0	0	3200	6400	0
123 (Hucker) Group A	Bovine mastitis	0	0	0	0	0	0	0	0	0	0	0
3 G Group A	Bovine mastitis	0	0	0	0	0	0	0	0	0	0	0
4 G Group A	Bovine mastitis	0	0	0	0	0	0	0	0	1600	0	0
1 A Group A	Bovine mastitis	0	0	0	0	0	0	0	0	0	0	6400
1 B Group B	Bovine mastitis	0	0	0	800	3200	200	0	0	0	0	0
90 (Saunders) Group B	Bovine mastitis	0	0	3200	100	0	400	800	0	0	0	0
91 (Saunders) Group B	Bovine mastitis	0	0	0	200	1600	0	800	0	0	0	0
AB-13 (Cecil)	Rheumatoid arthritis	0	200	0	800	100	0	800	3200	0	0	100
RB-5 (Cecil)	Rheumatic fever	0	0	0	0	800	0	0	0	200	800	0

* No agglutination at 1:100.

In 1927, Bargen[13] reported that 105 strains of the organism fall into two groups as regards mannitol fermentation; 41 were positive and 64 negative. In 1930, Bargen[13] stated that the organism fermented dextrose, lactose, saccharose, maltose, salicin and raffinose, but not inulin, was usually negative for mannitol and also did not clot milk. As regards resistance to heat, Bargen[13] reported the use of heating methods similar to those of Houston and McCoy, Dibble and Bagger (for the differentiation of enterococci), for the isolation of his organism because of its apparent resistance to heat.

The five strains investigated by us, agree with Bargen's description in that they all fermented raffinose. Three showed very marked resistance to heat (63 C. for 30 minutes). One resisted 60 C. but not 63 C. and one was heat sensitive. Bargen[14] believes his organism belongs in the Streptococcus viridans group rather than in the enterococcus group. One of his five strains (J.B.) however, conforms to all the characteristics of the type enterococcus (Dibble); mannitol and esculin bile positive and resistance to 60 C. for 30 minutes. Three strains (L.S., W.M., O.J.T.), although negative to mannitol and esculin bile, are unusually heat resistant (63 C. for 30 minutes) which is a distinctive characteristic of enterococcus. The one heat sensitive strain (H.D.) is serologically closely related to the enterococcus-like strain J B, as is shown later. All five strains grow well on McConkey agar medium, which is a differential characteristic of some value for the enterococcus group. All five strains also formed a solid clot in milk after four or five days incubation as does the enterococcus. The evidence indicates then that one strain certainly, and the other four strains probably fall within the streptococcal group designated enterococcus. Of 83 streptococcal strains isolated from the human intestine 83.1 per cent were reported by the writers[4] to be positive for esculin bile medium, but strains negative for this test could be shown by agglutination and agglutinin absorption to be closely related to those giving a positive reaction. The most distinctive and consistent cultural characteristic of the Bargen type is apparently fermentation of raffinose. Raffinose splitting enterococci, although not common, have been reported, Dibble[15] noting them in 13 per cent and Torrey and Montu[4] in thirty three per cent with a frequent correlation with heat sensitivity. Strains 3, 5, 13, 24 and 32, of our series, isolated over five years ago from ulcerative colitis, carried in semi-solid hormone agar, and originally negative for mannitol, gave positive reactions in 1935; also No. 5 had acquired the property of gelatin liquefaction. They differ from the Bargen series in not splitting raffinose.

The Saunders and the Bargen types have the reported cultural characteristics in common of predilection for reduced oxygen tension on first isolation, alpha prime hemolysis at first with frequent loss later of all hemolytic properties and similar morphology. They both produce a slight greenish zone on blood agar. The Saunders organism typically ferments lactose, sucrose, salicin and mannitol, but not raffinose or inulin. We,[4] believe it belongs in the enterococcus group. Among the ten which were tested, a good deal of diversity was found in fermentations but only one split raffinose,—a characteristic of the Bargen type. The Saunders type with three exceptions, produced H_2S and so did all the Bargen strains. As with the Bargen strains, the Saunders strains might or might not split esculin in bile salt medium and the same was true for reduction of methylene blue and resistance to 60 C. for 30 minutes. The three Bargen strains tested hydrolyzed sodium hippurate whereas four of ten Saunders strains failed to do so.

The ten strains from bovine mastitis have been divided into two groups A and B, in accordance with the recent study of Pastridge, Anderson, Brigham and Spaulding.[11] They reported that 87 per cent of 208 strains of udder streptococci from cases of bovine mastitis fell into a homogeneous group A on the basis of biochemical characteristics and conformed to the usual descriptions of Str. mastitidis (Str. agalactiae). Eleven per cent were placed in group B. This latter group was much more heterogenous but differed principally from group A in splitting mannitol and in reducing methylene blue in milk. Plastridge et al., reported this type as unable to establish itself permanently in the bovine udder and to be associated with a mild form of chronic mastitis of relatively short duration. Six of the strains in table 1 are definitely of group A type, one (3 G) is similar except for reduction of methylene blue in milk. All of these are chain

13. Collected Studies Mayo Clinic **19:** 351, 1927.
14. Arch. Int. Med. **45:** 559, 1930.
15. System of Bacteriology, London, 1929, vol. 2, p. 130.

forming, are killed at 60 C. and are mannitol and raffinose negative, and thus in one respect or another differ from the Saunders and Bargen types. The mastitis milk strains 90 and 91 resemble the Saunders type biochemically and were reported by him[3] to be serologically identical with his gastric ulcer type. They differ from Str. mastitidis in being positive for mannitol, in reduction of methylene blue and heat resistance. They are provisionally placed in group B. Strain 1 B is similar biochemically to the Str. inulinaceous as described by Sherman and Stark,[16] and as found in the milk and mouth of cows. The AB-13, a type strain, described by Cecil and associates as etiologically associated with rheumatoid arthritis, is much more actively hemolytic than any of the bovine mastitis strains, and on the other hand does not conform to the enterococcus type in biochemical reactions. The RB-5 type strain representative of the rheumatic fever group shows numerous biochemical characteristics in common with the Group B bovine mastitis and the enterococcus types.

AGGLUTINATION AND ABSORPTION RESULTS

The technics employed in the agglutination and agglutinin absorption tests have been described in a previous article.[4] Rabbits were used for the production of anti-serums and to prevent spontaneous clumping, the antigens were all homogenized according to the method of Dr. Anna Williams. Two of the Bargen strains (W.M. and O.J.T.) lacked agglutinogenic properties as did also strains 138, 140, 1 B, 90 and RB-5. In table 2, are recorded the agglutination results with 11 representative antiserums and in tables 3 to 8 absorption results with strains selected from the several groups.

In table 2, a close serological relation is indicated for the Bargen strains H.D. and J.B., and also a certain degree between L.S., W.M., and O.J.T. There is, however, no apparent relationship between these two groups except that absorption with the last three strains reduce slightly the specific agglutinins from H. D. serum (table 3). The evidence indicates accordingly a lack of serological homogeneity among authentic Bargen strains. On the other hand, two strains L.S. and W.M., show a close relationship with the type gastric ulcer strain 83 (tables 2 and 5) but not with the other gastric ulcer strains. Strains O.J.T., H.D., and J.B., show little or no relationship to the Saunders strains but O.J.T. agglutinated to full titer in strain 24 serum. This finding with absorption test, which is recorded in table 4, brings one of the Bargen strains into close serological relationship with an enterococcus type isolated from a stool specimen of an ulcerative colitis patient. There was no evidence of any relationship between the Bargen strains and streptococci from bovine mastitis.

Saunders[3] has reported a complete or nearly complete agglutinative relationship among strains isolated from 30 resected ulcers of the stomach and duodenum and also[2] with five strains isolated from gastric carcinoma, three from breast cancer and two from rectal cancer. Except for strains 66 and 83, the strains reported in this paper were not included in his series, having been isolated after his papers were published. In our hands, although a considerable degree of inter-agglutination occurred with the majority of these 10 Saunders strains, we were not able to confirm the claim of complete serological homogeneity. One strain, 143 from gastric carcinoma, in fact showed no agglutination in any of four serums immune to Saunders strains.

In view of Saunders report of identity of his streptococcal type with three strains isolated from bovine mastitis milk, we were particularly interested in a further investigation of this point in view of the fact that his strains 90, 91 and 100, are morphologically and biochemically unlike the Str. mastitidis type. As indicated in table 1, none of the four serums immune to Saunders strains (83, 142, 128 and 140) agglutinated any one of the seven Str. mastitidis strains (group A). Further, three serums immume to Str. mastitidis strains agglutinated no Saunders strains except 140, and that only in low dilutions. This 140 strain, although agglutinating only at low titer in Str. mastitidis 4784 serum absorbed nearly completely its specific agglutinins (table 6). On the other hand, the three strains from bovine mastitis milk (1 B, 90, 91) not conforming biochemically to the Str. mastitidis type agglutinated to varying degrees in three of the Saunders type serums and one (90) to titer in the ulcerative colitis strain 24 serum. Absorptions (table 4) indicate a very close serological relationship, if not identity, of strains 24 and 90,

16. J. Bact. **22:** 275, 1931.

and also of 1 B (mastitis milk) and 83 (gastric ulcer) (tables 2 and 5). Among the Str. mastitidis Group A strains themselves, 4784 an alpha prime hemolytic and 110 alpha, show complete reciprocal agglutinations and absorptions (tables 6 and 7) and 4787 and 1 A some agglutinative relationship.

The rheumatoid arthritis strain AB-13 (Cecil) agglutinated to titer in an antiserum to Saunders strain 140, but absorbed only 50 per cent of the specific agglutinins. It also agglutinated to some extent in 5 and 128 serums. Absorptions, however, indicated group but not specific relationships in these instances. The rheumatic fever strain RB-5 agglutinated in rather low titer in Str. mastitidis 4784 serum but completely absorbed the specific agglutinins (table 6). This result indicated a surprising serological relationship. This strain otherwise showed little or no serological relationship to the other strains listed in table 1.

DISCUSSION

In a recent publication Bargen[17] states that the diplo-streptococcus, which he is convinced is the primary etiological factor in so-called non-specific ulcerative colitis, can be recognized by its appearance, cultural characteristics and its biological reactions. By the latter term is apparently meant its capacity to produce lesions in experimental animal inoculations similar to those of human ulcerative colitis. These claims have given rise to much criticism and scepticism. Paulson has been particularly active in opposition and has submitted evidence[18] that lesions of the same character may be produced by intravenous inoculation not only of Bargen-like strains isolated from ulcerative colitis but also by streptococcal strains from other sources (alpha prime type from the normal throat, beta from the human uterus, puerperal sepsis, scarlatina throat) and by B. coli and B. dysenteriae; the lesions differing only in their location in the intestinal tract. One of us (Torrey)[19] in 1927 expressed the opinion that there is nothing distinctive in its morphology and examination of the strains dealt with in this paper, has confirmed this view. As regards cultural and biochemical characteristics, according to our observations of the strains received from Dr. Bargen, marked differences in heat resistance are exhibited as well as lack of uniformity in action on salicin, mannitol and esculin bile medium. The one consistent cultural characteristic of some differential value would seem to be the splitting of raffinose. The seven strains which we have examined were all positive and Bargen and Logan[12] in 1925 also reported 20 strains as raffinose positive. This finding would seem to lend some support to his view that his organism is not a member of the enterococcus, but rather of the Streptococcus viridans group. On the other hand, although raffinose splitting is not a usual finding for the enterococcus, Dibble[15] has stated that this is a characteristic of some strains (about 13 per cent), and Bagger[20] obtained a positive reaction in 11 per cent of 150 strains. In our series of isolations of enterococcus-like (esculin bile medium positive) organisms from ulcerative colitis cases, 10 of 23 (43.4 per cent) split raffinose. In 8 instances the strain was recovered from stool specimens and in 15 from swabbings of the lesion.

---

17. J. A. M. A. **101:** 1462, 1933.
18. Arch. Int. Med. **41:** 75, 1928.
19. Tr. Am. Gastro-Enterol. A. **30:** 125, 1928.
20. J. Path. & Bact. **29:** 225, 1926.

As indicated in a preceding section, the five Bargen strains seem to differ too greatly both biologically and serologically to warrant the view that they are representatives of any single specific streptococcal type. Furthermore, in our opinion, the evidence indicates that the so-called Bargen organism is a variant of that heterogeneous group of streptococci designated as enterococcus, and one which has the capacity of acting as a secondary invader of the large bowel wall when and where the tissues have been rendered susceptible by factors operative in initiating ulerative colitis as yet not thoroughly understood. In other words, although such strains may play an active rôle in the ulcerative process as secondary factors, as in fact may also representatives of other streptococcal groups, the so-called Bargen organism has not been established as the specific and essential agent in so-called ulcerative colitis.

In comparing the Bargen and the Saunders types, we note the reported characteristic in common of sensitivity to oxygen when first subjected to artificial conditions of cultivation. After repeated sub-culture under reduced oxygen tension they both acquire the capacity to grow on the surface of solid media. They also both exercise a slight hemolytic action (alpha prime) on blood agar and tend to lose this property on further cultivation. Morphologically they are similar, and in the main culturally, except that the Saunders type rarely splits raffinose (1 positive in 10). Little evidence of serological relationship was found. Only one Saunders strain (140) agglutinated in the Bargen J. B. serum and none in the H. D. serum. On the other hand, the serum immune to the Saunders strain 83 agglutinated Bargen strains L. S. and W. M. in high dilution (table 2) and these strains absorb the specific agglutinins (table 5). This indicates an occasional inter-relationship between these two groups.

TABLE 3.—*Absorptions of Bargen (Ulcerative colitis) Strain H D Antiserum*

Absorbing Antigen	Titer Before Absorption	Titer After Absorption	Homol. Antigen	Titer Before Absorption	Titer After Absorption
H. D	—	—	H. D.	800	<100
J. B	1600	200	H. D.	800	200
L. S	<100	<100	H. D.	800	400
W. M	<100	<100	H. D.	800	400
O. J. T.	<100	<100	H. D.	800	400

TABLE 4.—*Absorptions of (Ulcerative Colitis) Strain 24 Antiserum*

Absorbing Antigen	Titer Before Absorption	Titer After Absorption	Homol. Antigen	Titer Before Absorption	Titer After Absorption
24	—	—	24	3200	<100
13	800	<100	24	3200	<100
32	3200	<100	24	3200	<100
W. M	400	<100	24	3200	1600
O. J. T.	3200	200	24	3200	100
66	400	<100	24	3200	800
125	400	<100	24	3200	3200
90	3200	<100	24	3200	<100

Neither the Bargen nor Saunders types with one exception for the latter (140) show any definite relationship to bovine Str. mastitidis, group A.

This group according to Plastridge and associates[11] are associated with chronic mastitis of long duration. Members of this group tend to form chains, do not split mannitol or raffinose, and according to our finding do not resist a temperature of 60 C. for 30 minutes. No agglutination was obtained with the Bargen, enterococcus or Saunders serums. Saunders[3] reported an identity of bovine mastitis streptococci and his type, but it appears that he was not working with representatives of the true Str. mastitidis. His strains, 90 and 91, resemble in cultural features the group B type of Plastridge et al., and

TABLE 5.—*Absorptions of Gastric Ulcer Strain 83 Antiserum*

Absorbing Antigen	Titer Before Absorption	Titer After Absorption	Homol. Antigen	Titer Before Absorption	Titer After Absorption
83	—	—	83	6400	<100
J. B	<100	<100	83	6400	3200
L. S	3200	<100	83	6400	800
W. M	3200	<100	83	6400	200
H. D	<100	<100	83	6400	6400
O. J. T.	<100	<100	83	6400	6400
138	200	<100	83	6400	800
125	3200	400	83	6400	800
142	<100	<100	83	6400	3200
66	800	<100	83	6400	200
91	800	<100	83	6400	3200
1 B	3200	<100	83	6400	1600
AB-13	<100	<100	83	6400	3200
RB-5	800	<100	83	6400	3200

also the enterococcus of human origin. This group B type was reported to be associated with a mild type of chronic mastitis of relatively short duration. A related strain (1 B) isolated from mastitis milk is similar to Str. inulinaceous.[16]

One or more of these three strains showed agglutinative and agglutinin absorption relationships to enterococcus-like strains 5 and 24 from ulcerative

TABLE 6.—*Absorptions of Bovine Mastitis Strain 4784 Antiserum*

Absorbing Antigen	Titer Before Absorption	Titer After Absorption	Homol. Antigen	Titer Before Absorption	Titer After Absorption
4784	—	—	4784	3200	<100
110	3200	<100	4784	3200	<100
140	100	<100	4784	3200	200
RB-5	800	<100	4784	3200	<100

colitis and to Saunders strains 83 and 128, but not to the Bargen strains L. S. and J. B. (tables 2, 4, 5). The AB-13 strain, a Cecil type strain for rheumatoid arthritis, showed some agglutinative relationships to enterococcus 5 and to Saunders 83, 128 and 140, but absorbed none or very little

TABLE 7.—*Absorption of Bovine Mastitis Strain 110 Antiserum*

Absorbing Antigen	Titer Before Absorption	Titer After Absorption	Homol. Antigen	Titer Before Absorption	Titer After Absorption
110	—	—	110	3200	<100
4784	1600	<100	110	3200	<100
4-G	3200	<100	110	3200	800
140	200	<100	110	3200	3200
RB-5	200	<100	110	3200	3200

of the homologous agglutinins from these serums. The RB-5 (Cecil) streptococcus from rheumatic fever agglutinated in low titer in Saunders 83 serum and absorbed the agglutinins to a slight extent and to the same titer in Str. mastitis serum 4784 but here absorbed 100 per cent of the specific agglutinins (tables 2, 6). It would appear then that raw cows milk may be a vehicle of certain streptococci of bovine origin capable of invading the tissues of the human gastro-duodenal mucous membrane, but that they are rarely the Str. mastitidis of chronic bovine mastitis.

SUMMARY

A comparative study of authentic strains of the Bargen diplo-streptococcus of ulcerative colitis, of selected enterococci associated with the same disease, of representative strains of Saunders streptococcus of gastro-duodenal ulcers and of streptococci associated with bovine mastitis has led to the following conclusions:

The Bargen strains, although exhibiting certain features in common such as the splitting of raffinose, differed greatly in resistance to heat and in their antigenic constitution as indicated by agglutination and agglutinin absorptions. One strain exhibited all the biochemical attributes of an enterococcus and three others the marked resistance to heat characteristic of the enteric streptococci. It would seem proper to classify them as variants of the enterococcus.

The strains from gastric ulcers and gastric ulcer carcinoma tissue did not in our hands show as great a degree of cultural and serological homogeneity as has been reported by Saunders for other series of cultures isolated from these sources. A connecting link with the Bargen group was indicated by the close serological relationship of two of them to a type Saunders strain; the other three Bargen strains were agglutinated only to a slight degree, if at all, by the four Saunders strain serums. With one exception, none of the 10 Saunders strains split raffinose.

Biochemical and serological tests indicated only exceptionally any relationship between the streptococci associated with ulcerative processes in the human gastro-intestinal tract and Streptococcus mastitidis of bovine origin. On the other hand, three streptococcal strains from mastitis milk not related culturally or serologically to Streptococcus mastitidis, exhibited such relationships to two enterococcus strains from ulcerative colitis and to certain of the Saunders peptic ulcer and carcinoma strains. These and other findings suggest a bovine origin for certain enterococcus-like organisms capable of invading human tissues.

THE PATHOGENESIS OF ACTINOMYCOSIS

RECOVERY OF ACTINOMYCES-LIKE ORGANISMS FROM THE NORMAL MOUTH

FREDERICK T. LORD
AND
LAURENCE D. TREVETT
BOSTON

The pathogenesis of actinomycosis has recently been discussed and the following observations in part presented by one of us[1] (Lord). In view, however, of the difficulties encountered in isolating pure cultures of actinomyces of the Wolff-Israel type from the normal mouth, the importance of Naeslund's work and the desirability of further investigations in this field, it seems desirable to present the completed study of a strain of actinomyces-like organisms recovered from the normal mouth.

The experimental production in animals by Lord[2] and by Naeslund[3] of lesions histologically identical with actinomycotic tissue and containing typical club-bearing actinomyces granules by the inoculation of animals with material obtained from the normal mouth suggested the presence in the normal mouth of the actinomyces of the Wolff-Israel type. Inasmuch, however, as certain strains of the streptothrix are capable of forming similar compact, club-bearing colonies when inoculated into animals, identification of the mouth organisms with the actinomyces of the Wolff-Israel type by culture and animal inoculation is necessary before the relation of the disease to organisms harbored in the mouth can be regarded as established.

Naeslund's[4] success in isolating from the normal mouth organisms with morphologic and cultural peculiarities suggesting their close relationship to the actinomyces of the Wolff-Israel type and the production in animals[3] of typical actinomycotic lesions with club-bearing granules are, therefore, of special significance and go far toward unravelling the hitherto uncertain pathogenesis of the disease.

Of the three groups of organisms, (A) preferably aerobic actinomyces, (B) preferably anaerobic actinomyces and (C) actinomyces growing both aerobically and anaerobically, isolated by Naeslun from the normal mouth,

---

Received for publication, July 5, 1935.

From the Medical Laboratory of the Massachusetts General Hospital. This work was aided by a grant from the Proctor Fund of the Harvard Medical School for the Study of Chronic Disease.

1. M. Clin. North America **16:** 829, 1933.
2. Boston M. & S. J. **163:** 82, 1910; J. A. M. A. **55:** 1261, 1910.
3. Acta path. et microbiol. Scandinav. Suppl. 6, 1931.
4. Acta path. et microbiol. Scandinav. **2:** 110, 1925.

the preferably anaerobic organisms of Group B conform with unimportant exceptions in morphology and cultural peculiarities to the actinomyces of the Wolff-Israel type. The results of animal inoculation are also such as may be expected with the actinomyces. Many failures to produce typical lesions in the smaller laboratory animals are to be expected with the actinomyces as with Naeslund's preferably anaerobic actinomyces from the normal mouth. Actinomyces in successful inoculation experiments produces growths histologically like actinomycotic tissue and containing typical actinomyces colonies with radially-disposed, club-bearing filaments. In the illustrations accompanying Naeslund's article[3] the microscopic character of the lesions appears to be identical with actinomycotic tissue, but the colonies of organisms fail to show club-bearing filaments. There are club-shaped extremities to the radiating filaments, but no central filaments are shown. This is due to the photographic reproduction of the specimens as "the clubs were as well simple, club-shaped ends as quite typical eosin-staining clubs." (Personal communication from Naeslund.)

RECOVERY OF AEROBIC-ANAEROBIC ACTINOMYCES-LIKE ORGANISMS FROM THE NORMAL MOUTH

Lord isolated two strains of actinomyces-like organisms from the normal mouth in the spring of 1932 and Trevett isolated two more strains in the fall of the same year.

Material for cultivation was obtained from the dental scum or the contents of carious teeth of about 90 patients without actinomycosis in the medical wards of the Massachusetts General Hospital by scraping the teeth with a platinum loop. The material thus obtained was washed in bouillon, macerated and streaked on the surface of saliva agar plates. The plates were incubated in jars in an atmosphere of hydrogen by the McIntosh and Fildes method with electric or Bunsen flame heating of palladinized asbestos. After about five days in the incubator the plates were examined under a dissecting microscope for suspicious colonies. These were found in material obtained from about one in five patients, but sufficiently separated from other colonies to permit of isolation in only four instances. Suspicious colonies, cut from the agar with a spatula, were washed in bouillon or normal saline and planted on various media.

Smears from cultures show Gram-staining, non-acid fast, branched and unbranched, long and short filaments. The morphology is variable and includes short, bent rods, diphtheria-like forms, filaments with staining points and areas and filaments with club-shaped terminal portions. Much variability in morphology was observed in the same strains under different conditions of cultivation. Club-shaped terminal portions are usually gram-staining, but one strain in glucose bouillon showed abundant eosin-staining material about the filaments suggesting the formation of true clubs in culture.

The cultural peculiarities of the four strains are essentially the same. The organisms grow at incubator temperature under completely anaerobic conditions and equally well under access of air. Young colonies show radiating, branched rods and unbranched filaments. No aerial hyphae or spores are formed. Plain or dextrose bouillon cultures of three of the four strains show growth as a soft, friable, grayish-white, amorphous, slightly viscid sediment. In one of the four, the growth in bouillon is in the form of more compact masses. Cultures are without odor, clouding of the medium or surface colonies. At times growth extends upward along the sides of the tubes. Suspension dextrose agar cultures after several days in the incubator show colonies throughout the medium. In unstirred tubes the growth is most abundant in a narrow zone about one centimeter below the surface with few or no colonies just below the surface. In tubes stirred after inoculation, the growth is equally abundant throughout. Under the microscope the smaller colonies are seen to be composed of branching filaments radiating toward the periphery. The larger colonies are round, grayish-white, compact and sharply outlined without radiating filaments. On slanted medium growth occurs in the form of grayish-white, opaque, discrete or confluent, nodular, soft, moist, shiny colonies somewhat adherent to the surface. Growth occurs equally well on plain, saliva and glucose agar. No hemolysis is observed on blood agar and no proteolysis on Loeffier's blood serum. Gelatin is not liquefied. No growth is observed on potato, or in milk, pleural or ascitic fluid. Club-formation was not promoted by growth in pleural or ascitic fluid or human blood serum from patients with pneumonia.

Growth may occur on transplantation from surface cultures kept in the incubator in tubes with paraffined cotton plugs for as long as two to three weeks in dextrose agar and in plain and dextrose bouillon suspension cultures for about a month, but transplants should be made every week to insure preservation of the strain. Transplants grow only after fairly heavy inoculation. The range of temperature at which multiplication takes place was not definitely determined, but may be roughly approximated from the observation that growth occurs on all media at room temperature during the warmer months of the year at about 26–30 C. and no growth takes place during the colder months of the year when the room temperature is about 22 C. Resistance to drying was tested by placing portions of growth on the inner surface of sterile test tubes kept in the icebox. Transplants usually showed growth from such material after drying for a few days to a week and not after a longer interval.

Nine guinea pigs were inoculated intraperitoneally. Of these, seven were injected with organisms suspended in bouillon and two through a laparotomy wound with split colonies in pieces of sugar agar. Nine rabbits were inoculated, one intravenously, three into the testicle, three into the anterior chamber of the eye, one intraperitoneally and one both intra- and subcutaneously. A cow, a heifer and calf were inoculated subcutaneously. The inoculations were made with from one to ten cubic centimeters of a heavy suspension in bouillon of surface growth from young cultures. Each animal was injected in from four to twelve places along the side of the trunk. In one animal the injection was made deep into the tissue of the jaw.

Autopsy on the guinea pigs from 16 days to three months after inoculation was negative. The rabbit inoculated intravenously was negative at autopsy 7 weeks later. Following the testicular and the intra- and subcutaneous inoculations small suppurative lesions developed within a few days. These contained filamentous organisms without true clubs. Cultures from these lesions showed organisms similar to those with which the inoculations were made. The lesions healed and postmortem examination was negative. Inoculations with the assistance of Dr. Arturo Quevedo into the anterior chamber of the eye of rabbits gave rise to a local inflammatory reaction as in the following example: On enucleation of the eye 18 days after inoculation of the anterior chamber, the aqueous was slightly cloudy. There was marked ciliary injection. The cornea was opaque with intact epithelium. Through the cornea a yellowish-white mass could be seen about 7 mm. in diameter. Tension of the eye was about normal. Cultures from the anterior chamber fluid were sterile. Histological examination showed numerous filaments in loose clusters in the tissue neighboring the anterior chamber, but no clubs. The subcutaneous inoculation of cattle gave rise to local inflammatory lesions usually subsiding within a few days to weeks. Aspirated fluid 27 days after inoculation of the largest local lesion showed many pus cells and short, Gram-positive filaments with club-shaped ends, but no true clubs. The cow was disposed of after observation for 9 months and the calf and heifer after four and five months respectively.

COMPARISON OF MOUTH ORGANISMS ISOLATED BY US WITH THOSE ISOLATED BY NAESLUND

The organisms isolated by us correspond in general to those isolated by Naeslund[4] and described under "Group C, actinomyces growing both aerobically and anaerobically." Our organisms are uniformly Gram-positive, grow well in nutrient broth and show no diastatic or proteolytic action.

COMPARISON OF THE ORGANISMS ISOLATED BY US FROM THE NORMAL MOUTH WITH THE ACTINOMYCES OF THE WOLFF-ISRAEL TYPE

No difference is observed between the mouth organisms and the actinomyces of the Wolff-Israel type in morphology and staining reaction.

In their cultural peculiarities, the mouth organisms isolated in pure culture differ from the actinomyces of the Wolff-Israel type. Initial growth in bouillon of three of the four strains of the mouth organisms occurs as a soft, friable, amorphous and somewhat viscid sediment at the bottom of the tube. The initial growth in one of the strains is in the form of more compact, spherical masses. The initial growth of the actinomyces of the Wolff-Israel type is usually in the form of coherent, nodular, spherical, mulberry-like masses, with which only one of our strains corresponds. Under continued cultivation, however, the actinomyces of the Wolff-Israel type loses its coherent character and grows as a soft, friable, amorphous and somewhat viscid sediment, identical in appearance with the mouth organisms under similar conditions.

It is especially in their behavior with respect to the access of air that the mouth organisms differ in cultural peculiarities from the actinomyces of the Wolff-Israel type. The mouth organisms isolated by us grow equally well under aerobic and anaerobic conditions, while the actinomyces of the Wolff-

Israel type is essentially an anaerobe and not well adapted to surface growth.

The results of animal inoculation in our hands with pure cultures of the mouth organisms have been negative, so far as the production of lesions resembling actinomycosis is concerned. Transient local suppurative inflammation occurs with the presence in the abscesses of numerous branched and unbranched filaments in loose clusters. At times the filaments show club-shaped extremities. The experimental lesions in animals with the mouth organisms are in contrast to the results in a varying and often small proportion of animal experiments with the actinomyces of the Wolff-Israel type with which local abscesses containing compact colonies of branching filamentous organisms with radially-disposed, club-bearing filaments may be produced.

DISCUSSION

The etiologic relation of organisms of the Wolff-Israel type to actinomycosis must be regarded as established. The evidence has long suggested that the disease arises from organisms harbored in the normal mouth and this method of origin has now been established by Naeslund. Our own observations are in accord with his findings with respect to the presence in the normal mouth of a group of anaerobic-aerobic organisms closely related to the actinomyces of the Wolff-Israel type, but we have failed to isolate the actinomyces of the Wolff-Israel type. Confirmation of his findings is desirable and there are still unsolved problems in this connection, such as a more complete understanding of the relation of other branching filamentous organisms to those of the Wolff-Israel type and the importance, if any, of the synergistic action of other organisms in causing the disease.

THE RELATION OF ORGANISMS HARBORED IN THE NORMAL MOUTH TO ACTINOMYCOSIS

The experimental production in animals of lesions histologically identical with actinomycotic tissue and containing typical club-bearing actinomyces granules by the inoculation of animals with material obtained from the normal mouth suggests the presence in the normal mouth of the actinomyces of the Wolff-Israel type. Inasmuch, however, as certain strains of the streptothrix are capable of forming similar compact, club-bearing colonies when inoculated into animals it is necessary that pure cultures of the mouth organisms be obtained before the relation to the disease of organisms harbored in the normal mouth can be regarded as established.

Naeslund has succeeded in isolating from the normal mouth anaerobic organisms morphologically and culturally like the actinomyces of the Wolff Israel type and capable of giving rise in animals to characteristic actinomycotic lesions. The presence in the normal mouth of the actinomyces of the Wolff-Israel type has thus been established.

So far as our observations are concerned, the aerobic-anaerobic organisms isolated by us from the normal mouth appear to be identical with the actinomyces of the Wolff-Israel type in morphology and staining reaction. The character of their initial growth in bouillon, the readiness with which growth occurs under aerobic conditions and failure to produce lesions characteristic of actinomycosis in animals make it impossible to classify them as belonging to the group of the actinomyces of the Wolff-Israel type.

Organisms of the Wolff-Israel type have not been demonstrated outside the human or animal body and, in view of their biologic character, it is unlikely that multiplication takes place in the outside world under any ordinary conditions. Implantation of the parasite within the tissue through injury by a foreign body may be a factor. There are many instances recorded in the literature of the presence in the lesions of foreign bodies, mostly of vegetable nature, but in the majority of cases there is no history of a foreign body and none is found in the lesions. As the most common site of the disease is the region about the head and neck, with abdominal involvement next in frequency and the pulmonary form in a relatively small proportion of cases, the buccal cavity is to be regarded as the portal of entry with secondary invasion of the neighborhood by direct extension and the abdomen and lungs through swallowed or inhaled organisms.

STUDIES ON BACTERIAL NUTRITION

II. THE DISTRIBUTION OF A GROWTH STIMULATING FACTOR IN ANIMAL AND PLANT TISSUES

STEWART A. KOSER
FELIX SAUNDERS
ISADORE I. FINKLE
AND
RAYMOND C. SPOELSTRA
CHICAGO

In a previous study of the requirements for growth of the more exacting bacteria it was found that a growth stimulating factor[1] could be removed from veal infusion. This factor, when added to a simple culture medium, rendered the medium suitable for growth of some of the more fastidious organisms. In certain instances small amounts of added substance amounting to only 0.0006 to 0.00006 milligram of total solids per cubic centimeter of medium were sufficient to permit development in a synthetic medium in which the organisms ordinarily refused to grow.[2]

Additional study of the factor responsible for this effect seemed desirable. However, before attempting chemical purification of the growth substance obtained from veal infusion, it was considered best to take up first the question of its occurrence in various natural sources.

There is considerable evidence in bacteriological literature that growth stimulating substances can be found in a number of animal and plant tissues. In many of these reports, however, it is not clear whether the stimulating effect is due simply to a more abundant supply of readily available food or to the presence of accessory factors which may be required by certain types in addition to the ordinary nutritive material. While no attempt will be made to give a comprehensive survey of the literature, since this has been summarized by Peskett,[3] certain references which bear upon the present study should be mentioned. The important rôle of plant or animal tissue extracts in cultivation of Hemophilus influenzae has been emphasized especially by Davis,[4] Thjötta and Avery,[5] Fildes[6] and others. Substances of a supposedly vitamin-like nature which exerted a strong growth-stimulating activity on hemolytic streptococci and yeast were reported by Freedman and Funk[7] in

---

Submitted for publication, July 6, 1935.

From the Departments of Hygiene and Bacteriology and of Physiological Chemistry, the University of Chicago. This investigation was aided by a grant from the Logan fund.

1. It is uncertain whether one or more growth stimulating factors are concerned, but until more exact information is available it seems simpler to refer to the effect as that produced by one substance.
2. Koser, S. A., and Saunders, F.: J. Infect. Dis. **56**: 305, 1935.
3. Biol. Rev. **8**: 1, 1933.
4. J. Infect. Dis. **21**: 392, 1917.
5. J. Exper. Med. **34**: 97, 455, 1921.
6. Brit. J. Exper. Path. **4**: 265, 1923.
7. J. Metabolic Res. **1**: 457, 469, 1922.

beef muscle, beef heart and yeast. Leichtentritt and Zielaskowski[8] studied the growth-stimulating properties of lemon juice. Morgan and Avery[9] studied the effect of plant tissue, especially potato, upon growth of pneumococci and streptococci. Thompson[10] found that pneumococci and streptococci developed in plain broth after the addition of several plant extracts whereas these organisms refused to grow in the broth alone. Enhanced growth of the tubercle bacillus by the use of plant extracts, together with a study of the active principles of potato was reported by Uyei.[11] The stimulating effect of potato upon butyric acid bacteria noted by Tatum, Peterson and Fred was later reported to be due to asparagine.[12] Hoder and Breuer[13] tested the effect of various plant extracts upon growth of several pathogens and found coconut milk to be especially valuable for enhancing growth. According to Salle and Dunn[14] an extract of rice bran exerted a stimulating effect upon representative bacteria from many different genera. James[15] found that infusions of fish roe and quahaug when incorporated in ordinary culture medium produced a good growth of several of the more exacting pathogens. Knight and Fildes[16] reported that a vitamin-like substance necessary for growth of Clostridium sporogenes in a simple medium could be obtained from several animal tissues and yeast. There was also some evidence that this same factor facilitated the growth of certain strains of Eberthella typhosa.[17] Hughes[18] obtained an "activator" from meat extract which when added in very small amounts to Uschinsky's medium or casein hydrolysate permitted development of Staphylococci. Allison and Hoover[19] found a growth accessory factor for legume nodule bacteria (Rhizobium) in yeast, cane molasses, humic acid, commercial egg albumen, and commercial sucrose.

In many of the foregoing reports it is evident that the animal or plant tissue extract simply increased the rate of growth or luxuriance of growth in mediums in which the organisms were able to develop in the first place. In a few cases, however, notably the reports of Hughes, Knight and Fildes and of Allison and Hoover, the addition of the accessory factor permitted development in a very simple medium in which the organisms ordinarily produced no appreciable growth.

In addition to the foregoing studies on bacteria, the "bios" or yeast growth stimulant of Wildiers has received much attention. The literature of this subject has been covered by others and need not be reviewed here

8. Biochem. Ztschr. **131:** 499, 513, 1922.
9. J. Exper. Med. **38:** 207, 1923.
10. J. Bact. **17:** 379, 1929.
11. J. Infect. Dis. **40:** 433, 1927. Am. Rev. Tuberc. **22:** 203, 1930.
12. J. Bact. **27:** 207, 1934; **29:** 563, 1935.
13. Ztschr. f. Immunitätsforsch. u. exper. Therap. **70:** 279, 1931.
14. Proc. Soc. Exper. Biol. and Med. **32:** 939, 1935.
15. J. Bact. **28:** 323, 1934.
16. Brit. J. Exper. Path. **14:** 112, 1933.
17. Fildes, P., Gladstone, G. P., and Knight, B. C. J. G.: Brit. J. Exper. Path. **14:** 189 1933.
18. J. Bact. **23:** 437, 1932.
19. J. Bact. **27:** 561, 1934.

except to mention several recent studies regarding the occurrence and nature of this growth stimulant. Williams and associates[20] found that growth of the "Gebrüde Mayer" strain of Saccharomyces cerevisiae was accelerated by extracts from widely different sources. The effect was regarded as being due to a single acidic substance to which the name "pantothenic acid" was applied. It was later reported to be present, as judged by the stimulating effect, in most animal tissues.[21] Autolyzed liver was found to be especially rich in this substance.

The purpose of our present study was to gain some additional knowledge concerning the distribution of the bacterial growth stimulating factor, and also to determine which sources appeared the most promising for preparation of the larger amounts of the factor required for further chemical studies and purification. The study included an examination of over thirty extracts which were obtained from various plant and animal tissues.

The following procedure was used for preparation of the tissue extracts. Five kilograms of tissue were finely ground and added to 30 liters of water. Where it was necessary to start with smaller amounts of tissue a proportionate volume of water was added. The tissue was extracted 24 hours or longer and the water and tissue together were heated to boiling. The coagulum was removed by filtration. If the filtrate was turbid, washed Supercel was added to remove the turbidity. Previous work had shown that Supercel did not remove the growth factor. The adsorbant was then filtered off and washed with 3 liters of water. Charcoal was stirred into the combined filtrates in small portions until 50 grams had been added. The charcoal was removed by filtration and the process was then repeated, using only 25 grams of charcoal. The combined charcoal was suspended in two liters of water and collected by filtration. The charcoal was now placed in thimbles while still wet. It was extracted 24 hours with hot ethyl alcohol. About 50 cubic centimeters of water were added to the alcohol during the extraction. After extraction the alcohol was removed in vacuo. The residue was taken up in 200 cubic centimeters of water and after thorough shaking the aqueous solution was cooled in the refrigerator for 12 hours. Any undissolved solid material was removed by filtration. The filtrate was the first crude preparation.

For bacteriological tests the extracts prepared in this way were sterilized in the autoclave at 15 pounds extra pressure for 15 or 20 minutes and then added aseptically to tubes of synthetic medium.

The presence of growth promoting principle in these extracts was determined by adding them in several different dilutions to a synthetic medium[22] and noting the effect upon development of several different types of bacteria. Organisms which ordinarily refused to develop in the synthetic medium were used for these tests so that the stimulating effect of any added substance would be shown more clearly. Ten different cultures were selected so as to

20. J. Am. Chem. Soc. **55:** 2912, 1933.

21. Rohrman, E., Burget, G. E., and Williams, R. J.: Proc. Soc. Exper. Biol. and Med. **32:** 473, 1934.

22. The synthetic medium was similar to that previously employed and consisted of 1.4 grams Na_2HPO_4, 1.0 gram KH_2PO_4, 2.0 grams NaCl, 0.1 gram $MgSO_4$, 3.0 grams asparagine, 0.1 gram cystine, 0.2 gram tryptophane and 2.0 grams dextrose in 1000 cc. of distilled water.

include organisms representative of both the positive and negative results secured in our earlier work with growth factor from veal infusion. Of the ten organisms, it was known that four developed readily in the synthetic medium containing added growth factor from veal infusion, three usually developed sparsely or slowly, and the remaining three were negative. The inclusion of a few organisms which had been uniformly negative in the previous tests seemed desirable, since it was considered that growth factors affecting different organisms might be encountered in the various preparations and that organisms which did not respond to one substance might do so to another.

Throughout the experiments care was taken to avoid carrying over a heavy inoculum when testing for the presence of growth-promoting factor. Light suspensions of each of the 10 organisms were first made in 5 cc. of a buffered salt solution by transferring a small bit of growth from a 24 or 48-hour agar slant of the culture. These suspensions showed no evident turbidity. After thorough distribution, 0.1 cc. of the suspension was then pipetted to each tube of synthetic medium containing the added extract and also to controls of synthetic medium alone and to veal infusion broth. All tests were carried out at 37 C.

Observations of growth were made at several different intervals for a period of 10 days and occasionally longer. The rapidity of development of the organisms as well as the dilution in which growth occurred served to give a general idea of the potency of the preparations. Altogether over 30 preparations were tested in this manner for the presence of growth factor.

Tables 1 and 2 show the results obtained with several of the more promising extracts in comparison with a preparation made from veal infusion. It will be seen that in each case the microörganisms failed to develop in the synthetic medium alone (see footnote of table 1 for statement of a few exceptions to this). Several of them, however, were able to initiate growth and to develop at least fairly rapidly when small amounts of the various preparations were added. In our previous communication[2] reasons were presented for believing this growth factor to be in the nature of a growth accessory substance.

Certain of our preparations appeared either to be especially rich in this substance or else they contained several factors. Thus, the calf spleen preparation appeared the most promising because when added to the synthetic medium all of the organisms developed, at least to some extent. The liver preparation also gave very good results, while several extracts of plant origin exhibited results quite comparable to those secured with veal infusion. Throughout the work the purity of cultures developing in the various tests was often checked by gram stains together with whatever further study appeared desirable.

It is unnecessary to give the detailed results for each of the thirty or more preparations which were tested. A summary and comparison is presented in table 3. In this outline each statement expresses the composite result of a series of tests with the 10 organisms similar in every way to each of those presented in the first two tables.

Calf spleen, calf liver, and yeast gave the most promising results, although many of the other tissues were good sources of the growth stimulating factor. In considering this summary it should be pointed out that the results are only roughly comparable. They do not necessarily give a true picture of the amount of growth factor actually in the tissue, since extraction

TABLE 1.—*The Occurrence of Growth Stimulating Factor in Several Typical Extracts of Animal Origin*

	Amount of Extract Added* cc.	Development in Synthetic Medium with Addition of Extract from								
		Veal Infusion days			Calf Liver days			Calf Spleen days		
		1	2	5	1	2	5	1	2	5
Streptococcus scarlatinae	0.1	0	0	0	0	0	+	+	2+	3+
	0.01	0	0	0	0	0	0	0	0	0
	0.001	0	0	0	0	0	0	0	0	0
	none	0	0	0	0	0	0	0	0	0
Streptococcus lactis	0.1	0	0	0	0	?	+	2+	3+	3+
	0.01	0	0	0	0	0	0	?	?	?
	0.001	0	0	0	0	0	0	0	0	0
	none	0	0	0	0	0	0	0	0	0
Staphylococcus aureus	0.1	0	+	+	+	2+	3+	0	3+	3+
	0.01	0	0	+	0	+	+	0	0	+
	0.001	0	0	0	0	0	0**	0	0	0
	none	0	0	0	0	0	0	0	0	0
Staphylococcus albus	0.1	+	2+	3+	2+	3+	3+	3+	3+	3+
	0.01	0	+	2+	+	2+	3+	2+	2+	3+
	0.001	0	0	0	0	+	2+	+	+	2+
	none	0	0	0	0	0	0	0	0	0
Corynebacterium diphtheriae (Park 8)	0.1	0	+	3+	+	3+	3+	+	2+	3+
	0.01	0	+	3+	?	2+	3+	?	+	3+
	0.001	0	0	+	0	+	2+	0	+	2+
	none	0	0	0	0	0	0	0	0	0
Brucella abortus	0.1	0	0	+**	0	+	2+	+	+	2+
	0.01	0	0	0**	0	0	0	?	+	+
	0.001	0	0	0	0	0	0	0	0	0
	none	0	0	0	0	0	0	0	0	0
Pasteurella avicida	0.1	0	0	0	0	0	0	+	+	2+
	0.01	0	0	0	0	0	0	+	+	+
	0.001	0	0	0	0	0	0	0	0	0
	none	0	0	0	0	0	0	0	0	0
Salmonella pullorum	0.1	+	+	2+	+	+	2+	+	2+	2+
	0.01	0	0	+	+	+	+	+	2+	2+
	0.001	0	0	0	0	0	0	0	0	0
	none	0	0	0	0	0	0	0	0	0
Shigella dysenteriae (Shiga)	0.1	2+	3+	3+	3+	3+	3+	3+	3+	3+
	0.01	+	3+	3+	3+	3+	3+	3+	3+	3+
	0.001	0	+	3+	2+	3+	3+	+	3+	3+
	none	0	0	0	0	0	0	0	0	0
Eberthella typhosa	0.1	2+	3+	3+	3+	3+	3+	2+	3+	3+
	0.01	+	3+	3+	+	2+	3+	2+	3+	3+
	0.001	0	0	2+	+	2+	2+	+	3+	3+
	none	0	0	0	0	0	0	0	0	0

Certain strains of C. diphtheriae, S. dysenteriae, and E. typhosa will develop in the synthetic medium itself without added growth factor. The particular strains chosen for our work were unable as a general rule to develop to the point of showing visible turbidity in the synthetic medium. However, occasional exceptions to this were noted in the control tubes of these organisms and a delayed growth occurred in a few instances.

The luxuriance of growth, varying from light to heavy turbidity is represented by the number of plus signs. Absence of visible turbidity is shown by the zero, 0. An occasional doubtful result is recorded with a question mark.

* Amount of extract added to each 5 cc. tube of synthetic medium.

** Growth apparent, or heavier growth, at 10 days.

might be accomplished much more readily from some sources than from others. There is the added possibility that substances which inhibit growth might also be present or that conditions tending to inactivate the growth factor might at times be encountered. Also, the various preparations contained somewhat different amounts of total solids. However, comparison on the basis of total solids does not necessarily afford better grounds for judging potency, since in each case it is not known how much extraneous material is present in the total solids along with the growth factor. Despite these uncertainties the results appear to have some value in showing the general distribution of growth-promoting principle and also in affording some idea of those products which might be used as sources of material for further attempts at chemical separation and purification.

TABLE 2.—*The Occurrence of Growth Stimulating Factor in Several Typical Extracts of Plant Origin*

	Amount of Extract Added* cc.	Development in Synthetic Medium with Addition of Extract from								
		Tomato days			Potato (white) days			Rice Bran days		
		1	2	5	1	2	5	1	2	5
Streptococcus scarlatinae	0.1	0	0	+	0	0	0	0	0	0
	0.01	0	0	0	0	0	0	0	0	0
	0.001	0	0	0	0	0	0	0	0	0
	none	0	0	0	0	0	0	0	0	0
Streptococcus lactis	0.1	0	0	0	0	0	0	0	0	0
	0.01	0	0	0	0	0	0	0	0	0
	0.001	0	0	0	0	0	0	0	0	0
	none	0	0	0	0	0	0	0	0	0
Staphylococcus aureus	0.1	0	2+	3+	0	2+	3+	0	+	2+
	0.01	0	0	0	0	0	2+	0	0	+
	0.001	0	0	0	0	0	0	0	0	0
	none	0	0	0	0	0	0	0	0	0
Staphylococcus albus	0.1	2+	3+	3+	2+	3+	3+	+	3+	3+
	0.01	+	+	3+	0	+	2+	?	2+	3+
	0.001	0	0	0**	0	0	0**	0	0	+
	none	0	0	0	0	0	0	0	0	0
Corynebacterium diphtheriae (Park 8)	0.1	?	2+	3+	0	2+	3+	0	+	3+
	0.01	0	+	3+	0	+	3+	0	0	2+
	0.001	0	0	2+	0	0	0	0	0	+
	none	0	0	0	0	0	0	0	0	0
Brucella abortus	0.1	+	2+	2+	0	+	2+	0	0	+
	0.01	0	0	+	0	0	+	0	0	0
	0.001	0	0	0	0	0	0	0	0	0
	none	0	0	0	0	0	0	0	0	0
Pasteurella avicida	0.1	0	0	0	0	0	0	0	0	0
	0.01	0	0	0	0	0	0	0	0	0
	0.001	0	0	0	0	0	0	0	0	0
	none	0	0	0	0	0	0	0	0	0
Salmonella pullorum	0.1	+	2+	2+	+	2+	2+	+	+	2+
	0.01	0	+	+	?	+	+	0	?	+
	0.001	0	0	0	0	0	0	0	0	0
	none	0	0	0	0	0	0	0	0	0
Shigella dysenteriae (Shiga)	0.1	2+	3+	3+	2+	3+	3+	2+	3+	3+
	0.01	2+	3+	3+	0	3+	3+	+	3+	3+
	0.001	+	3+	3+	0	0	0	0	0	3+
	none	0	0	0	0	0	0	0	0	0
Eberthella typhosa	0.1	2+	3+	3+	2+	2+	3+	2+	3+	3+
	0.01	+	3+	3+	+	2+	3+	+	3+	3+
	0.001	0	0	0	0	0	0**	0	0	0
	none	0	0	0	0	0	0	0	0	0

* Amount of extract added to each 5 cc. tube of synthetic medium.
** Growth apparent, or heavier growth, at 10 days.
See also footnote of table 1.

Several requirements must be considered in the selection of material for this further work. The tissue should be readily available, inexpensive, and relatively free from toxic substances and from compounds which interfere with ultimate purification. Several tissues such as blood and brain, which are not included in table 3, were tried and abandoned for one or more of the above-mentioned reasons. Further work is being done on these tissues using a modified extraction technic. Even yeast, which gave excellent results in our tests, had at least one decided disadvantage in that gummy substances accompanied the growth factor and interfered with attempts at purification.

A few tissues such as cancerous liver were included in the list for purposes of comparison even though they were not seriously considered as sources for the ultimate preparation of large amounts.

TABLE 3.—*Comparison of Various Animal and Plant Tissue Extracts as Sources of Growth Factor*

Animal Sources		Higher Plants	
Veal infusion	+++	Oat sprouts	++
Skim milk	+++	Wheat germ	++±
Calf liver	+++±	Rice bran	+++
Calf liver ash	–	Tea, Lipton's (yellow label)	–
Calf thymus	+++	Lettuce	++±
Calf heart	++	Soy beans	++±
Calf spleen	++++	Tomato juice	+++
Calf kidney	+++	Turnips	+++
Calf lung	++±	White potatoes, whole	+++
Pig embryo	++	White potatoes, ash	–
Chicken liver	+++	White potatoes, sprouts	+±
Shad roe	+++	White potatoes, tuber left after removal of sprouts	++±
Human liver with carcinoma	++±	Carrots	++
Human placenta	+++	Coconut milk	+++
Human urine	+		
		Microörganisms	
		Yeast, bakers'	+++±
		Pseudomonas fluorescens*	+
		Molds, mixture**	++
		Molds, several pure cultures of Aspergillus and Penicillium**	+ or ++

* Ps. fluorescens was grown in veal infusion after removal of growth factor with charcoal.
** The molds were grown in Czapek-Dox liquid synthetic medium.

In most of the tests where growth stimulating principle was demonstrated, the response of the microörganisms was very similar in a qualitative way. Usually the same organisms developed. S. dysenteriae, E. typhosa, S. albus, and C. diphtheriae developed readily. S. aureus, Br. abortus, and S. pullorum developed somewhat more slowly and sparsely. Moreover, these results were much the same whether the extract was prepared from a plant or animal tissue. In the presumably more potent preparations these organisms developed more rapidly and in somewhat higher dilutions. In a few instances where the best development of the foregoing types occurred, the streptococci and P. avicida were also able to produce a slow growth. This is shown best with the spleen extract and to some extent with liver in table 1. It was also observed with yeast extract. Aside from this, there was no real difference in the types of bacteria which were able to grow as a result of the addition of the various extracts to the synthetic medium. These results suggest that the growth factor in the various preparations was quite similar and that some organisms required greater concentrations of the factor than others.

SUMMARY

A growth stimulating factor which permits development of some of the more fastidious bacteria in a synthetic medium was found to be widely distributed in animal and plant tissues.

Of the various sources tested by our method, calf spleen, calf liver and yeast were the richest, although many tissues gave good results.

On the basis of the qualitatively similar responses of the organisms it appears that there is a marked similarity in the growth factor secured from widely different sources.

NOTE ON THE LIQUEFACTION OF GELATIN BY SALMONELLA, TYPE DAR-ES-SALAAM

EDWIN O. JORDAN

CHICAGO

In all descriptions of the paratyphoid bacilli or genus Salmonella[1] inability to liquefy gelatin is registered as a characteristic. It seems worth recording that the free lance Salmonella type Dar-es-Salaam[2] liquefies gelatin, albeit slowly. The Dar-es-Salaam type, according to the Kauffmann-White schema,[3] belongs in "Group D" of the Salmonella genus (somatic antigen IX) and is monophasic, with the specific H-antigenic constitution enlw. The three cultures that I have tested have behaved entirely alike in their cultural characteristics, which agree with those described in tabulations by English writers[4] and in the recent tabulation by Kauffmann.[1] Inosite is not fermented and d-tartrate not attacked.[5]

All these cultures have liquefied gelatin. The tests of two cultures have been made at intervals over a period of some four years and a third culture obtained more recently has given similar results. On several occasions the cultures have been plated out and five or more colonies picked. In every case these subcultures have liquefied gelatin. In stab cultures at 22 C. the liquefaction usually appears between the second and third weeks as a slight crateriform cupping which varies in depth and is followed by more pronounced liquefaction, usually within four weeks. Incubation of inoculated gelatin tubes at 37 C. followed by cooling in ice water has also demonstrated the occurrence of liquefaction.

From the Department of Hygiene and Bacteriology, University of Chicago.

1. White, P. B.: A System of Bacteriology, Medical Research Council, London, His Majesty's Stationery Office **4:** 86, 1929; Lovell, R.: Bull. Hyg. **7:** 405, 1932, Kauffmann, F.: Ergebn. d. Hyg., Bakt., Immunitätsforsch. u. exper. Therap. **115:** 219, 1934.

2. The organism given this name was isolated by Butler in 1922 from the urine (not blood as stated by Kauffmann: Zentralbl. f. d. ges. Hyg. **25:** 273, 1931) of a patient with pyrexia of about two weeks' duration (White, P. B.: Further Studies of the Salmonella Group, Medical Research Council, Special Report, Series 103, London, His Majesty's Stationery Office, 1926, p. 107). It has been preserved in the National Collection of Type Cultures—"No. 2206," and I have obtained two cultures at different times from this source and one from Dr. W. M. Scott. No other strain of this organism seems yet to have been isolated.

3. J. Hyg. **34:** 333, 1934.

4. See, e.g., Lovell.[1]

5. White[1] (p. 100) records the Dar-es-Salaam strain as fermenting salicin slowly (not until the third to fifth day), but none of my cultures have given any indication of attacking this glucoside within a period of 14 days' incubation.

PSITTACOSIS

A REVIEW OF THE LITERATURE ON THE LESIONS OF THE CENTRAL NERVOUS SYSTEM WITH A REPORT OF A CASE

DOUGLAS H. SPRUNT
AND
GEORGE P. BERRY
DURHAM, NORTH CAROLINA

Since 1880, when psittacosis was first described as a clinical entity in man, many papers have appeared dealing with various phases of the subject. Interest in the disease has been stimulated during the last few years by the epidemic and endemic cases of the malady that have occurred in this country and in Europe. Lillie[1] in a recent paper summarized the morbid anatomy in 52 cases. Since then no other pathologic reports have appeared. In reviewing these papers and in studying the work of Rivers and Berry[2] and others who have produced the disease experimentally in monkeys, it is apparent that the lesions in the lung and the other viscera have been well described. Although patients with psittacosis evidence symptoms and signs of involvement of the central nervous system, few reports of detailed studies of the changes in the brain and cord have appeared. In this paper an attempt is made to evaluate previous findings recorded in the literature and to report a case in which the brain was studied in detail.

In 21 of the 52 cases discussed by Lillie,[1] the brain was at least mentioned. In the majority of instances, the brain was dismissed with a few words; in some, no histological studies were made. Of these 21 cases, 6 had meningeal congestion and cerebral hyperemia; 3, pial edema; 4, no lesions; and 8, ring hemorrhages. In addition to these 8 cases with ring hemorrhages, Russell[3] cites 2 in which she found a similar condition. The hemorrhages were microscopic in all but two instances. If the other cases had been studied with more care, small hemorrhages would probably have been found.

Freeman[4] reported that he found vascular nodules associated with perivascular cellular collections. The intima was damaged, many of the cells multiplying and others undergoing necrosis. The staining reactions of the myelin in the region of the hemorrhages was altered, but the axis cylinders were not damaged. He did not see any increase of fat. Besides vascular changes, Scholte[5] described neuronophagia and glial rosette formation. His case, however, had extensive arteriosclerosis. Polayes and Lederer[6] described

Received for publication, March 19, 1935.

From the Hospital of Rockefeller Institute for Medical Research and the Department of Pathology of the Duke University School of Medicine.

1. Nat. Inst. Health Bull. **161:** 1, 1933.
2. J. Exper. Med. **54:** 129, 1931.
3. Brit. M. J. **1:** 888, 1931.
4. Freeman, Walter: Neuropathology, W. B. Saunders Co., Philadelphia, p. 162, 1933.
5. Nederl. tijdschr. v. geneesk. **74:** 2741, 1930.
6. Arch. Int. Med. **49:** 253, 1932.

swelling of the ganglion cells, increase of fat, tigrolysis and increase in glial cells.

REPORT OF CASE

A white man, aged 31, contracted psittacosis through contact at a bird store with parrots and parrakeets which were later shown (by G. P. B.) to have the disease. His first association with the birds occurred 17 days before the onset of his illness, so that the incubation period did not exceed this time.

Until the onset of the present illness, the patient's health had been excellent, and his family history was also irrelevant. The illness began October 29, 1931, with drowsiness and excessive fatigue. These symptoms were soon followed by severe headache and a fever which reached 104 F. (40 C) on the second day. During the first week, several chills followed by profuse sweating occurred. The patient developed a sustained mild delirium. There was a slight cough but no expectoration, and at no time was there any hemoptysis or pain in the chest. Anorexia was complete. Severe abdominal cramps were a daily complaint. A dull aching pain in the back and flanks was constantly present. The patient was admitted to the service of Dr. Henry S. Patterson at Saint Luke's Hospital, November 4, 1931, on the seventh day of illness.

On admission the rectal temperature was 104.4 F. (40.2 C.); the pulse rate, 100 per minute; the respiratory rate, 24 per minute. The patient was acutely ill. Marked injection of the tonsils and pharynx was noted. Evidences of consolidation were found in the lower and middle lobes of the right lung. A roentgenogram showed a moderately dense shadow throughout the lower right chest field. There was some tenderness on pressure upon the abdomen and in the region of the left kidney. Except for a trace of albumin, the urine was negative. The leucocytes numbered 10,200 per cu. mm., of which 80 per cent were polymorphonuclear neutrophilic elements. There was no anemia. The chemical constituents of the blood were normal.

The stay in the hospital was characterized by progressive decline, high continuous fever, relative bradycardia and bradypnea, delirium, and a spread in the pneumonic consolidation to the right upper and left lower lobes. There was no dyspnea or pain in the chest at any time. Some coughing developed as the pneumonia increased, but only small amounts of tenacious yellowish-white sputum were produced. On culture of the sputum, the predominant organism was a staphylococcus; in addition only a few colonies of group IV pneumococci appeared in the plates, along with a few of Neisseria catarrhalis and Haemophilus influenzae. Four blood cultures made during the course of the illness remained sterile. A typhoid agglutination test on the eighth day of the disease was negative. On the tenth day the leucocytes numbered 6,100 with 68 per cent polymorphonuclear neutrophilic elements; on the thirteenth day, 5,400 with 76 per cent polymorphonuclear neutrophilic elements. The patient died on November 13, 1931, 16 days after the onset of symptoms.

Demonstration of the Virus of Psittacosis.—Sputum collected from the patient on the tenth day of illness and the sixth day before death was passed through a Berkefeld V filter and inoculated intraperitoneally into 6 mice, 1 cc. into each mouse on 3 successive days. Two mice were sick on the seventh day after inoculation. They were killed and psittacosis bodies were demonstrated in impression smears. The virus was successfully passed to 6 more mice. Of the remaining 4 mice inoculated with sputum, one died and psittacosis bodies were demonstrated. The other 3 were shown to be immune when reinoculated with a known strain of psittacosis virus.

Blood from the patient on the tenth day, at the time the sputum was collected, was also injected intraperitoneally into 6 mice. None of the mice sickened or died and none evidenced an immune reaction when tested a month later with a known strain of psittacosis virus. This finding, i.e., the presence of the virus of psittacosis in the sputum but its absence simultaneously from the blood, has been noted by one of us (G. P. B.) in 2 other instances of human psittacosis.

Necropsy.—A necropsy was performed 13.5 hours after death. Since the nature of the changes in the viscera have been frequently described elsewhere, only a brief account is given here.

The body is slightly obese and well developed. Aside from edema of the external genitalia, nothing of interest is seen. The peritoneal surfaces are smooth and glistening. The liver edge extends 1 cm. below the costal margin in the right midclavicular line and 3 cm. below the xiphoid process. The intestines are slightly distended. The pleural cavities contain about 10 cc. of blood-tinged fluid. There are no adhesions in either chest.

The right lung weighs 820 grams. Only the anterior portion of the upper lobe contains air. The pleura is smooth, glistening and dark purplish-red. The parenchyma of the lung is non-air-containing. On section, the cut surface is smoothly consolidated in the lower and middle lobes, while the upper lobe is consolidated in patches. The consolidated areas have a waxy appearance and yield a slight amount of dark red frothy fluid when scraped. The left lung weighs 660 gm. and is similar to the right in other respects.

The spleen weighs 250 gm. The capsule is slightly wrinkled. The splenic pulp is friable and hemorrhagic.

The heart, liver, kidneys, pancreas, bladder, and intestines are essentially negative.

The marrow from the femur is dark red.

On removing the calvarium the dura mater is only slightly adherent. The venous sinuses are free from thrombi, and the bony sinuses show no gross abnormalities. The pia arachnoid is smooth and glistening. The blood vessels are slightly injected. On section nothing is noted except congestion of the blood vessels.

Small pieces of tissue from the viscera were fixed in Zenker's fluid and sections of them were stained with hematoxylin and eosin. The whole brain was fixed in 10 per cent formalin. After fixation, portions of the brain were placed in several successive lots of fresh 95 per cent alcohol for a period of several months. Then they were embedded in celloidin and stained after the technique of Nissl. Sections from other portions of the brain were stained with hematoxylin and eosin, according to the Kulschitsky method for myelin, Perl's stain for iron, and for fat according to the Marchi method. For all of the stains on sections from the brain numerous blocks of tissue were taken from the cortex, internal capsule, basal ganglia, cerebellum and cord.

Brain.—There is no swelling of the neurons, no neuronophagia and no tigrolysis. Many of the ganglion cells contain slightly more fat than usual. There is no increase in any of the glial elements.

The vascular system reveals small hemorrhages surrounding a few of the capillaries and smaller arterioles. The endothelium of the blood vessels both in the neighborhood of the hemorrhages and elsewhere is not proliferative, swollen, or necrotic. The hemorrhages are confined entirely to the Virchow-Robbins space. Around some vessels are accumulations of large phagocytic cells which contain fat and hemosiderin, probably as a result of earlier hemorrhages.

Lungs.—The alveoli are filled with a mixture of red blood cells, mononuclear cells, and occasional polymorphonuclear neutrophilic elements. The mononuclear cells consist of the following types: a few large phagocytic cells containing pigment, many lymphocytes, a moderate number of monocytes and plasma cells. Only a small amount of fibrin is seen. One microscopic preparation shows part of a hemorrhagic infarct.

Bronchi.—The mucosa and submucosa of the bronchi are infiltrated with many lymphocytes and plasma cells and a few polymorphonuclear neutrophilic leucocytes.

Hilic Lymph Nodes.—The lymph nodes contain a large amount of pigment which fails to give an iron reaction and is thought to be coal dust. The peripheral sinuses are filled with large mononuclear cells which contain small quantities of iron.

Spleen.—The splenic pulp is filled with red blood cells. The Malpighian corpuscles are small and inactive.

Liver.—The sinusoids are slightly dilated around the central veins. The hepatic cells, especially in the region of the central vein, contain large vacuoles in the cytoplasm which are probably due to fat. Many of the nuclei of the hepatic cells are represented as clear nuclear rings. This is probably due to glycogen. There are no cellular infiltrations, no areas of necrosis, and no increase in the number of Kupffer cells.

Kidneys.—Neither the glomeruli nor the tubules show any lesions.

Aorta.—No changes are seen in the intima or media, but in the adventitia there are a few lymphocytes around some of the vasa vasorum.

Bone Marrow.—The microscopic preparations show a slight hyperplasia. The cells are of both myeloid and lymphoid types. A few eosinophils are present but not more than normally seen.

Psittacosis Virus.—In none of the organs are the psittacosis bodies found. This, however, is not unusual as they have been seen in only a few human beings. We have searched for these elements in sections from a large number of monkeys and several human beings known to have had psittacosis with success in only one instance.

An unsuccessful attempt was made to demonstrate the presence of psittacosis virus in various organs removed at autopsy. These included the brain (tissue from each cerebral hemisphere and from the brain stem), the lungs (tissue from both early and advanced lesions from each lung), the liver and the spleen. In each case, the tissue was triturated in a mortar with an abrasive and Locke's solution to prepare a ten per cent suspension. From the lungs, in addition, a five per cent suspension in p_H 7.8 meat infusion broth was prepared and filtered through a Berkefeld V candle. Each of the tissue suspensions, and the filtrate of lung as well, was injected intraperitoneally into 6 mice. In no instance did the mice show any evidence of the activity of psittacosis virus nor of any immunity against this agent when tested a month later with a known strain. All of the mice receiving unfiltered lung suspension died within 2 days of bacterial infection; all of the other mice survived until the test for active immunity.

Bacterial Cultures.—The tissue suspensions, prepared for the mouse inoculations just described, were cultured on blood agar and in meat infusion broth under aerobic and anaerobic conditions. Since the bits of the various organs had not been obtained at autopsy with a sterile technique, these cultures showed the presence of a wide variety of contaminating bacteria. From the lungs pneumococci belonging to group IV, staphylococci, indifferent streptococci, influenza bacilli and diphtheroids were obtained. From the other organs a similar type of mixed growth was recovered. While the presence of these bacteria is without significance, the absence of specific pathogenic organisms, especially in the case of the lungs, is important. One may conclude that bacteria were not playing a role in engendering the pathological processes detailed above.

DISCUSSION

Psittacosis virus in man causes an extensive mononuclear cell pneumonia. It acts in a similar manner in monkeys, but in birds and mice the liver and spleen are principally involved. In this paper, as stated, we are primarily concerned with the nature of the lesions in the brain. A review of the literature shows that in almost every instance in which the brain was studied in detail, small hemorrhages around the blood vessels were found. We have verified these findings and also pointed out that many of the vessels may be surrounded by large phagocytic cells which contain hemosiderin and fat as a result of previous hemorrhages.

The small hemorrhages just described are spoken of as cerebral purpura and are associated with a number of morbid conditions. Kuczynski and Wolff[7] give a good review of the literature of this condition on page 1106 of their article. They summarize numerous theories in regard to the origin of the hemorrhages, but endorse none further than to say that the cause may be infectious, toxic, or traumatic. According to them the cerebral purpura caused by trauma evidences at times as much perivascular proliferation as do the infectious and toxic. Thus the perivascular changes are entirely secondary to the hemorrhages. They also state that the hemorrhages do not necessarily result from damage to the vessel walls, but may be due only to diapedesis. In this they agree with Polayes and Lederer[6] and ourselves who found no damage to the vascular walls.

The findings in our case lend support to the idea that the cerebral purpura in psittacosis is a toxic change secondary to the pneumonia. The more fre-

7. Ergebn. d. allg. Path. u path. Anat. **19:** Part 2, 947, 1921.

quent occurrence of this type of lesion in psittacosis than in the other forms of pneumonia is probably due to the severity and duration of the psittacotic pneumonia. Thus, the condition is most likely to occur in such maladies as smallpox or typhoid fever, diseases with a protracted course. This is in agreement with Russell.[3]

The other changes reported, particularly the increase of fat in neurons, may also be attributed to toxemia. The vascular nodules that have been described may be the result of hemorrhage and not proliferative lesions similar to the typhus nodules in which rickettsia are found. The demylinization noted by Peterson[8] and his coworkers, mentioned by Freeman,[4] is probably the result of a changed myelin reaction due to the large perivascular hemorrhages present in that case and is not to be considered similar to the perivascular demyelinization seen after vaccination against smallpox and after virus diseases.

SUMMARY

The literature on the lesions found in the central nervous system of cases of psittacosis are reviewed and the findings in an additional case are reported. Cerebral purpura occurs frequently in psittacosis because of the severity of the disease and is thought to be non-specific.

8. J. A. M. A. **95:** 171, 1930.

CYTOPLASMIC INCLUSION BODIES IN THE HUMAN THROAT

JEAN BROADHURST
ROSAMOND M. LIMING
MARGARET ESTELLE MACLEAN
AND
INEZ TAYLOR
NEW YORK CITY

The inclusion bodies, which are the subject of this paper, occur in the cytoplasm of the squamous epithelial cells of the upper respiratory tract. Because of their abundance (figure 1) in affected persons, they provide a ready means of studying inclusion bodies in the fresh, living state, and we, therefore, offer at this stage of our investigations the accompanying report of these bodies with regard to the three following points:

Their incidence, particularly in the throat area.
Morphological and staining characteristics.
Successful methods of cultivation.

INCIDENCE IN THE UPPER RESPIRATORY AREA

Our investigations have been limited, on the whole, to the epithelial tissue of the upper respiratory areas, especially the throat, but these bodies have also been observed in two other regions: the eye and the genital area. Two of our subjects who were throat carriers of these bodies, showed the same bodies in smears taken from the lining of the lower eye lid; one of these positive eye cases was being treated for a "chronic, low-grade infection" of the eyes, but the other "had not noticed any difficulty with her eyes." The examination of 100 routine maternity clinic smears of the genital area (cervical, vaginal) showed these bodies present in at least 10 per cent of the individuals. So far, however, our studies have been limited to the presence and characteristics of the bodies as found in the upper respiratory areas, especially the throat. No real attempt has yet been made to correlate the presence of these bodies in the throat with their presence in other areas of the body.

Our findings, with regard to the incidence of these bodies in the upper respiratory region, may be briefly reported under four headings:

(1) The incidence of such inclusion bodies in groups of (so-called) normal persons.
(2) Their incidence in persons reporting respiratory irritations.
(3) The changes observed during continued serial examinations of carriers.

Received for publication, September 16, 1935.

From the Institute of Practical Science Research, Teachers College, Columbia University.

These investigations have been aided materially by a grant from the Milbank Memorial Fund.

(4) The "incompatibility" of these inclusion bodies and bacteria, as indicated by their infrequent coincident presence in epithelial cells.

Our findings indicate that there has been among our students in the last few years a marked increase in the number positive for these inclusion bodies. We observed them in November, 1930,[1] in the throat smear of a student complaining of a chronic sore throat. Though distinctly visible in the routine methylene blue stained slides, they were not numerous in any given throat smear—only four or five cells in any smear containing any of these bodies. Having failed to cultivate them on any of the special culture mediums containing blood or serum by the time the student left college, we were quite definitely on the lookout for these bodies in the succeeding months. In the fall of 1933 we began to find them rather frequently; and at the present time they are easily demonstrated in at least one of every student group of 15 to 20.

The incidence of these inclusion bodies in the throats of groups of normal or "run-of-the-mill" individuals is apparently affected by the degree of contact within such groups. In groups with little inter-association, such as compose our bacteriology classes (mainly day students and representing widely distributed geographical areas), the incidence is low—about 8 per cent in the 250-odd students whose throats were examined this past school year. In smaller, closely associated groups, such as student-nurses housed in a dormitory, we have obtained 30 per cent or more positives for groups of 20 to 30 students on a given day.[2]

The percentage of positive findings is even higher when we consider only those reporting throat or other respiratory irritations. These bodies are, as might be expected, often absent from specimens taken from severe sore throats, e.g., where streptococci are numerous, but they are present in suprisingly high percentages of samples taken from many of the milder affections. Having found these bodies in several samples taken from individuals who complained of chronic coughs, chronic sore throats and "little sore throats" we made a special effort to secure throat specimens from ambulatory throat cases, especially the "acute but mild sore throats without fever" frequently reported in the winter-spring season of 1933–34. In this series we included also chronic irritations, described by the various subjects as "a chronic sinus" and "a post-nasal drip."

In the first three months of 1934 we collected, in round numbers, 130 such samples, over 100 of which proved to be positive, some of them to a surprising degree, several affected cells being present in many of the oil-immersion fields on a given slide. One very interesting subject, a student nurse whose hospital record showed seven colds or sore throats demanding nursing care during a period of 14 months, had by far the largest and most distinctly capsulated bodies which we found in the whole series of 100 positives. Her tonsils were

1. Broadhurst, Jean: Am. J. Nursing **34**: 985, 1934.

2. Serial throat examinations, carried out by L. Deimler and H. Porter, independently in Pennsylvania and Ohio in 1934–35, which will be reported later, indicate an increasing incidence in such groups throughout the first ten or twelve weeks of association.

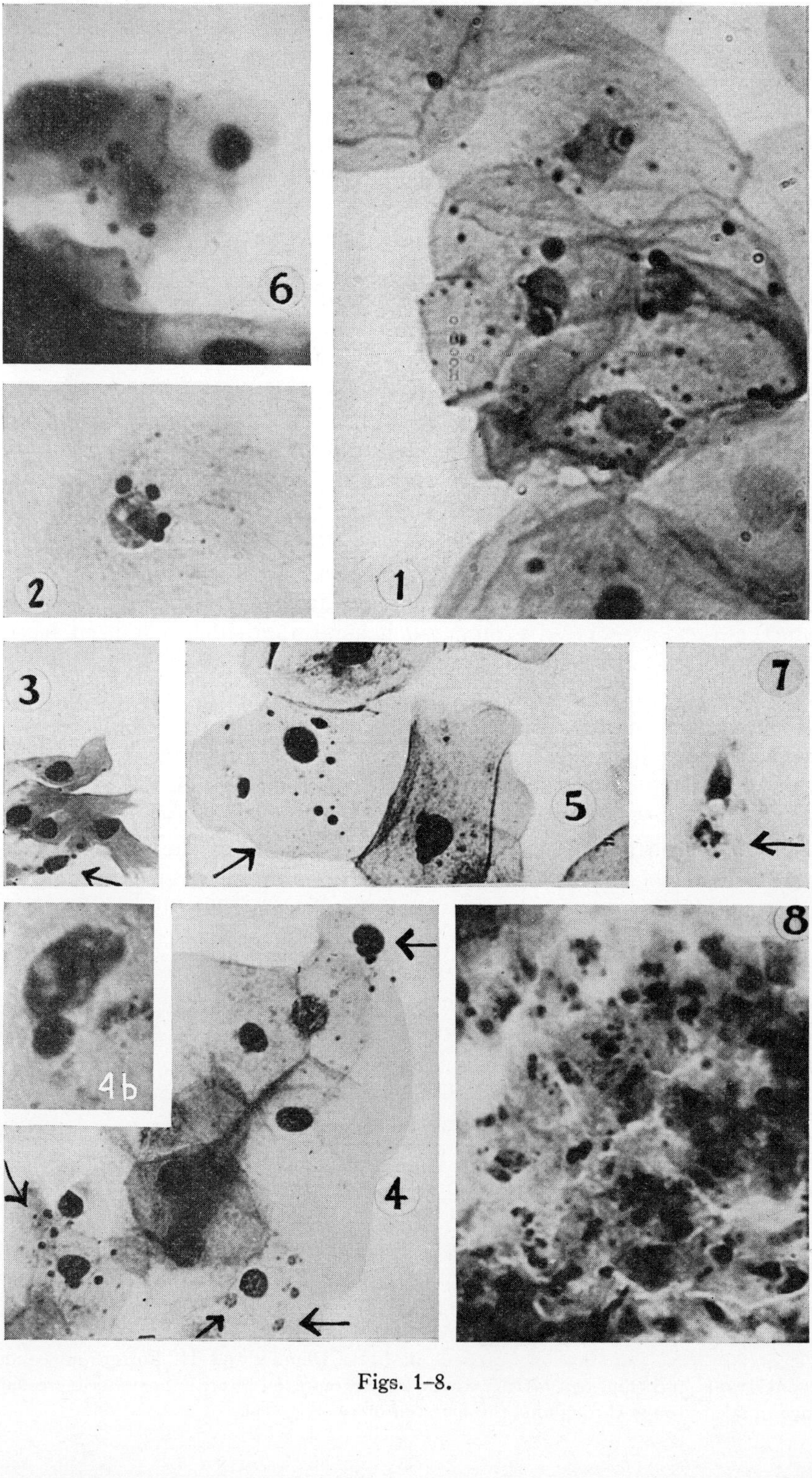

Figs. 1–8.

removed after her fourth illness, but three more of the series of seven respiratory illnesses occurred after that operation.[3] A second individual, with unusually distinct and well-developed bodies (figure 2) was a tuberculosis suspect, a young man who was being sent west as a remedial measure, although all tests for tuberculosis had been negative.

In a few cases we have found these inclusion bodies in throats of persons who claim that they never have colds or sore throats; this does not militate against their possible relation to throat affections, as definite evidences of irritation may be seen in the throats of such persons; for example, one young man, an interne in a medical laboratory, who had a large number of inclusion bodies in his throat sample, emphatically denied having any throat irritation, though there were eroded, red areas, about the size of a dime, on each side of his throat.

Smears made from the persons reporting chronic sinus conditions sometimes show unusually large numbers of inclusion bodies. In one quiescent sinus case, in which material taken repeatedly from an opening made for drainage usually showed few or no bacteria, inclusion bodies were uniformly present. These samples were all scanty, owing to the small size of the area available; but the quite uniform presence of these bodies and the frequent absence of bacteria in such samples at least raises the question whether or

---

EXPLANATION OF FIGURES

Figs. 1–8

All photographs were taken with dry objectives with variations in eyepieces and tube length.

Fig. 1.—Smear from throat of a human carrier; stained with acetic acid-Nucplascoll; magnification approximately ×1000.

Fig. 2.—Four inclusion bodies lying close to the nucleus in a disintegrating epithelial cell; stained with methylene blue; magnification approximately ×1000.

Fig. 3.—Inclusion bodies lying at the poles of a nucleus; stained with gram-stain, but under-bleached to preserve purple color; magnification approximately ×750.

Fig. 4.—Throat smear of individual having a chronic cough; stained with methylene blue; magnification approximately ×900. At the upper right are shown two inclusion bodies impinging upon the nucleus; at the lower left may be seen an inclusion body similarly placed and several other bodies distributed in the cytoplasm; and at the lower right are two bodies showing faintly an aggregate structure.

Fig. 4b.—Inclusion body, lying next to the nucleus, in a human epithelial cell, showing the stippled character seen in Negri bodies; Sellers stain, followed by a dip in alcohol; magnification ×1500, oil immersion.

Fig. 5.—The nucleus of the epithelial cell and the cytoplasmic bodies of the cell on the left have retained their integrity, although the cytoplasm of the cell has practically disappeared; Gentian violet stain; magnification approximately ×900.

Fig. 6.—Epithelial cells from throat of inoculated monkey, J, showing six bodies grouped around the nucleus, much as in Fig. 2; stained with nigrosin, followed by a dip in methylene blue; magnification ×1200.

Fig. 7.—Chick tissue showing a cluster of inclusion bodies in the cytoplasm; stained with methylene blue; magnification approximately ×1000.

Fig. 8.—A mass of chick tissue showing numerous nuclei with one or more inclusion bodies in the cytoplasm surrounding them; stained with methylene blue; magnification approximately ×1000.

---

3. While the tonsils and larynx are usually good positive sources, the roof of the mouth and soft palate may be equally good.

not these bodies may be "primary invaders" if not themselves the cause of irritation of such tissues.

Continued examination of carriers may reveal a decrease or an increase in these bodies as time goes on. One very positive carrier has become so nearly negative during the latter part of the past ten months that her throat specimens can no longer be used to test new staining procedures. On the other hand, four who 15 to 18 months ago rarely showed more than 1 or 2 bodies in any oil immersion field are now so positive that there are many fields on every smear as thickly spattered with inclusion bodies as the one shown in figure 1.

Carriers usually show increased numbers during and following any slight nose or throat irritations. The type of throat irritation most often experienced by them is described as a slight fullness, a "thickened or stuck-together feeling," lasting one to three days. In four carriers under observation, these attacks recur frequently. Occasionally a definitely sore throat occurs, demanding the use of gargles, etc. One of these four carriers loses two to five days of work every two or three months because of "sore throat."

There seems to be what might be called, for lack of a better term, a definite "incompatibility" between bacteria and these inclusion bodies, for both are rarely present in the same epithelial cell. This fact was remarked independently by each of the authors. It must be recognized, of course, that the epithelial cells of the throat are so thin and flat that it may not always be possible to determine beyond doubt whether or not a given bacterium is on the surface of the cell or just within its delicate, limiting membrane. But the simultaneous presence of inclusion bodies and bacteria in or on the same epithelial cell is most infrequent—so infrequent that the question as to whether or not the bacteria are in the cell with the inclusion body or bodies rarely has to be decided. It is much more common to find two or more kinds of bacteria associated with a given epithelial cell than to find bacteria and these cytoplasmic inclusion bodies so associated.

MORPHOLOGICAL AND STAINING CHARACTERISTICS

These throat inclusion bodies are strictly cytoplasmic, never nuclear. In this they resemble the bodies figured more or less incidentally by Thom-

---

Plate 1.—Human epithelial cells containing cytoplasmic inclusion bodies, differentially stained, magnification approximately ×1500, except in figure 3, which is approximately ×3000.

See table 1 for differential staining results; see also the procedures described in the Appendix to this article.

Fig. 1.—Nigrosin-Nucplascoll-magenta.

Fig. 2.—Acetic acid-Nucplascoll (nigrosin omitted); note the clear, capsule-like margin of the inclusion bodies and the margination of stain on the adjacent surfaces of the nucleus.

Fig. 3.—Acetic acid-nigrosin-magenta (nigrosin omitted, and bodies brown rather than black); note the aggregate structure of the larger bodies in the upper cell.

Fig. 4.—Sellers-alcohol.

Fig. 5.—Acetic acid-pyronin-methyl green.

Fig. 6.—Nigrosin-Feulgen magenta; note especially the blue color of the nucleus in some of the epithelial cells.

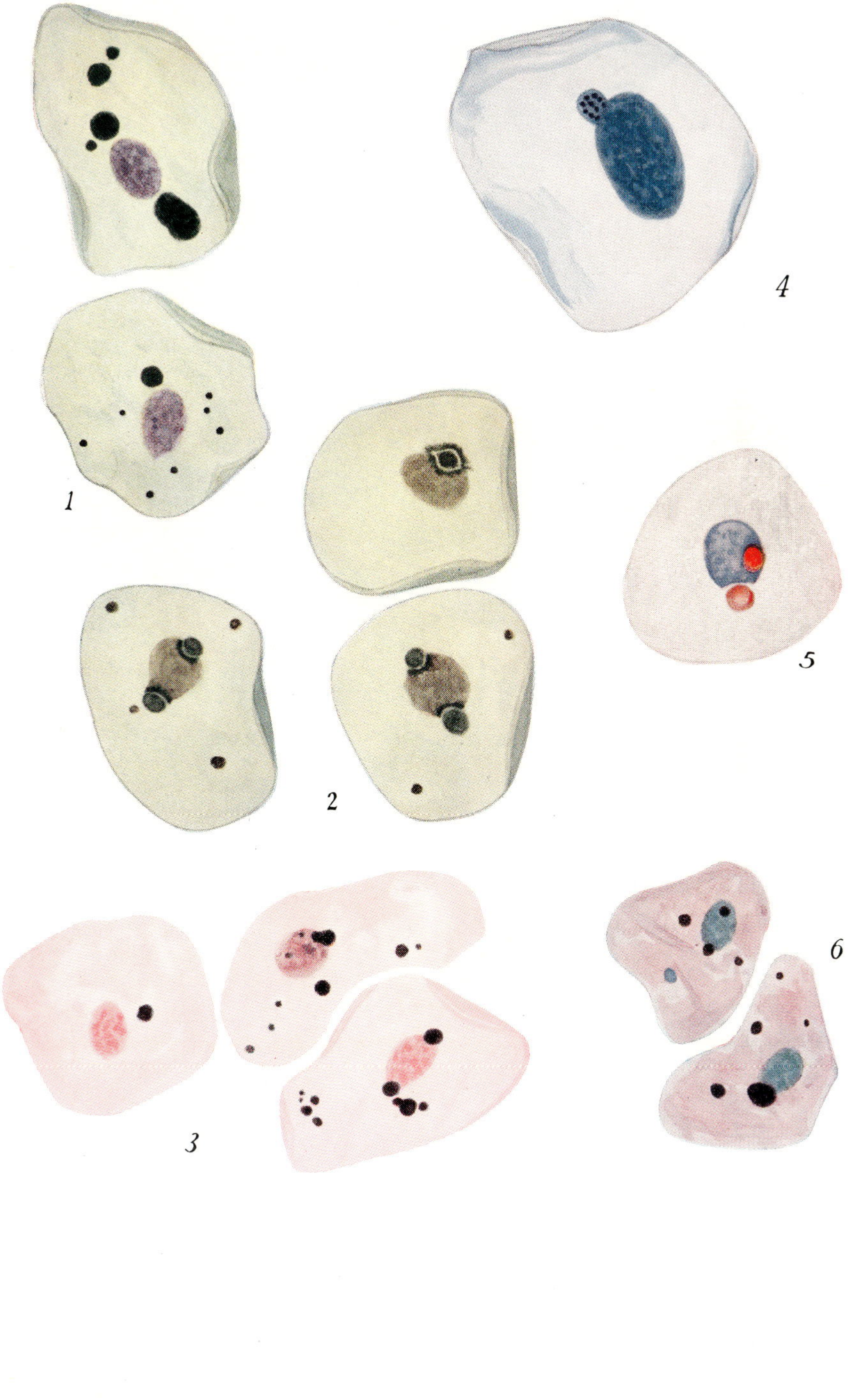
1
2
3
4
5
6

son and Thomson[4] in their reports on colds, tonsillitis and influenza. Their non-nuclear character differentiates them from the nuclear inclusion bodies of herpes and from the giant nuclear inclusions reported by Goodpasture and Talbot[5] and by Farber and Wolbach[6] in the salivary glands of infants and by Covell[7] in the respiratory tissues of monkeys; it also differentiates them from the bodies described by Pearson[8] in the sub-maxillary glands of guinea pigs.

These cytoplasmic inclusion bodies may lie in close proximity to the nucleus of the epithelial cell or they may be distributed through the cytoplasm. When close to the nucleus, they are sometimes polar in position (figure 3), occurring at one or both ends of the long axis of the nucleus. Such a position is apt to catch the eye, and lead one to overemphasize that relationship. They are just as often irregularly grouped around the nucleus (figures 1 and 6) and they may be quite distant from it. Occasionally these inclusion bodies develop as flattened or appressed masses, lying against the nucleus. When the bodies lie close to the nucleus, it may be indented or at least flattened at the line of contact. The bodies are never confluent with the nucleus and are easily distinguishable from the nucleus or possible buds or proliferations from it, by differences in intensity with almost any bacterial or nuclear stain. Overstaining, e.g., with mercurochrome, quite uniformly stains these bodies more than the nuclei and decolorizing affects them less rapidly.

---

4. Thomson, David, and Thomson, Robert: Ann. Pickett-Thomson Res. Lab. **5**: p. 184–5, pl. 44, 1929; **8**: p. 294–5, pl. 36, 1932; and **9**: pl. 28, 1933. These authors picture in three places what are apparently these same bodies seen in epithelial cells of a throat specimen taken from one of the authors in 1928 "during a mild coryzal attack which passed off in a day or two" and later, 1933, in a brief cold. The very incidental treatment accorded these bodies (less than two pages in the 800-odd pages of text of the first two reports and no text discussion in the third two-volume report of over 1,300 pages and about one full plate in the combined total of over 120 full page plates) is doubtless explained by the fact that the findings so extensively illustrated deal with cultures rather than direct examinations of the specimens collected in tonsillitis, colds, and influenza. Doubt as to the significance of the observed bodies is expressed by the authors following their detection "in the sputum of a normal healthy individual," and they make "a guarded statement that the bodies might, perhaps, play some part in the causation of colds" and suggest that "they should be looked for by other workers on the subject"; they also state that they are "unable to decide whether or not they might be a large species of a gram-negative coccus of the *Micrococcus catarrhalis type*," and again, that they are "inclined to the belief that they are masses of the true *Micrococcus catarrhalis* which at times show large swollen forms." In 1934, however, David Thomson, in a personal communication to one of the authors of this article, refers again to the probable filterable virus explanation of these bodies, adding, "I have not done any further work on them but I alway keep a lookout for them in cases of colds, and I often find them."

5. Am. J. Dis. Child. **21**: 415, 1921.

6. Am. J. Path. **8**: 123, 1932.

7. Am. J. Path. **8**: 151, 1932. These large intra-nuclear bodies of the nasal mucous membranes, trachea, etc., are described as having a halo and a margination of basophilic material on the inner surface of the nuclear membrane, quite similar apparently to the condition shown in our figure 2, pl. 1.

8. Am. J. Path. **6**: 261, 1930. Despite the title, Cytoplasmic Inclusions Produced by the Sub-Maxillary Virus, these bodies are primarily nuclear; they are also much larger than ours (3 to 8 microns) and the illustrations show very different structure.

The inclusion bodies are, so far as we have observed, foreign to the cytoplasm and imbedded in it (until released by the disappearance of the cell membrane), except as occasionally seen in mucoid matter present between cells in deeper throat scrapings. When appropriately stained, a transparent or capsule-like area (figure 1) is visible between the nucleus and the inclusion body. Such capsule-like margins are sometimes also fully visible around bodies lying in the paler or less-stained cytoplasm and distant from the nucleus.

In size the bodies vary greatly. They may be mere points, much smaller than the staphylococcus and streptococcus cells present in the same throat smear; they vary in size from these minute bodies up to bodies fully one-third and occasionally one-half the long diameter of the nucleus of the cell in which they lie.

When small, they seem perfectly spherical. The larger forms may be either spherical or somewhat ellipsoidal. Occasionally they appear as elongated bodies, convexly rounded on their free side, but appressed against the nucleus making a cap-like body. Only rarely are they distinctly elongated when lying in the cytoplasm distant from the nucleus. They somewhat infrequently occur in pairs; in such cases, one part is often smaller than the other, suggesting budding yeast cells. (This is a wholly superficial comparison; for, as shown later, these bodies are not at all like yeasts in their staining reactions, especially when nigrosin is used as a stain.)

When alcohol or acetic acid is used as an aid in differential staining, the capsular margin previously mentioned may be clearly seen. This capsule may show in relatively small bodies, but is usually distinct only in the larger bodies. These capsules are not ordinarily seen in the milder single stains, nor are they very marked even with Nucplascoll or Pinacyanol used as a single stain. With acetic acid and Nucplascoll, however, the capsule is very distinct and the adjacent nuclear margin may be heavily darkened, as shown in plate 1, figure 2.

When decolorizing and dehydrating agents such as alcohol and acetic acid are used, we often obtain definite indications of the aggregate character of the larger bodies, although this character is occasionally seen with plain methylene blue staining of the larger, older bodies. Those seen in figure 4 suggest an ultimate separation into smaller units, possibly the globoids mentioned later in this paper.

The aggregate character of these bodies may be demonstrated by bleaching with alcohol, after using either the Williams or the Sellers rabies stain (figure 4b; plate 1, figure 4); but it is sometimes shown where treatment with acetic acid precedes staining. The stippled character of these bodies when alcohol decolorizing follows a stain treatment, is strongly suggestive of the stippled magenta Negri bodies which are obtained by the usual Williams or Sellers rabies stains, without final alcohol decolorization. The essential likeness of our stippled bodies to Negri bodies has been verified by two experienced workers in rabies; and there is, of course, no reason to expect that any one stain will invariably give exactly the same result with all inclusion bodies, any more than any selected stain would give identical results with all bacteria. This difference, however, was one of the reasons for experimenting with the large variety of stains described later in this report.

We are not able to confirm wholly the free "elementary bodies" reported in trachoma by Thygeson[9] and Craigie[10] for vaccinia. The great range in size and age of the inclusion bodies found in the throat samples taken from "heavy carriers" (figure 1) would lead us to expect to find such cyclic phases in our continuous observations of these cases. The few free, minute bodies we have observed have seemed gram-positive rather than negative as described by Thygeson. Occasionally, a clump of a few unstained globoids, each with a minute central point, may be found in the area apparently formerly occupied by an epithelial cell. These globoids appear mucoid in character and much less substantial than the capsules of the inclusion bodies. Unless they do represent a phase in the development of these inclusion bodies, we have no extracellular phase to report at this time.

Well-developed inclusion bodies are present in epithelial cells which are surprisingly normal in appearance, with deeply-staining, well-delimited nuclei, and little or no indication of cytoplasmic disintegration, such as vacuolation and irregularly staining granules or areas. The change that characteristically occurs in the cells containing these bodies seems to be a gradual and general decrease in cytoplasmic material, shown by the decrease in staining power, accompanied by a gradual disappearance of the limiting cell membrane. At this stage, the nucleus (which may still show little apparent change in morphological integrity and in affinity for stains) and the accompanying inclusion bodies appear as definitely staining bodies on a wholly unstained background the size of the original epithelial cell (figure 5), suggesting that the bodies are finally freed by the dissolution of its membrane.

To forestall the objection that the inclusion bodies are themselves disintegration products or, as has been claimed, artifacts, Golgi bodies, Nissl granules, mitochondria, as well as fat and other cell accumulations, it seemed desirable to establish the integrity of these throat inclusion bodies by generally accepted stains and tests, especially as no specific clinical condition invariably accompanies their presence, even when found in great numbers.

We may state, in the beginning, that to the trained observer the inclusion bodies are distinctly visible in fresh unstained material, even with the low power objective. This one characteristic prevents them from being dismissed as artifacts; and it also prevents them from being classed with Nissl granules, Golgi apparatus bodies and mitochondria. Furthermore, unlike the Golgi bodies,[11] these inclusion bodies do stain after fixation in Bouin's solution, staining much more deeply with Delafield's hematoxylin, for example, than the nucleus and cytoplasm of the cells containing them.

To further differentiate these bodies from mitochondria we may state that they may be vitally stained in very weak dilutions of neutral red, using

9. Arch. Ophth. **12:** 307, 1934.

10. J. Path. and Bact. **3:** 185, 1933.

11. Lee, A. B.: The Micromotist's Vade Mecum. eighth edition, p. 316, 1921. P. Blakiston's Sons, Philadelphia.

dilutions as weak as 1:10,000. With Janus Green B (specific for mitochondria, 1:10,000 and 1:500,000)[12] these bodies are not stained or show but the faintest tinge of color. Further evidence that these bodies are not mitochondria is shown by the fact that they are not destroyed by acetic acid[13] nor "by any fluid with a p_H lower than 4.2";[14] they resist even 5 per cent acetic acid for 24 hours without losing their integrity. In fact, as already stated, pre-treatment with acetic acid may be used advantageously to bring out these bodies, as in our acetic acid-nigrosin-magenta stain (plate 1, figure 3).

Confusion with metabolic accumulations such as fat, glycogen and volutin may be eliminated by various accepted tests. Such fat stains as osmic acid, sudan III, sudan IV and Nile blue sulphate do not stain these inclusion bodies. Glycogen tests are also negative, whether made with iodine and weak NaCl on fresh material or with Best's glycogen stain on fixed preparations. Volutin tests too are negative: (a) These inclusion bodies do not stain with Calkins' modification[15] of Feulgen's stain in which the fuchsin-sulphurous acid component is used alone. (b) These bodies, unlike volutin, are not destroyed by heat (80 C.) for 5 minutes or by treatment with a 5 per cent solution of sodium carbonate for 5 minutes;[16] after either treatment the bodies stain readily and distinctly with Heidenhain's hematoxylin. (c) Volutin is not stained[16] by eosin-borax-carmine or by nigrosin; but both of these stains are very positive for our bodies, nigrosin being the one single stain which is most helpfully differential for them.

The possible vacuolar nature of these bodies is not supported by staining, by plasmolyzing conditions or by long-continued observations of them under conditions favoring disintegration changes. These bodies are definite, dense-appearing bodies and in no way resemble the pale-staining, often irregular vacuolar areas sometimes seen in cast-off epithelial cells. Strong salt solutions, even 20 per cent NaCl for 30 minutes, do not cause plasmolysis or other visible changes in fresh, unstained material. Fresh, epithelial cells, containing one to several inclusion bodies, have been kept under observation in hanging drops for prolonged periods (15 days) to see if these refractile bodies increase in size or in number, as they might be expected to do if they represented disintegration changes; but we found no indication in our carefully charted hanging drops to support this view—either in the unstained condition or after careful drying and staining of the drops.

In our staining studies some sixty stains or combinations of stains have been tried: with and without a variety of preparatory procedures, such as treatment with sodium chloride, sodium hydroxide, acetic acid, ether and

---

12. Cowdry, E. V.: General Cytology, p. 411, 1924. University of Chicago Press, Chicago.

13. Lowther, F. de L.: On the Cytoplasmic Constituents of Uroleptus Mobilis, p. 207, 1925. Mack Printing Co., Easton, Pa.

14. Sharp, L. W.: Introduction to Cytology, pp. 73–93, 1934. McGraw-Hill, New York.

15. Calkins, G. N.: Biology of the Protozoa, second edition, p. 68, 1933. Lea and Febiger, Philadelphia.

16. Baumgartel, T.: Jordon, E. O. and Falk, I. K.: Newer Knowledge of Bacteriology and Immunology, p. 16, 1929. University of Chicago Press, Chicago.

Zenker's fluid; and with and without final decolorizing by alcohol. The stains we found most helpful for differentiation of these bodies in throat smears and in chick tissues are listed in tables 1 and 2.

TABLE 1.—*Results Obtained with the Eight Staining Procedures Most Markedly and Consistently Helpful in Differentiating the Throat Inclusion Bodies from Accompanying Bacteria, Yeasts, Epithelial Cells and White Corpuscles*

Staining Procedure	Throat Epithelial Cells		Cytoplasmic Inclusion Bodies	Bacteria	Yeasts	Nuclei of White Corpuscles
	Nuclei	Cytoplasm				
Acetic acid-pyronin-methyl green	Blue	Light purple	Red	Red	Purple to Blue	Dark blue
Nigrosin-Feulgen-magenta	Pale blue to purple or red	Pink	Black	Red	Pink	Pink purple
Sellers-alcohol	Purple	Pink	Pale to azure blue	Blue to purple	Bluish purple	Blue
Sodium chloride-nigrosin	Light gray to gray	Unstained to light gray	Black	Unstained	Unstained	Gray black
Sodium chloride-nigrosin-magenta	Pink	Pink	Black	Red	Red	Pink
Sodium chloride-nigrosin-Nucplascoll	Pink	Pale gray-green	Green	Dark green	Dark green	Pink
Williams-alcohol	Red	Pink	Pale to azure blue	Blue	Blue	Blue
Zenker-Giemsa	Blue	Pale purplish	Pink	Blue to purple	Purple	Blue

TABLE 2.—*Results Obtained with the Five Staining Procedures Most Helpful in Differentiating the Inclusion Bodies from Chick Tissue. We Prefer the Simple Sodium chloride-Nigrosin or the Complex Nigrosin-Feulgen-Magenta*

Staining Procedure	Throat		Chick Tissue		
	Cytoplasmic Inclusion Bodies	Bacteria	Background	Cell nuclei	Cytoplasmic granules
Acetic acid-pyronin-methyl green	Red	Red	Pale purplish	Blue	Blue
Nigrosin-Feulgen-magenta	Black	Red	Pale red	Red	Pale red
Sellers-alcohol	Pale to azure blue	Dark blue	Red	Blue	Red
Sodium chloride-nigrosin	Black	Unstained	Purplish	Purplish	Unstained
Williams-alcohol	Blue	Purple	Red	Deep red	Deep red

Having been greatly hampered in our work by the lack of specific staining directions in some of the more important contributions in these fields, we have given in detail in the staining discussion at the end of this paper, the procedures we found most successful—in consistency of result as well as in the degree of differentiation, especially when associated confusing materials are abundant.

These bodies take all the nuclear stains ordinarily used in bacteriology.[17] They stain quite readily also with many so-called cytoplasmic stains, such as acid-fuchsin and nigrosin. The cytoplasmic stains, as well as nuclear stains, usually stain the bodies more quickly or more deeply than the cytoplasm itself. Their affinity for cytoplasmic stains does not necessarily affect

17. These bodies remain unstained with Feulgen's nuclear stain, specific for animal nucleic acid. This fact does not militate against their nuclear nature, however, as some of the Sarcodina, e.g., Amoeba dubia react very slightly, if at all, to Feulgen's stain. (Dawson, J. A., College of the City of New York. Unpublished work on Amoeba dubia.) Pearson (loc. cit.) reports similarly for his guinea pig inclusion bodies.

their status as inclusion bodies, since it is recognized that we do not know how much cytoplasmic reactions have to do with the formation and composition of inclusion bodies.

These inclusion bodies stain pink with Grubler's Giemsa[18] stain, being more uniformly pink when Zenker's fluid precedes the Giemsa stain; the smaller bodies are sometimes purplish and occasionally definitely purple. The most valuable single stain for showing these bodies in throat samples is nigrosin. With this stain bacteria, yeasts and other fungi remain unstained and extraneous food particles practically so, while the inclusion bodies are distinctly black, especially when the slide is first treated with sodium chloride. This stain is especially helpful in throat examinations of laboratory animals, particularly monkeys. Without it searching for inclusion bodies in their throat smears is more difficult than finding the proverbial haystack needle, for transverse-splitting fungi which adhere to the epithelial cells are often present in large numbers and there are always innumerable, confusing masses of bacteria and partly masticated food.

SUCCESSFUL METHODS OF CULTIVATION

These cytoplasmic bodies have been successfully cultivated in (1) monkeys and in (2) embryo chick tissues.

(1) Our first experiments, with young guinea pigs, rabbits and kittens, proved quite disappointing. Four kittens inoculated by mouth three times, at two-week intervals, with a 1 per cent acetic acid suspension of material taken by swab from a carrier with a sore throat failed to yield positive smears. Six guinea pigs and seven rabbits also failed to give positive results with swab suspensions. After three unsuccessful mouth inoculations, the six guinea pigs and four of the rabbits were each given vaginal and eye inoculations, two inoculations each, one week apart, using as before a 24-hour suspension of human material in 1 per cent acetic acid. Examinations made every second day for two weeks were negative for all ten animals. On the 15th day, inclusion bodies were seen in eye smears of two guinea pigs and in vaginal smears of two rabbits. These positive findings were not heavy—only two or three affected cells being found in any given smear. In the eye examinations this sparsity may be related to the limited amount of material available, especially from the eyes of guinea pigs. It is not improbable that more positive results might have been obtained if definite tissue injury had attended the inoculations. It seemed to us, however, desirable to avoid irritation of the various sites of inoculation, as Gifford and Lazar[19] had reported chemical irritation as a causal factor in the production of inclusion bodies in the conjunctiva. By the end of 3 to 4 weeks after the first positive findings in the guinea pigs and rabbits, all eye and vaginal smears were again negative; they remained so for three weeks when observation of these animals ceased.

18. We tried two lots of the National Commission Giemsa stain repeatedly, with and without Zenker's fluid, but obtained only purple bodies.

19. Arch. Ophth. **4:** 468, 1930.

During this same period these cytoplasmic inclusion bodies were found in the throat of a small, pet dog, a constant companion of two human carriers. The bodies were not numerous in any given smear; but they were repeatedly noted, although a series of weekly examinations of two other dogs in the same household were consistently negative. A young puppy, about 6 weeks old, shown to be negative for these inclusion bodies, was then placed with the positive dog; but, during the 20 weeks he was under observation, he remained negative, despite the fact that both dogs ate and drank from the same dishes and chewed the same bones and playthings. Later, this negative puppy was inoculated directly by mouth from a chronic human carrier but remained negative.

At this time four rhesus monkeys were placed at our disposal by Dr. W. H. Park and Dr. M. Brodie.

Preliminary examinations of the throats of twenty monkeys in the animal rooms being negative, four of these negative monkeys were inoculated by mouth with fresh saline suspensions made from specimens taken from four persons strongly positive for these inclusion bodies: three chronic carriers who at the time had no accompanying clinical symptoms and one individual who was at the time in a Brooklyn hospital under nursing care.

Rubber-bulb medicine droppers were used to expel the suspensions into the throat and both nostrils of each monkey. No mechanical injury accompanied transfer of material, the only preparatory step being the swabbing of each monkey's throat, with a large cotton swab moistened in sterile water, to help remove the masses of food material which were present and so facilitate the contact of the injected material with the epithelial tissues.

Examinations of the four monkeys one week later were all negative. Two were positive when examined at the end of the second week: the monkey receiving an inoculation from the ill carrier and one receiving an inoculation from one of the carriers who evinced no accompanying clinical symptoms. By the third week, monkey 116 inoculated from the ill-carrier had become more strongly positive; but, unfortunately, the other three monkeys had, through a misunderstanding, been transferred to a poliomyelitis experiment, and no report could be obtained for them.

Monkey 116 was then used to determine if further monkey passage could be secured by contact and by throat inoculation (figure 9). He was placed in a small cage with two negative monkeys (56 and B); at the same time, a swab from his throat was used to inoculate another negative monkey (529). All three of these monkeys were positive when examined three weeks, and again four weeks, later. The mouth-transfer monkey (529) was then placed in a cage with a negative monkey (J). Two weeks later, this monkey was found to be positive (figure 6). At this time, all the other positive monkeys were still positive, but not strongly so. We have, therefore, two serial passages of two monkeys each, and one serial passage of three monkeys.

No other examinations of these monkeys were made until four months had passed. At that time only monkeys J and B were available. Both of these monkeys were still positive, but not strongly so.

When these last samples of J and B monkeys were taken, samples were also taken of five other monkeys selected, at random, from the monkeys in the same general animal room. Each of these five was negative for the inclusion bodies. In all, 29 uninoculated monkeys were examined (1 to 4 times each) during this study and no uninoculated monkey was found to be positive. Since these inclusion bodies may develop in both monkeys and persons, it may, however, be but a matter of time, before the incidence in uninoculated monkeys approaches that in man, depending upon the degree of contact between the attendants and the monkeys.

(2) In the embryo chick cultures, the technic used was similar to that described by Goodpasture, Woodruff and Buddingh.[20] Fertile eggs incubated at a temperature of 100–102 F. for periods varying from 2 to 15 days before inoculation, were used in these experiments. As the work progressed it was

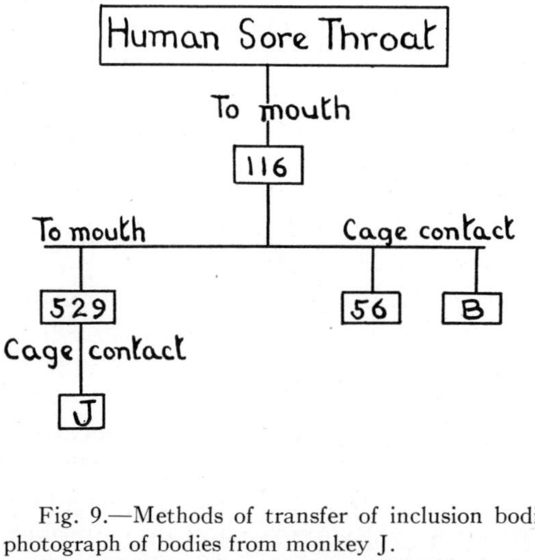

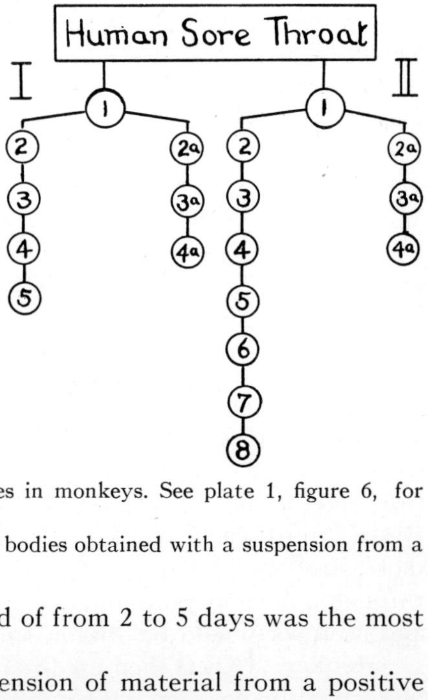

Fig. 9.—Methods of transfer of inclusion bodies in monkeys. See plate 1, figure 6, for photograph of bodies from monkey J.

Fig. 10.—Four lines of egg transfer of inclusion bodies obtained with a suspension from a positive human throat.

found that a preliminary incubation period of from 2 to 5 days was the most satisfactory.

The eggs were inoculated with a suspension of material from a positive human throat. Each suspension was made by rinsing the throat swab thoroughly in about 3 cc. of sterile, physiological salt solution (0.85 per cent). Afterward, an equal amount of 1 per cent acetic acid was added to the tube and the tube was shaken to mix the contents thoroughly and allowed to stand over night at room temperature. It was then centrifuged (International Centrifuge, No. 2 speed) for 10 minutes. Drops of the supernatant fluids taken just below the surface of the fluid were first stained and examined to insure securing material probably free from bacteria; and then similar drops, from the tubes in which bacteria were not found, were used to inoculate the incubated eggs.

The coverslip was temporarily removed from the opening in the egg

20. Am J. Path. 8: 271, 1932.

previously prepared and the shell membrane punctured or torn off carefully with sterile forceps. The inoculum was introduced by means of a sterile pipette and delivered as near as possible to the chorio-allantoic membrane. The coverslip was then replaced, warming it enough to remelt the paraffin along the shell edges and insure a good seal, and the egg was returned to the incubator.

The inoculated eggs were incubated for 7 to 10 days and at the end of that period the inoculated membrane and adjacent embryonic tissue examined for inclusion bodies. If the material was found to be positive, it was used to inoculate a second set of fertile, incubated eggs. The material for the second and all following inoculations was occasionally transferred directly from one egg to the next in the series; more often a suspension in physiological salt solution was used as the inoculum. Several eggs were inoculated at each transfer, the most strongly positive (figures 7 and 8) being selected for continuing the series, as pictured in figure 10.

From one positive throat which had a history of several recurrences of sore throat within a few months we obtained two eggs which proved to be positive; from them, two culture lines, 1 and 2, were started. Each line was carried on from one egg generation to another until the last inoculation failed to give a positive result. While this ultimate failure to give positive results was apparently in great part due to the fact that eggs are not a wholly satisfactory medium, it was also partly due to the condition of the eggs used during the latter part of the work. A large percentage of them proved to be not fertile as summer approached; more of the eggs, too, were found to be contaminated with bacteria. The work finally ceased (June, 1934) after four lines of four to eight successive or serial transfers in embryo chick tissue had been obtained (figure 10).

SUMMARY

Cytoplasmic inclusion bodies may be demonstrated in human throats and other parts of the upper respiratory area.

A relatively high proportion of persons with certain of the milder respiratory irritations are positive for these inclusion bodies.

Carriers of these inclusion bodies may show an increasingly heavy incidence in the throat epithelial cells—both in the number of cells affected and in the number of bodies per cell.

These inclusion bodies are rarely present in epithelial cells which contain bacteria.

They are easily demonstrated in epithelial cells of affected persons; but they do not persist, in the same form at least, outside the host cells.

These epithelial inclusion bodies seem acceptably classified as inclusion bodies: they multiply only when living tissue is available. They stain pink with Giemsa's stain (after Zenker's fluid). An aggregate structure (as in Negri bodies of rabies) and a capsule may be demonstrated by appropriate stains.

Special stains have been developed for their ready differentiation from other cell parts and constituents and extraneous material: notably, nigrosin

—sodium chloride for throat specimens and methyl green—pyronin for embryo chick cultures.

These cytoplasmic inclusion bodies have been cultivated in throats of monkeys and in embryo chick tissues.

APPENDIX

While at least a dozen of the sixty-odd staining procedures tested in this investigation are uniformly differential for these inclusion bodies in human throat specimens, but seven of them are wholly satisfactory differential stains under the conditions met in dealing with throat specimens from laboratory animals or with chick-egg tissues.

It may be of value, therefore, especially to teaching institutions where other types of inclusion bodies are not available for comparative study, to have in detail these seven staining procedures, in addition to the established Giemsa stain.

1. *Preparation of Slides.*—A throat swab is transferred to a tube containing about 5 cc. sterile salt solution (0.9 per cent) or water, thoroughly rinsed in it and discarded. The tube is then centrifuged (5–10 minutes) or allowed to settle by gravity. The sediment is then drawn up into a pipette, deposited on a slide, and dried at room or incubator temperature.

Chick tissue is placed with sterile forceps into a tube of sterile salt solution (or water); the tissue is broken or separated somewhat by repeated pressure with the rough edges of a broken-tipped sterile pipette. The suspension is then centrifuged, etc., as described in the preceding paragraph.

2. *Fixation.*—Throat smears are fixed by heat flaming two to three times, as usually done in bacteriological work.

Chick tissue is fixed by immersion in 95 per cent ethyl alcohol for 30 seconds. (Treatment to remove fat (ether; alcohol, xylol, chloroform, or 5 per cent NaCl for 10 min. to "break the protein film") does remove a great deal of confusing material, but such treatment is not necessary with the stains described below.)

3. *Staining.*—Our preferred stains all begin with or end with treatment with sodium cloride, acetic acid or alcohol. The steps are always indicated by the sequence in the title, e.g., sodium chloride—nigrosin.

Alcohol is 95 per cent ethyl alcohol, unless otherwise indicated. Washing after a staining step means a good "swishing" in water until all free stain is removed and is always done in tap water unless otherwise indicated. Draining does not necessarily mean a perfectly dry smear; the smear may be dry or still moist when the next step is undertaken.

After the last drying, slides may be examined directly with the oil-immersion lens; or these thin smears may be satisfactorily mounted while still dry in balsam, without clearing in xylol, etc.

1. Acetic acid—Nucplascoll
   - Acetic acid, 5 per cent, 1 dip
   - Wash; drain
   - Nucplascoll, 2 per cent aqueous, 30 min.
   - Wash; drain
2. Acetic acid—pyronin—methyl green
   - 1 part 1 per cent aqueous methyl green
   - 2 parts 1 per cent aqueous pyronin
   - Acetic acid, 5 per cent, 1 dip
   - Wash; drain
   - Pyronin-methyl green, flood or immerse, 1 to 2 min.
   - Wash; drain
3. Nigrosin—Feulgen—Magenta
   - Nigrosin, 1 per cent, flood or immerse, 10–15 minutes
     - Wash; drain
   - Feulgen (modified) Dilute these three solutions or decrease the time, if necessary, to obtain blue nuclei as in fig. 6, plate 1.

Feulgen (modified)
Sol. 1. Normal HCl (82.5 cc. Sp. Gr. 1.19, to 1 liter distilled water)
Immerse, 8–12 min. at 60 C.
Wash; transfer immediately to sol. 2.
Sol. 2. Fuchsin sulphurous acid (To 200 cc. boiling distilled water, add 1 gm. basic fuchsin, cool to 50 C., filter, add 20 cc. N–HCl; cool to 25 C., add 1 gm. anhydrous sodium sulphite).
Keep in dark.
Immerse, 60–90 min. at room temperature.
Sol. 3. Sodium bisulphite solution (To 200 cc. of distilled water add 10 cc. of 10 per cent sol. of anhydrous sodium bisulphite and 10 cc. of N–HCl). Rinse 2–3 times.
Wash; drain
Magenta, 0.2 per cent, aqueous, 1 dip
Wash; drain

4. Nigrosin—Nucplascoll
(Omit sodium chloride of No. 6)
5. Sellers—alcohol
1 cc. sat. methyl alcohol solution basic fuchsin
15 cc. sat. methyl alcohol solution methylene blue
25 cc. methyl alcohol (absolute, acetone free)
Sellers stain, immerse, 5 min.
Wash; drain
Alcohol, 95 per cent, 1 dip
Wash; drain
6. Sodium chloride—nigrosin (with counter stain)
Sodium chloride, 1 per cent, 10 min.
Drain without washing
Nigrosin, 1 per cent, flood or immerse, 10–15 min.
Wash; drain
Counter stain
Any dilute stain, e.g., 1 per cent mercurochrome, 1 dip
Magenta, 0.2 per cent aqueous, 1 dip
Nucplascoll, 2 per cent aqueous, 30 min. (figure 1, plate 1)
Wash; drain
7. Williams—alcohol
0.5 cc. saturated alcoholic solution basic fuchsin
10 cc. saturated alcoholic solution—methylene blue
30 cc. distilled water
Fix, as usual (heat or 95 per cent alcohol)
Methyl alcohol (absolute), 2–3 dips
Williams stain, flood slide; heat gently until steam rises
Wash; drain
Alcohol, 95 per cent, 1 dip
Wash; drain
8. Zenker—Lugol—Giemsa
Zenker's Fluid (Add 5 per cent glacial acetic acid to a stock solution containing 5 per cent sat. bichloride of mercury in the following: potassium bichromate, 2–2½ parts; sodium sulphate, 1 part and water 100 parts).
Immerse, 30 min.
Transfer directly to Lugol's solution
Lugol's solution (Iodine, 1 gm.; potassium iodide, 2 gms.; distilled water, 300 cc.)
Immerse, 5 min.
Giemsa (To 1 part of stock solution (Grubler's Giemsa, 1 gm.; glycerine, 50 cc.; methyl alcohol, 50 cc.) add 4 parts distilled water and 5 parts methyl alcohol).
Immerse, 1–2 hrs.
Wash; drain

ON THE MECHANISM OF IMMUNITY IN EXPERIMENTAL POLIOMYELITIS

CLAUS W. JUNGEBLUT

NEW YORK

It is a well known fact that recovery from a paralyzing attack of poliomyelitis leaves experimental animals uniformly with a high degree of resistance against the disease so that reintroduction into the central nervous system of large amounts of the same passage strain of virus fails to produce infection.[1] It has also been claimed that active immunization with virus, apparently killed by chemical treatment (phenol, formalin), brings about essentially the same results, in that such immunized animals develop not only circulating anti-bodies but also prove insusceptible to intracerebral injection of virus.[2] These experimental facts have been drawn upon to substantiate an epidemiological hypothesis according to which contact with subinfectious doses of virus leads to the production of virucidal substances and, pari passu, to the development of general resistance, which, in turn, is said to explain the gradual disappearance of infantile paralysis with the advance of age.[3]

In all three cases, it is assumed that the presence of virucidal substances in the circulating blood coincides with the presence of tissue resistance. So firm is this belief that the conclusion has been drawn that the serological titer may serve as a reliable index of the degree of general bodily or central nervous system resistance to poliomyelitic infection. One may take exception to these statements on several grounds. First, it has been shown that the number of convalescent human and monkey serums which contain appreciable quantities of virucidal substances is not nearly as high as one might expect from the regular occurrence of solid resistance to natural or artificial reinfection.[4] Second, active immunization with formalin-inactivated virus in our hands and in the experience of three other investigators[5] has failed to protect monkeys against intracerebral infection even though the serum may occasionally

---

Received for publication, June 27, 1935.

From the Department of Bacteriology, College of Physicians and Surgeons, Columbia University.

Aided by a grant from the Rockefeller Foundation.

1. Poliomyelitis, International Committee for the Study of Infantile Paralysis, Baltimore, Williams & Wilkins Company, 1932.

2. Brodie, M.: Am. J. Pub. Health **25:** 54, 1935; Cowie, D. M.: Proc. Soc. Exper. Biol. & Med. **32:** 632, 1935.

3. Wernstedt, W.: Ergebn. d. inn. Med. u. Kinderh. **26:** 248, 1924; Aycock, W. L.: J. A. M. A. **97:** 1199, 1931.

4. Jungeblut, C. W., and Smith, L. W.: J. Immunol. **23:** 35, 1932; Jungeblut, C. W.: J. Immunol. **27:** 17, 1934; Howitt, F. B.: J. Infect. Dis. **51:** 565, 1932; Brodie, M.: J. Exper. Med. **56:** 493, 1932.

5. Abramson, H. L., and Gerber, H.: J. Immunol. **3:** 435, 1918; Roemer, P. H.: Epidemic Infantile Paralysis, New York, Wood, 1913; Jungeblut, C. W., and Engle, E. T.: J. Exper. Med. **59:** 43, 1934; Schultz, E. W. and Sebhardt, L. P.: California and West. Med. **43:** 111, 1935.

contain virucidal substances. Third, the application of these experimental facts to the epidemiology of the human disease is, in our opinion, open to question because of numerous observations which seem to account for the age incidence and the mass development of virucidal substances on a non-specific, physiological basis.[6]

In view of the conflicting data which affect our concept of the nature of immunity in poliomyelitis, particularly with regard to the balance of tissue resistance and serological phenomena, it seemed important to undertake some experiments in an attempt to clarify the issue. It was also hoped that such experiments would throw new light on the relationship between typical acquired immunity in the monkey and the mechanism of natural insusceptibility in man. In the first place, it was necessary to investigate more systematically than has hitherto been possible, the appearance of virucidal substances in infected monkeys during the course of the disease, how long they persist in convalescence, and, last but not least, whether any correlation may be demonstrated between the refractory state in convalescent monkeys and the absence or presence of virucidal substances in the serum. In the second place, an opportunity arose for submitting to experimental verification an important auxiliary hypothesis of the theory of latent immunization which postulates that the quantitative increase of virucidal substances in the serum of growing children represents the summation of serological responses to secondary antigenic stimuli which fall on immune soil. A partial answer to this question could be given by determining whether or not reinoculation of convalescent monkeys with large doses of virus, which fails to induce a new attack of the disease, is followed by any increase in the titer of virucidal substances as compared with the titer existing before reinoculation.

The experiments outlined are presented in two separate parts.

RATE OF DEVELOPMENT AND PERSISTENCE OF VIRUCIDAL SUBSTANCES AFTER PRIMARY INFECTION OF MONKEYS AND CORRELATION BETWEEN SEROLOGICAL PHENOMENA AND TISSUE RESISTANCE IN CONVALESCENCE

This work includes virucidal tests on a total of 40 samples of serum obtained from 21 monkeys infected with poliomyelitic virus. These samples were taken throughout the incubation period, the phase of the active disease, and at certain intervals after recovery. In some instances, samples were obtained from the same animal at several intervals. Specimens were secured as early as during the preparalytic stage and as late as in the fourth month of convalescence. All serums were tested in amounts of 0.8 cc. against 0.2 cc. of a 10 per cent suspension of virus, the technic of the neutralization test being the same as described in previous papers. The results of these experiments together with the accompanying controls are brought together in table 1.

---

6. Jungeblut, C. W., and Engle, E. T.: J. A. M. A. **99:** 2091, 1932; J. Exper. Med. **59:** 43, 1934; Jungeblut, C. W.; Meyer, K., and Engle, E. T.: J. Immunol. **27:** 43, 1934; Jungeblut, C. W.: Arch. Neurol. a. Psych. **33:** 1367, 1935; Jungeblut, C. W.: Schweiz. Med. Woch. **65:** 650, 1935.

Table 1 reveals a remarkable irregularity among different convalescent monkeys with respect to their ability to produce virucidal substances, the speed of their formation and the degree of their persistence. There are apparently some animals that never show any appreciable neutralizing substances at any time during convalescence. Others, again, possess this property early after the attack of the disease but lose it rapidly by the end of the second month while another group seems to be very slow in antibody production. There is still another type of convalescent which maintains a measurable

TABLE 1.—*Development of Virucidal Substances in the Serum of Monkeys after Primary Infection with Poliomyelitic Virus*

Monkeys	Preparalytic Stage	Acute Paralytic Stage	Convalescence 2 weeks	Convalescence 1 month	Convalescence 2 months	Convalescence 3 months	Convalescence 4 months
M1	0	0					
M97	0	0					
N50	0	0					
O62	0	0					
M32	±	0					
M2	+	0					
M79	+	0					
O33	+	0					
M95	+	±					
K52		0					
K65		+					
K55				+	+		
K56		0		+			
K29			+	±	0		
K5			0		+		
J100			0				
K26				0	0		
K57				0			
K79				+			
K60					+	+	+
K63					+	+	+

Technique: 0.8 cc. serum + 0.2 cc. 10% virus, contact one and one-half hour 37 C., overnight icebox, mixture injected intracerebrally into individual monkeys.
+ = neutralization (no paralysis)
± = partial neutralization (paralysis after incubation period over 14 days)
0 = no neutralization (complete or partial paralysis within 5–10 days)
Controls for virucidal tests: Of 17 monkeys injected with 0.2 cc. of 10% virus + 0.8 cc. saline or normal monkey serum, 16 developed complete paralysis within 6–10 days and 1 developed partial paralysis after 11 days.

antibody titer for as long as 3 and 4 months after recovery, this being the longest interval tested for in our experiments. On checking our autopsy records it was found that animals of the latter type, without exception, were suffering from very extensive visceral tuberculosis, while those in which the neutralizing property had either not developed at all, or was rapidly fading, seemed to be free from this complication as far as can be told from a macroscopic examination of the organs. It seems to us, therefore, that intercurrent tuberculosis which occurs so frequently with monkeys in captivity, may constitute an important factor that has to be reckoned with in work of this kind. In view of the observations of Lewis and Loomis[7] who have shown that tuberculous rabbits are better antibody producers than normal rabbits, the suggestion is offered that the unusually long persistence of the neutralizing property may have been due to the stimulating effect of the current tuberculous infection on the antibody-producing tissues.

Another phenomenon recorded in table 1 is of great interest, namely the frequent presence during the preparalytic stage of a transient spurt in neutralizing substances of the serum which is followed immediately upon the

7. Lewis, P. A., and Loomis, D.: J. Exper. Med. **40:** 503, 1924; **43:** 263, 1926.

onset of paralysis by a disappearance of this property. This sudden release of virucidal substances, synchronously with the first rise of the fever, probably reflects a critical stage in the development of the disease when the body is making a futile attempt to limit the infection by a mobilization of all the forces which might check further progress of the virus (Draper[8]).

The question whether or not there is any correlation between the presence of neutralizing substances in the serum of convalescents and the results of reinoculation, was tested by reinoculating intracerebrally, with a heavy dose

TABLE 2.—*Results of Intracerebral Reinoculation of Monkeys Convalescing from a Paralytic Attack of Poliomyelitis with Respect to the Reactivity of the Serum*

Monkeys	Degree of Residual Paralysis	Virucidal Test with Serum at Time of Reinoculation (0.8 cc. Serum + 0.2 cc. 10 Per Cent Virus)	Result of Reinoculation (1 cc. 10 Per Cent Virus)
K29	Complete paralysis one leg and one arm	No neutralization	No renewed paralytic attack
J100	Complete paralysis both legs	No neutralization	No renewed paralytic attack
K26	Partial paralysis one arm	No neutralization	No renewed paralytic attack
K57	Complete paralysis both arms	No neutralization	No renewed paralytic attack
N47	Complete paralysis both arms	No neutralization	No renewed paralytic attack
N26	Complete paralysis both legs and one arm	Partial neutralization	No renewed paralytic attack
K5	Complete paralysis both legs	Neutralization	No renewed paralytic attack
K56	Complete paralysis both legs	Neutralization	No renewed paralytic attack
L69	Partial paralysis one arm	Neutralization	No renewed paralytic attack
N8	Complete paralysis both legs	Neutralization	No renewed paralytic attack
N39	Complete paralysis both legs	Neutralization	No renewed paralytic attack

Neutralization—No paralysis.
Partial neutralization—Complete or partial paralysis after incubation period over 14 days.
No neutralization—Complete or partial paralysis within 5–10 days.
Controls (for virucidal tests and for reinoculation): 11 monkeys injected intracerebrally with 0.2 cc. 10 per cent virus plus 0.8 cc. saline developed complete paralysis within 6–11 days.

TABLE 3.—*Results of Reinoculation of Monkeys Convalescing from a Paralytic Attack of Poliomyelitis with Respect to Extent and Duration of Paralysis*

Number of Monkeys	Degree of Residual Paralysis	Interval Since Onset of Paralysis	Results of Intracerebral Reinoculation with 1 cc. of 10 Per Cent Virus
6	Partial paralysis of one limb	2 to 6 weeks	No renewed paralytic attack
13	Partial or complete paralysis of two limbs	1 to 12 weeks	No renewed paralytic attack
4	Complete paralysis of more than two limbs; animal still able to sit up	1 to 6 weeks	No renewed paralytic attack

Controls for reinoculation: 9 monkeys injected with either 0.1 cc. or 0.2 cc. of 10 per cent virus developed complete paralysis within 6–10 days.

of virus, 11 recovered monkeys, 5 of which had no demonstrable virucidal serum titer at this time, while the serum of the remaining 6 animals possessed either partial or definite neutralizing power. For purpose of general information, a group of 23 convalescent monkeys with various degrees of residual paralysis, the serum of which was not tested individually for neutralizing power, were reinoculated at different intervals after the onset of paralysis. In order to compare the immunizing effect of a preceding paralyzing and nonparalyzing attack of the disease, we have, finally, carried out reinoculations with a series of 20 monkeys all of which had passed through a distinct febrile cycle following intracerebral inoculation with poliomyelitis virus mixed with certain inactivating agents, but had failed at any time to develop manifest paralysis. The results obtained in these experiments are listed in tables 2, 3 and 4.

8. Draper, G.: Infantile Paralysis, New York, Appleton-Century Company, 1935.

As can be seen from table 2, all of the monkeys convalescing from a paralytic attack of poliomyelitis were insusceptible to reintroduction of the virus, irrespective of whether or not their serum contained demonstrable virucidal substances. It follows therefore that there is no relation whatsoever between the degree of resistance to massive intracerebral reinoculation with poliomyelitis virus and the prevailing reactivity of the serum of the recovered animal. It can also be safely said that tissue immunity, induced by a paralytic attack of poliomyelitis, shows no correlation with either the extent or the duration of paralysis (table 3). In marked contrast herewith, the data recorded

TABLE 4.—*Results of Reinoculation of Monkeys which had Passed through a Febrile Episode without Paralysis Following Intracerebral Injection with Poliomyelitis Virus in Combination with Certain Inactivating Agents*

Number of Monkeys	Result of Intracerebral Reinoculation with 1 cc. of 10% Virus	
	Partial Paralysis (7–11 days)	Complete Paralysis (4–11 days)
20	5	15

Controls for reinoculation: of 12 monkeys injected with amounts of 10% virus ranging from 0.1 cc. to 0.6 cc., 10 developed complete paralysis within 6–9 days and 2 developed partial paralysis within 7–8 days.

in table 4 reveal clearly that non-paralyzing attacks suggestive of poliomyelitis which are characterized by fever and occasionally even by an episode of general weakness and awkwardness in movements, fail to leave such animals with any demonstrable resistance to intracerebral reinoculation with the same strain of virus. The infection produced in these cases differed in no way, be it in length of the incubation period or severity of the symptoms, from the course of events commonly observed in controls.

HAS REINOCULATION OF CONVALESCENT MONKEYS ANY EFFECT ON THE TITER OF VIRUCIDAL SUBSTANCES IN THE SERUM?

It was stated in the introduction that it seemed highly desirable to ascertain whether intracerebral reinoculation of recovered monkeys with a massive dose of poliomyelitis virus would lead to any appreciable change in the concentration of virucidal substances in the serum of the animal. To answer this question, we selected five recovered monkeys with partial paralysis in various stages of convalescence, four of which showed definite virucidal power of the serum while the last animal possessed no demonstrable virucidal titer. All these animals were re-injected intracerebrally with 1 cc. of a 10% suspension of virus. None showed any signs of renewed paralysis at any time following reinoculation. Two weeks later, samples of blood were obtained and the serum was tested again for virucidal properties. The results of this work are given in table 5.

It appears from table 5 that in no instance was there any significant change in the reactivity of the serum following symptomless reinoculation. This is to say, when the serum failed to neutralize before reinoculation it failed to acquire such property after reinoculation and when the serum did neutralize before reinoculation, quantitative titrations of both sets of serums failed to reveal any increase in the amounts of such substances present. The one variable result in monkey N47 is evidently offset by an opposite variation in monkey N39.

TABLE 5.—*Experiments on the Virucidal Titer of the Serum of Recovered Monkeys Before and After Reinoculation with Poliomyelitis Virus*

Monkeys	Type of Serum	Result of Virucidal Test (0.2 cc. 10 Per Cent +0.8 cc. of Serum)	Controls (0.2 cc. 10 Per Cent Virus+0.8 cc. Saline)
L69	Before reinoculation, undiluted	Neutralization	M78 Complete paralysis, 11 days; M79 complete paralysis, 8 days
	Before reinoculation, 1:2	Partial neutralization	N26 Complete paralysis, 7 days
	After reinoculation, undiluted	Neutralization	M78 Complete paralysis, 11 days; M79 complete paralysis, 8 days
	After reinoculation, 1:2	Partial neutralization	N26 Complete paralysis, 7 days
N8	Before reinoculation, undiluted	Neutralization	N26 Complete paralysis, 7 days
	Before reinoculation, 1:2	Neutralization	O2 Complete paralysis, 6 days
	Before reinoculation, 1:5	Partial neutralization	O20 Complete paralysis 7 days; O21 complete paralysis, 5 days
	After reinoculation, undiluted	Neutralization	N26 Complete paralysis, 7 days
	After reinoculation, 1:2	Neutralization	O2 Complete paralysis, 6 days
	After reinoculation, 1:5	Partial neutralization	O20 Complete paralysis, 7 days; O21 complete paralysis, 5 days
N26	Before reinoculation, undiluted	Partial neutralization	O2 Complete paralysis, 6 days
	After reinoculation, undiluted	Partial neutralization	O20 Complete paralysis, 7 days; O21 complete paralysis, 5 days
N39	Before reinoculation, undiluted	Neutralization	O2 Complete paralysis, 6 days
	After reinoculation, undiluted	Partial neutralization	O20 Complete paralysis, 7 days; O21 complete paralysis, 5 days
N47	Before reinoculation, undiluted	No neutralization	O2 Complete paralysis, 6 days
	After reinoculation, undiluted	Partial neutralization	O20 Complete paralysis, 7 days; O2 complete paralysis, 5 days

Neutralization—no paralysis
Partial neutralization—complete or partial paralysis after incubation period over 14 days.
No neutralization—complete or partial paralysis within 5–10 days.

DISCUSSION

The experiments reported in this paper seem to indicate that the development of virucidal substances in the serum of monkeys recovering from a paralytic attack of poliomyelitis follows no set rules but that considerable irregularities exist between different animals with respect to their ability to form such substances and to retain them. In marked contrast to the irregular character of the serological phenomena it was found that all monkeys which had passed through a definite paralyzing attack of the disease were uniformily insusceptible to intracerebral reinoculation with massive doses of virus. The failure of such animals to develop a renewed attack of paralysis upon reinoculation was in no way related to the presence or absence of virucidal substances in the serum at the time of reinoculation. It was also shown conclusively that monkeys, which had previously been injected intracerebrally with poliomyelitis virus in combination with certain inactivating agents and had passed through a distinct cycle of fever, without, however, developing at any time any manifest paralysis, were fully susceptible to intracerebral reintroduction of the virus. It was finally demonstrated that reinoculation of recovered paralytic monkeys, which did not lead to a renewed attack of the disease, failed to produce any demonstrable change in the power of the serum to inactivate the virus in vitro.

We believe that these data taken together suggest that the formation of circulating antibodies is a by-product of poliomyelitic infection and that the presence or absence of virucidal substances in the serum shows little if any correlation with the resistance of the central nervous system to reintroduction of the virus. This is also indicated by the fact that monkeys suffering from experimental poliomyelitis, whose serum is tested during the preparalytic stage, frequently possess an appreciable concentration of such substances in the circulating blood even though the infectious process continues to proceed to paralysis. If it is further considered that a non-paralyzing febrile episode in monkeys, which may bear a certain resemblance to so-called abortive attacks in man, fails to induce tissue immunity, one is led to believe that resistance of the nerve cells to invasion of the virus is intimately linked with the production of an actual lesion in the central nervous system. Acquired immunity therefore, as seen in its purest form in the insusceptibility of recovered monkeys, appears to depend essentially upon the presence of an immunity factor in the nervous tissue itself which, in all probability, is predominantly cellular in nature.[9]

If these deductions are correct, it follows that active immunization with dead virus although capable of provoking an immunological response to the antigen, must fail to induce that type of tissue resistance which determines protection of the susceptible nerve cells. It would seem that immunity of this sort can be accomplished only by recovery from actual paralysis or, possibly, by active immunization with live virus. We suspect that the occasional resistence to intracerebral infection of monkeys, actively immunized with live virus, really rests upon the production of an active, though mild, lesion in the central nervous system. This is fully in accord with the fact that repeated injections of live virus into monkeys, by circumvention of the intracerebral route, are followed in a considerable number of instances by the development of manifest paralysis. If the experimental facts are at all applicable to the problem of prevention of the human disease, it would seem that neither the use of dead nor of live virus guarantees that degree of efficacy and of safety which are indispensable for the general use of such a procedure in children.

The data also demonstrate that symptomless reinoculation of convalescent monkeys leads to no increase in the virucidal titer of the serum. The analogy between this experimental observation and the epidemiology of the human disease is not altogether clear since it is unknown to what extent virus entering the body by natural exposure actually reaches the central nervous system. While therefore not invalidating the possibility of extraneural antigenic stimulation, the data fail to support the assumption that the gradual increase in the quantity of neutralizing substances in the serum of growing normal children represents the summary response to a series of immunizing, non-infectious stimuli received by the central nervous system. If these natural virucidal substances are really specific antibodies, they would have to be formed without implication of the central nervous system, by purely subclinical immunization.

CONCLUSIONS

The occurrence of virucidal antibodies in the serum of monkeys convalescing from a paralytic attack of poliomyelitis is very irregular with re-

9. Jungeblut, C. W.: J. Immunol. **22:** 99, 1932.

respect to the formation of such substance, the speed of their development and their maintenance over long periods of time.

Monkeys convalescing from a paralytic attack of poliomyelitis are uniformly insusceptible to intracerebral reinoculation with the same strain of poliomyelitis virus, irrespective of whether the serum does or does not contain a demonstrable virucidal titer at the time of reinoculation.

Monkeys which have passed through a febrile cycle but have failed to develop manifest paralysis following intracerebral injection of poliomyelitis virus in combination with certain inactivating agents are fully susceptible to intracerebral reintroduction of the virus.

Monkeys convalescing from a paralytic attack of poliomyelitis whose serum is tested before and after reinoculation fail to show any evidence of an increase in the serological titer of virucidal substances following reintroduction of the virus into the central nervous system.

These data are discussed in their relation to the mechanism of acquired immunity in the experimental infection and to the epidemiology of the human disease.

VACCINATION AGAINST TUBERCULOSIS—A COMPARATIVE STUDY IN MAN AND ANIMALS

H. J. CORPER
A. P. DAMEROW
M. L. COHN
AND
C. B. VIDAL
DENVER

The correlative problems of immunity and vaccination in tuberculosis are encumbered with conflicting viewpoints which warrant further experimental investigation. The earlier studies by Calmette, Krause,[1] Birkhaug,[2] and others[3] point to a beneficial effect of previous contact with tubercle bacilli, and another school[4] stresses only the detrimental subsequent effects of such first association with the bacilli. Our own results favor the former viewpoint. It is the purpose of this paper to present briefly the findings on which this conclusion is based. It is not generally recognized that tubercle bacilli, viable or nonviable (heat or chemically killed), possess a definite and immediate quantitative tissue destructive action. This action with viable bacilli is influenced by the factor of the ability of the bacilli to multiply in the tissues of the host. We have found[5,6] that viable avirulent human or avirulent bovine tubercle bacilli produce no more local tuberculous skin lesion, when injected intracutaneously into a species of animal susceptible to the type of tuberculosis in question, than an equivalent amount of nonviable tubercle bacilli of the same strain. Such viable avirulent tubercle bacilli when injected intracutaneously in small amounts disappear in viable form from the site of inoculation and possess little tendency to disseminate to internal organs. In contrast, the virulent tubercle bacillus, pathogenic for the species of animal in question, produces a chronologically progressive skin lesion with multiplication of tubercle bacilli at the site of inoculation as well as at the site of dissemination to the organs.

Relatively large amounts (five milligrams in fine suspension) of avirulent tubercle bacilli injected intravenously into the guinea pig result in a transient acute splenomegaly without producing ultimate gross tuberculous changes in any of the organs. This amount of avirulent bacilli given intravenously

---

Received for publication, July 16, 1935.

From the Research Department, National Jewish Hospital.

1. Krause, A. K., and Willis, H. S.: Am. Rev. Tuberc. **14:** 316, 1926.
2. Am. Rev. Tuberc., **27:** 6, 1933.
3. Zeyland, J., and Piasecka-Zeyland E.: Beitr. z. Klin. d. Tuberk. **85:** 369, 1934.
4. Myers, J. A., and Harrington, F. E.: J. A. M. A. **103:** 1530, 1934; Steward, Chester A.: Tubercle **15:** 123, 1933.
5. Corper, H. J., and Cohn, Maurice L.: Am. Rev. Tuberc., in press.
6. Corper, H. J.; Cohn, M. L., and Damerow, A. P.: Am. Rev. Tuberc., in press.

to dogs or rabbits produces no evident gross changes in the organs of these animals.[7]

When suspensions of virulent tubercle bacilli are artificially mixed with suspensions of avirulent tubercle bacilli so that the relative amounts are in proportion of one to one hundred millionth (0.000,000,01 mg. to 1 mg.), the virulent bacilli can be detected by intravenous injection into the guinea pig, since gross tuberculous organic changes result. From the above and additional observations by ourselves and others,[8] it appears that dissociation of these avirulent strains of tubercle bacilli cannot occur in the animal economy even though dissociation might be possible in vitro.

That first contact with virulent tubercle bacilli leads to an immunity in the sense of a changed or protective reaction to subsequent infection which benefits the reinfected animal, has been qualitatively demonstrated before[9] With cutaneous infection we have found that there is a definite chronological development of the tuberculous skin lesion following the first intracutaneous infection with virulent human or bovine tubercle bacilli in the guinea pig, dependent upon the amount of bacilli and their relative virulence for this animal. The chronological sequence of development of the tuberculous skin lesion resulting from the second and subsequent intracutaneous injections of the same virulent human or bovine tubercle bacilli and in the same quantity shows a definite retardation. With small infections, there may occur in the second and following infection a complete absence of reaction or lesion at the site of the intracutaneous injection as compared with the normal animal.

The original first virulent inoculation pursues its progressive course, and such virulent immunization, although tried,[10] obviously would be dangerous and impractical. In guinea pigs, appropriate previous injections with avirulent human or bovine tubercle bacilli given intracutaneously, subcutaneously, or intravenously (but not enterally), retard the development of subsequent infection with virulent human or bovine tubercle bacilli.[6] The effect is evident in the retardation of the disease in the local intracutaneous lesions, the tributary glands, and in the metastatic organic disease developed. The immune effect develops definitely at the point where local macroscopic tubercles are produced by the intracutaneous injection of the avirulent tubercle bacilli. Findings in the dog verified those in guinea pigs so far as comparisons could be made.

In the rabbit, however, evidences of biological specificity of the strains in the immune relation was noted. Calmette[11] hinted at such specificity but never reported on the use of a human avirulent strain of tubercle bacilli for immunologic purposes. The guinea pig and dog are about equally susceptible to virulent human and bovine tubercle bacilli, while the rabbit shows a

---

7. Corper, H. J.; Damerow, A. P., and Cohn, M. L.: Am. Rev. Tuberc., in press.

8. Park, W. H.; Kereszturi, C., and Mishulow, L.: J. A. M. A. **101:** 1619, 1933; Behner, Dorothy M.: Am. Rev. Tuberc. **31:** 174, 1935.

9. Krause, A. K., and Peters, Dorothy: Am. Rev. Tuberc. **4:** 551, 1920–21.

10. Webb, G. B., and Williams, W. W.: J. A. M. A. **57:** 1431, 1911.

11. Tubercle Bacillus Infections and Tuberculosis in Man and Animals, Baltimore, Williams and Wilkins Co., 1923.

striking relative insusceptibility to virulent human tubercle bacilli as compared with virulent bovine tubercle bacilli; a fact Theobald Smith first used for biologic differentiation. It was for this reason and the fact that an avirulent human strain of tubercle bacilli had never been tested before in viable form on human beings that we considered the study of avirulent human strains.[12]

Although there are those who view clinical immunization with BCG—as do Park[13] and his colleagues, Heimbeck[14] and Ustvedt[15]—as being harmless, there are, as far as we are aware, no definite observations in man which would compare with those in animals and which would disclose the quantitative relation of the injections of avirulent tubercle bacilli with immunity. It was also desirable to determine in man the type of skin lesion developed with relation to the dose used, since numerous investigators have reported on the troublesome cold abscess which developed even from the use of dead bacilli in vaccination.[16] As human strains of tubercle bacilli are biologically acknowledged to be more pathogenic to man than bovine strains, the criteria of pathogenicity of avirulent strains required determination on the basis of lesion production and multiplication of bacilli at the site of inoculation. Finally, it was also desirable to determine whether the reaction in man paralleled that in animals.

In earlier experiments in animals, it was found that the intracutaneous injection of avirulent human or bovine tubercle bacilli produced gross tubercles in amounts as low as 0.01 milligram in fine suspension. The maximum effect was consummated in about three to four weeks and resolution, dependent on the dose, usually occurred within ten weeks.

The human subjects chosen for the tests were thoroughly examined clinically and roentgenologically to exclude evidences of clinical tuberculosis, and were given intracutaneous tuberculin tests to gain an insight into their relative tuberculin reacting power. For the latter purpose, the purified tuberculin P. P. D., kindly supplied by Dr. W. W. King of Parke, Davis and Company, was used. All evidences of other diseases were excluded. Thus the subjects were grouped as being relatively tuberculin negative or positive. Both types were studied. There was noted, as in the animals, a macroscopic reaction ranging in the smaller doses from a small just palpable nodule (tubercle) in concentrations as low as 0.001 mg. (0.1 cc. being injected) per cc. of avirulent human or bovine tubercle bacilli to a large purulent ulcer which discharged and finally healed in about six months when concentrations of 1 to 10 mg. of fine suspension per cc. were injected intracutaneously. There was no marked difference between the reactions resulting from the first injections of either the human or bovine (BCG) avirulent strains (see figure 1). Coincident with the large intracutaneous injection of these avirulent tubercle bacilli, there occurred a transient pyrexia (temperature eleva-

12. Corper, H. J., and Cohn, Maurice L.: Am. Rev. Tuberc. **28:** 856, 1933.
13. Am. J. Dis. Child. **48:** 507, 1934.
14. Med. Klin. **29:** 1731, 1933; and Tidskr. f. d. Norske Laegeforening. **53:** 529, 1933.
15. J. A. M. A. **104:** 851, 1935.
16. Goodwin, Campbell T., and Schwentker, Francis F.: J. Pediat. **5:** 475, 1934.

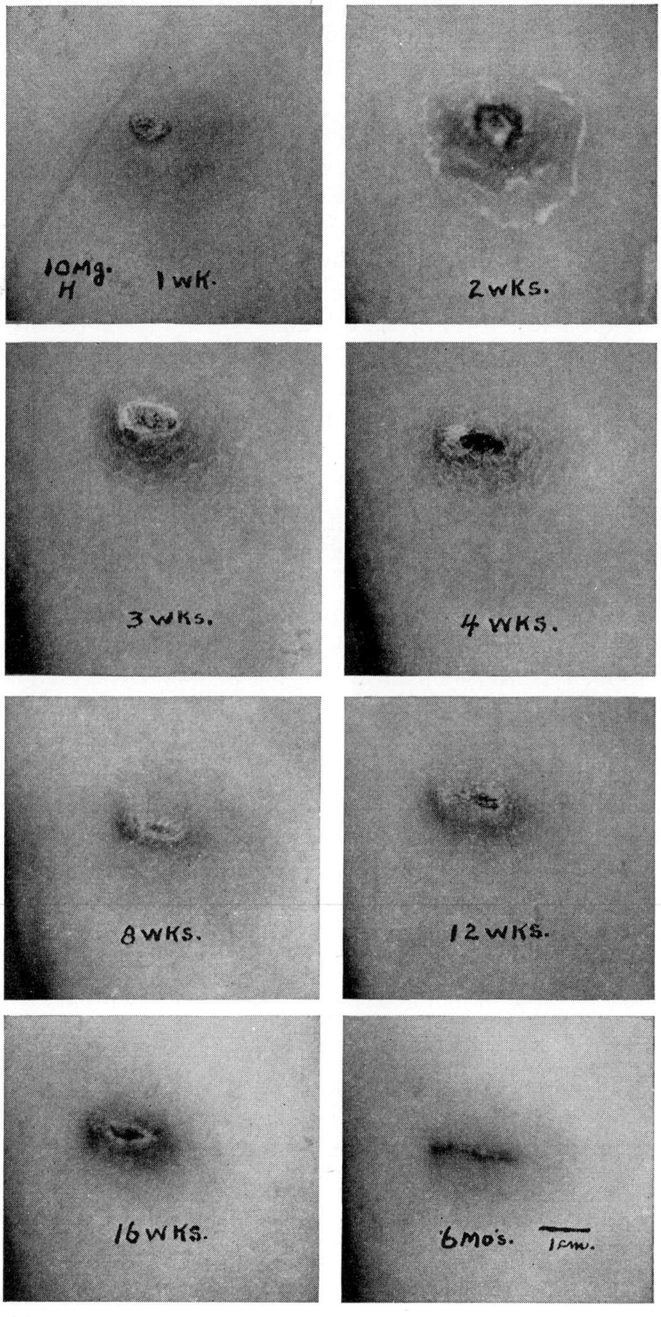

Fig. 1.—The reaction to avirulent human tubercle bacilli injected in relatively large amounts (0.1 cc. of a fine suspension containing 10 mg. per cc.) intracutaneously in man relatively tuberculin negative. Note the large ulcerating lesion which required over six months to heal. Avirulent bovine tubercle bacilli (BCG) cause similar lesion in this amount.

tion of several degrees Fahrenheit), an increased pulse count, and a transient leukocytosis which subsided within several days to a week. At the same time there occurred a slight transient local lymph adenopathy which also subsided before the retrogression and healing of the local lesion had occurred. The local glands at times, especially following large injections, were tender to the touch.

The reaction to the live avirulent human or bovine (BCG) tubercle bacilli did not appreciably differ from that occurring with non-viable (heat or chemically killed) bacilli. Regardless whether the bacilli were viable or not (heat or chemically killed) or whether they were avirulent human or bovine tubercle bacilli, the intracutaneous lesions produced with concentrations ranging from 0.001 mg. of bacilli in fine suspension to 1.0 mg. per cc. paralleled each other in man as well as in animals. For example, during the first three days the lesion to the 0.1 milligram per cubic centimeter concentration develops a small nodule about seven millimeters in diameter with an erythematous peripheral zone extending to a diameter of about ten to twelve millimeters. This lesion tends to suppurate in about one week and either forms a dry eschar or ulcerates and discharges during the second to fourth week, resulting in complete healing with depressed scar formation after two or three months to six months. The smaller injections (0.01 and 0.001 mg. per cc.), which do not suppurate, form a transient nodule which resolves in about six months usually leaving a small depressed or contracted scar.

Thus, in the human being, one of the criterions for avirulent tubercle bacilli has been fulfilled. The second criterion of avirulence as demonstrated by previous animal experiment was that these bacilli should not reproduce but should gradually lose their viability. For the purpose of determining this in man, subjects who were relatively tuberculin negative to P. P. D. were given intracutaneous injections of fine suspensions of the avirulent tubercle bacilli in 0.1 cc. amounts, the site being marked by the addition of a small amount of pure sterile India ink added to the suspension. The concentration of bacilli injected was chosen so that complicating ulceration would not interfere with the findings (0.01 mg. per cc. being used). After injection, the lesions were excised completely under procain local anesthesia, which had proven in control and in vitro tests to exert no influence on the viability of the bacilli. Sample specimens were removed and cultured (by culture methods capable of demonstrating the presence of 0.000,000,01 mg. per cc. of tubercle bacilli),[5] and it was found that the bacilli could be recovered by this delicate method up to four months but not six months after inoculation. This substantiates the animal findings and establishes the second criterion for the absence of virulence for man for both the human avirulent and the bovine avirulent strain (BCG) of tubercle bacilli.

In animals which have received a first injection of 0.001 milligram or more of viable avirulent tubercle bacilli, there has been demonstrated a definite retardation of subsequent infection with virulent tubercle bacilli. When the same amount (0.001 mg. or more) of viable avirulent tubercle bacilli are injected intracutaneously at semi-monthly or monthly intervals, there is noted a changed reaction to these avirulent bacilli which expresses itself as a more pronounced acute reaction with resultant larger and more extensive lesion. This occurs in spite of the fact that the bacilli are not capable of multiplying in the tissues. If, for example, a guinea pig is given a single or double intracutaneous injection of 0.1 or 0.2 cc. of the 0.01 mg. per cc. concentration of fine suspension of avirulent human tubercle bacilli, the first injection results in a small just appreciable nodule developing at the site of injection at one week and gradually subsiding after about five to seven or eight weeks. The second lesion at the site of the second injection of the same amount of bacilli, given intracutaneously four weeks after the first injection, develops more rapidly and to a perceptibly larger size nodule which persists for a longer time after injection. A third and fourth intracutaneous injection of the same bacilli in the same amount likewise show a still greater nodule development when the 0.01 milligram suspension is used than that occurring respectively after the first or second injections at four-week intervals. The same findings are noted for smaller and larger amounts of bacilli when within the range in which conflicting ulceration does not interfere markedly with the sequence of the chronological results obtained. All records were made photographically at the same magnification and were again read side by side to obviate individual reading errors and as a check on the regular measurement readings made during the course of the experiment.

In order to determine whether this change in reaction to avirulent human tubercle bacilli also occurs in man, the same tests were conducted on human subjects by giving intracutaneous injections of 0.1 cc. of 0.01 mg. per cc. of fine suspensions of young cultures (about 3 to 4 weeks old) of avirulent human tubercle bacilli; the injections being given at monthly intervals and photographic records being made at regular intervals at the same magnification so that comparative readings of the successive injections could be made. The reactions paralleled those noted in animals. If, for example, we compare the findings at the two week interval after the intracutaneous injection, spaced four weeks apart, of 0.1 cc. of a fine suspension of viable avirulent human tubercle bacilli containing 0.01 mg. per cc., the respective readings in diameter of the lesions and surrounding erythema were as follows: first, three mm. and five mm.; second, five mm. and eight mm.; third, six mm. and nine mm.; and fourth, eight mm. and twelve mm. These effects are strikingly shown when photographs of the various lesions taken at weekly intervals are compared.

SUMMARY AND CONCLUSIONS

It has been demonstrated that in animals there is a retardation of virulent tuberculous infection resulting from a previous vaccination with viable avirulent human and bovine tubercle bacilli.

Avirulent tubercle bacilli in amounts exceeding one-thousandth of a milligram of fine suspension per cc. produce in man and animals definite intracutaneous local lesions similar to those resulting from the injection of the same non-viable tubercle bacilli.

The extent of such local lesions in man and the slow retrogression of these would not seem to warrant the use of excessive amounts of these bacilli as has been done in the past for producing immunity.

Avirulent human or bovine (BCG) tubercle bacilli do not produce progressive lesions when injected intracutaneously in man and when injected in amounts capable of causing tubercle without ulceration (0.01 mg.) lose their viability in these lesions within about six months as tested by delicate methods for discerning the presence of viable tubercle bacilli in tissues. Likewise, even large cutaneous local ulcers produced by avirulent human or bovine tubercle bacilli completely heal with scar formation in approximately six months.

The reactions to viable avirulent tubercle bacilli in man, used in amounts revealing visible changes, show a sequence of changed reaction upon repeated monthly injections similar to the changes noted in animals and occurring coincidently with the development of artificial immunity in these animals. There is an apparent paradox resulting from this reaction in that the lesions produced by small or large numbers of virulent tubercle bacilli are retarded by the immune reaction as a result of preventing or retarding the multiplication of virulent bacilli—less lesion to virulent infection—and on the other hand, there is a greater tissue reaction in the immune organism as compared with the non-immune, to large numbers of avirulent bacilli incapable of multiplying in the tissues—more tissue reaction to avirulent bacilli. When this is realized, it becomes obvious that conclusions drawn from pathological findings alone, without knowing definitely the quantity of either one of these two decisive factors concerned and necessary for such interpretation, the number of bacilli producing the reaction or the existing immune condition present, can be of no practical value.

There exists a biological specificity of the immune reaction in animals with avirulent bovine tubercle bacilli against virulent bovine infection which would suggest a greater efficiency from the use of avirulent human tubercle bacilli against virulent human infection. For this reason perhaps a mixed vaccine for human purposes deserves consideration.

When viable avirulent tubercle bacilli are to be used for vaccinating, it would appear advisable to use intracutaneous injections for this purpose and to use an amount of bacilli well within the range of producing a visible reaction and yet not excessive to the point of producing large abscesses and ulcers with consequent necrosis and slow healing. It also appears that two or more intracutaneous injections at semimonthly or monthly intervals would serve to reinforce the desired effect.

DISSOCIATION OF SACCHAROMYCES ACERIS-SACCHARI FABIAN AND HALL AND PICHIA ALCOHOLOPHILA KLÖCKER

L. J. WICKERHAM
AND
F. W. FABIAN
EAST LANSING

INTRODUCTION

Dissociation in yeasts has been studied extensively by Fabian and McCullough.[1] Henrici[2] has also reported variations in colonies of a species of Torula. As morphological changes of the dissociating yeasts have not been studied in detail, an investigation to do this was undertaken. The large size of the yeast cell, as compared to the size of the bacterial cell, makes the changes in internal structure as well as the changes in shape more clearly apparent. The novel forms which the cells assumed as they passed from one stage in their dissociation cycle to another made their study interesting. Of the six yeasts with which we worked, only two responded to the dissociating agent used. They were Saccharomyces aceris-sacchari Fabian and Hall, and Pichia alcoholophila Klöcker.

DISSOCIATION OF SACCHAROMYCES ACERIS-SACCHARI

Saccharomyces aceris-sacchari in the normal or smooth form produces glistening colonies on agar plates (figure 1). No scum is produced in young broth cultures, but after a few days' growth a thin pellicle appears. The cells are round and show little, if any, internal structure. When rapidly growing in liquid medium the budding cells tend to remain attached, thus forming small clumps, or "colonies," a common condition among S yeasts. The cells range from 3.5 to 7 microns in diameter (figure 2).

The dissociating mediums used contained lithium chloride as the dissociating agent. Yeast extract broth with two different concentrations of lithium chloride; i.e., 0.10 per cent and 0.25 per cent were used. Yeast extract broth is in itself a mild dissociation agent and promotes the growth of yeasts. This medium consisted of 0.1 per cent of digested yeast cells, 0.5 per cent tryptophane broth and 0.5 per cent glucose. Plain broth containing 0.25 per cent lithium chloride was also used because Fabian and McCullough[1] used it to induce dissociation in many species of yeasts.

Received for publication, July 17, 1935.
From the Department of Bacteriology, Michigan State College.
1. J. Bact. **27:** 583, 1934.
2. J. Bact. **26:** 125, 1933.

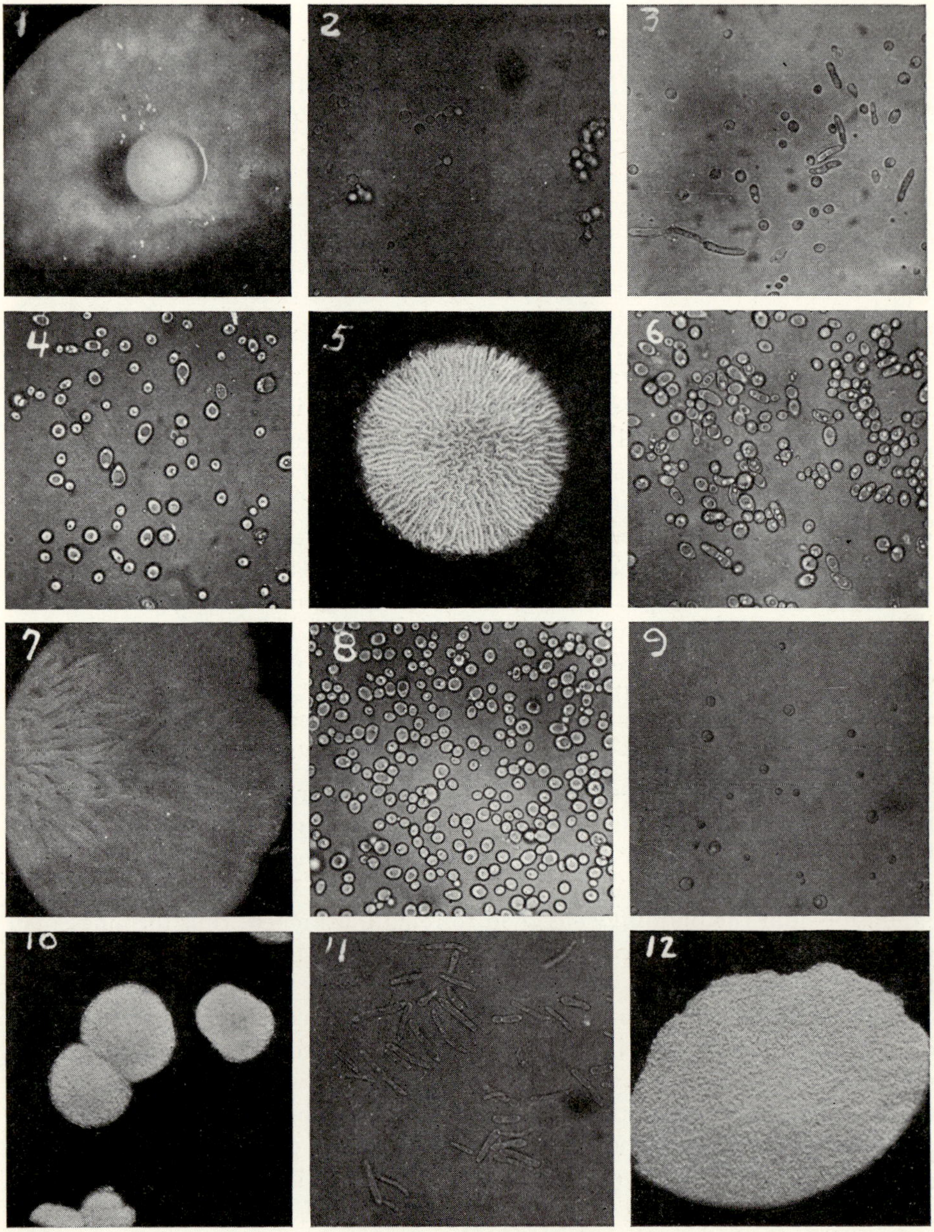

Figs. 1–12.

A rapidly growing culture of the S strain of S. aceris-sacchari was inoculated into culture tubes of the 0.10 per cent lithium chloride yeast extract broth and serially transferred daily. Platings and microscopic examinations were made at each transfer in order to note any changes which might occur. The mediums used for plating were malt extract agar and dextrose agar. The first transfer produced a variation from the S form, for many of the cells instead of producing round buds produced elongated buds having large central vacuoles. There were some clumps of cells in which the mother, or primary, cell was round and in which each succeeding generation became more elongated. These elongated buds had large central vacuoles. They were common by the sixth transfer, by which time most of the cells, whether elongated or round, contained vacuoles and small, highly refractive bodies which gave the characteristics of fat when stained by Sudan III or osmic acid. These refractive globules, or oil drops, appear in the photographs either as very light or very dark spots, depending upon the focus when the pictures were taken (figure 3).

The seventh transfer in the 0.10 per cent lithium chloride yeast extract broth, when examined microscopically, appeared to be composed of more or less rounded cells of various sizes. The central vacuole was very large and constituted most of the interior of the cell. The oil drops had become larger and were usually two in number. They were located around the periphery of the vacuole into which they sometimes escaped and showed Brownian movement (figure 4).

When plated these cells gave rise to colonies which had an outer band that was dull and wrinkled and a center which was smooth and glistening. The next, or eighth, transfer produced colonies which, when plated, were completely rough. These R colonies were two or three times as large as the smooth colonies; they were snow-white, and consisted of many radial ridges

---

Figs. 1–12.

Fig. 1.—A typical S colony of S. aceris-sacchari. ×8.

Fig. 2.—Typical cells from an S colony of S. aceris-sacchari. ×460.

Fig. 3.—Elongated and round cells from a colony of S. aceris-sacchari showing the first signs of turning rough, after six daily transfers in 0.1 LiCl broth. Note the presence of vacuoles and numerous small oil drops. ×460.

Fig. 4.—Same cells at end of seven daily transfers in 0.1 per cent LiCl broth showing large round cells. The oil drops are much larger. ×460.

Fig. 5.—A typical R colony of S. aceris-sacchari. ×8.

Fig. 6.—Typical cells from the R colony in figure 5. ×460.

Fig. 7.—Spreader colony of S. aceris-sacchari which results when cells from an R colony are transferred into maltose extract broth for 24 hours. This is the first step in the conversion of an R to an S colony. ×8.

Fig. 8.—Cells from the R spreader colony in figure 7. ×460.

Fig. 9.—A recently reverted S type colony that still retains the oil drops which are fewer and larger. ×460.

Fig. 10.—An evenly contoured R colony of S. aceris-sacchari which results when cells from 0.1 per LiCl broth are transferred into 0.25 per cent LiCl broth. ×8.

Fig. 11.—Cells from the R colony in figure 10. ×460.

Fig. 12.—Evenly contoured R spreader colony which results when cells from colony shown in figure 10 is inoculated into maltose broth and grown 24 hrs. ×8.

extending from the center to the edge of the colony. Between the ridges was a lacy network (figure 5). The cells forming these colonies produced a heavy growth at the surface of liquid mediums and moderate growth at the bottom. Microscopically the cells varied greatly in size and morphology. Some were elongated and some were spherical. The oil drops were large and vacuoles were prominent. When the cells of a young rough colony were suspended in a drop of water and examined microscopically the preparation showed a great many oil drops which had escaped from the cells and were moving about by Brownian movement. Many such oil drops were present when the microphotograph labeled figure 6 was taken; however, only those that were adhering to the surface of the yeast cells show in the photograph since they were not moving. The cells do not form clumps as the S cells do, but appear as single individuals (figure 6). No further change occurred on continued transfer in the 0.1 per cent lithium chloride.

For further study this R form was inoculated into malt extract broth and also into a medium containing 0.25 per cent lithium chloride in yeast extract broth. The former medium is very favorable for yeasts and aids in the reversion of the R form into the S form. It was prepared by adding 3.0 per cent Trommer's malt extract and 1.0 per cent glucose to nutrient broth. The latter medium was used to learn whether any further change would occur in the R form.

After one to three daily transfers of the rough in malt extract broth the cells became rounded (figure 8), and when plated on malt extract agar produced spreading colonies which reached 70 to 80 millimeters in diameter after a few days' growth. These colonies were rugose and the periphery was somewhat irregular. This type was designated the spreader form (figure 7).

A single transfer of the spreader in yeast extract broth caused its return to the R type. When the spreader colony was allowed to age a few days on the malt extract agar plate and was then directly plated on the same medium, the resulting colonies were of the R type. However, after continued daily serial transfers of the spreader type in malt extract broth, it was converted into the S form after approximately four transfers. The growth was almost completely at the bottom of the culture tube. The colonies were smooth and glistening, and the cells were round and homogeneous except for the presence of a large oil drop in many of the cells. After four more transfers the oil drops disappeared. It was found that unless the newly reverted S form was rapidly transferred in malt extract broth, it tended to revert to the spreader or R type (figure 9).

In order to study the effect of an increased amount of lithium chloride in the medium, the rough form was inoculated into a tube of 0.25 per cent lithium chloride yeast extract broth. The culture was set aside for 9 days and was then plated. About 50 per cent of the resulting colonies were of the type from which the culture was originally made; the other 50 per cent did not show the characteristic radial ridges, but had an even contour. Slender filaments extended outward from the edge of the colonies into the medium (figure 10). Both types of colonies were snow-white and both types were of the same size, i.e., 4 to 10 millimeters in diameter. The cells of this new R type were all narrow rods having large vacuoles, but only a few small oil drops. Many of the cells had no oil drops whatever (figure 11).

When this R was grown twenty-four hours in malt extract broth and then plated on the corresponding agar, a spreading type of colony was produced. The spreader likewise was not rugose. It had the same surface texture as the R from which it was derived. The colonies grew to a size equal to that

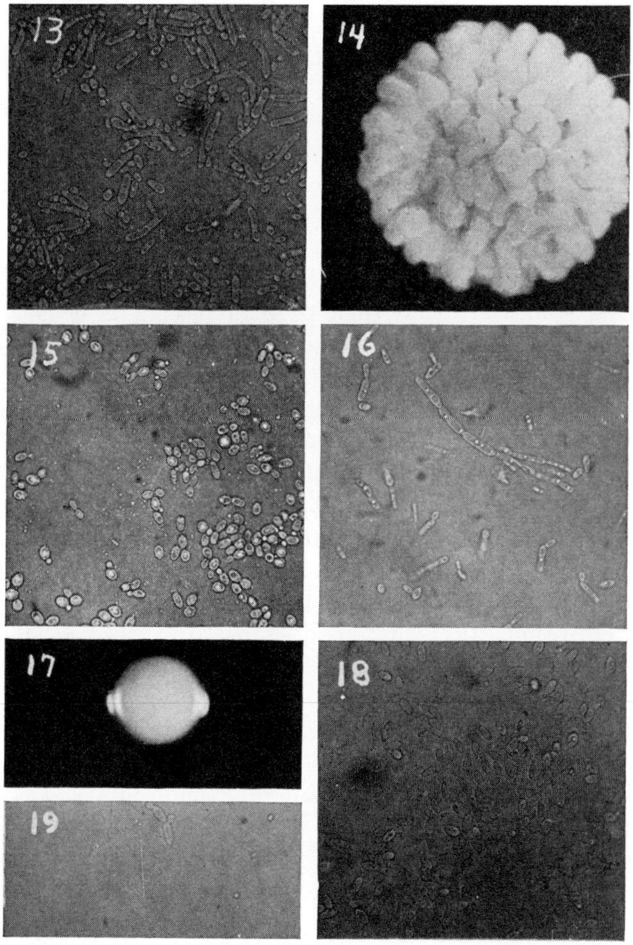

Fig. 13.—Cells from R spreader colony shown in figure 12. ×460.

Fig. 14.—Typical R colony of Pichia alcoholophila. ×8. Colonies of this yeast are normally rough.

Fig. 15.—Cells from 4 day old R colony shown in figure 14. ×460.

Fig. 16.—Cells from a 7 day old R colony shown in figure 14. Cells are greatly enlongated and show vacuoles and oil drops. ×460.

Fig. 17.—Typical S colony of Pichia alcoholophila. (The light, slightly bulging spots on the periphery of the colony are artifacts due to reflected light.)

Fig. 18.—Cells from 4 day old S colony shown in figure 17 showing oil drops. ×460.

Fig. 19.—Cells from S colony shown in figure 17 after they had been transferred daily in malt extract broth for two weeks. It takes about this long for the oil drops to disappear. ×460.

of the rugose spreader referred to previously, and similarly had an irregular periphery (figure 12). The cells were mainly rods, although some round cells were present. Vacuoles were common, but oil drops were small and scarce (figure 13). This evenly contoured spreader was just as unstable as the rugose spreader. On continued transfer in malt extract broth, it reverted to the S form.

At the same time that the first inoculation of the S form was made into the 0.10 per cent lithium chloride yeast extract broth, another transfer from the same culture was inoculated into 0.25 per cent lithium chloride plain broth and serially transferred. The growth in this medium was very slow. None of the serial transfers showed any variation, and at the end of 30 days the colonies that were produced still glistened. The cells were of the S type, but were dwarfed in size.

DISSOCIATION OF PICHIA ALCOHOLOPHILA KLÖCKER

The S form of Pichia alcoholophila Klöcker grows at the bottom in liquid mediums. The colonies are smooth and glistening. The cells are round to slightly elongated in shape and frequently produce pseudo-mycelia. They average about six microns in length. A stock culture showing a wrinkled growth typical of R yeasts was examined and was found to contain cells with small oil drops and no vacuoles. An attempt was made to dissociate this yeast by growing it in 0.10 per cent lithium chloride yeast extract broth, but this yeast could not tolerate it. Even 0.05 per cent lithium chloride inhibited its growth. It was found that yeast extract broth is in itself a mild dissociating agent, and after a few transfers in it colonies were produced which were extremely rugose (figure 14). Colonies two to six days old were composed of cells which were round to elongated in shape. All cells had small vacuoles, and a few contained small oil drops (figure 15). They approximated the S cells in size. When the colonies were six days old or older, the cells became much larger, averaging 10 to 16 microns, with vacuoles constituting most of the interior. Metachromatic granules were easily visible in most of the cells, and oil drops became very prominent. Pseudo-mycelial formation was also common at this stage (figure 16).

When giant colonies of this R form were grown on malt extract agar and incubated for 10 to 15 days, secondary S colonies appeared at several points on the periphery. When these were subplated, they produced smooth colonies, the cells of which had the appearance of the true S cells except for the presence of small oil drops (figures 17 and 18). The oil drops disappeared only after many rapid transfers in malt extract broth. As long as the S cells retained the oil drops they could be brought back to the R form by aging in malt extract broth for two weeks, at the end of which time a thin pellicle formed on the surface of the medium. It was found that the R form remains stable in yeast extract broth.

DISCUSSION

When the S form of S. aceris-sacchari was grown in yeast extract broth containing 0.10 per cent lithium chloride the cells lost their homogeneous appearance. Oil drops were numerous, nearly all of the interior of the cell was a vacuole, and the cells grew mainly at the surface of liquid mediums rather than at the bottom, as obtained with the S form. This R form produced a rugose, opaque colony. When grown in yeast extract broth containing 0.25 per cent lithium chloride, this rugose R further changed into long slender rods having large vacuoles and the oil drops had practically disappeared. When plated, these cells produced opaque, evenly contoured colonies in contrast to the rugose colonies previously produced. Both types of the R form when rapidly transferred in malt extract broth soon produced unstable spreading colonies and later the S form of the yeast.

A stock culture of Pichia alcoholophila which was intermediate between the S and R form was made thoroughly R by transferring it in yeast extract broth. The cells composing the R colony underwent a change in morphology, became larger and developed more and larger oil drops as the colony became older. When giant R colonies were grown and incubated for 10 to 15 days, secondary S colonies appeared around the periphery. The cells of the secondary colonies contained oil drops, but after several transfers in malt extract broth the cells were typical of the S form.

SUMMARY AND CONCLUSIONS

A detailed study of the characteristics of the S and R forms of the two yeasts, Saccharomyces aceris-sacchari and Pichia alcoholophila, show that dissociation in yeasts is a gradual process and that none of the various stages arise spontaneously. There is a gradual transition from one type of cell or colony to another.

There is a marked tendency for the dissociants to revert to the form from which they were derived.

A comparative study of the S and R forms under identical condition show that rough yeasts have certain characteristics in common which distinguish them from smooth yeasts. The most common ones are:

Large oil drops are usually present in the R yeasts. Sometimes S cells show oil drops, but they are small in size and few in number as compared to the oil drops present in the R forms.

The R cells have very large vacuoles. When vacuoles are present in S cells they are much smaller than those in the R cells.

The R cell is larger than the corresponding S cell.

The R colony is larger than the corresponding S colony.

The R colony is opaque and rough, the S colony is smooth and glistening.

The R cells do not tend to form "colonies" in liquid mediums as do the S forms. The R daughter cells separate immediately from the mother cell.

The R cells come to the top of a hanging drop and adhere to the coverglass, making it possible to photograph them readily. Smooth cells go to the bottom of a hanging drop and show Brownian movement, which makes it difficult to photograph them.

These characteristics were determined by observations made on R yeasts produced by Fabian and McCullough, on naturally occurring R yeasts, and on the R yeasts which the writers have produced.

VARIATION OF SALMONELLA PULLORUM

H. VAN ROEKEL

AND

LEO F. RETTGER

NEW HAVEN, CONNETICUT

Bacterial variation has received but little attention in the study of pullorum disease of fowl. This is due, in part, to the long-prevailing impression that the etiological agent, S. pullorum, is stable in its morphological, cultural and serological properties. However, epidemics of pullorum disease have been known to occur in varying degrees of intensity, and we must assume that the causative organism fluctuates widely in its pathogenicity. Plastridge and Rettger[1] observed a very unusual outbreak of the disease in young and adult fowl. The mature stock suffered rather heavy losses, which is rare in natural outbreaks. Considerable difficulty was experienced in determining the etiological agent, due to the marked pleomorphic tendencies which it exhibited.

In the control and eradication of pullorum disease by means of the agglutination test, the doubtful or suspicious reactor presents a rather perplexing problem. To what extent bacterial variation enters into this problem is an important question. While much progress has been made in perfecting and standardizing the methods and technique employed in the macroscopic agglutination test, certain contributing factors require further elucidation. Bacterial variation of the causative agent may play a not insignificant rôle.

The present investigation had as its main purpose a determination of the extent to which variants of this organism occur in nature, and in the laboratory under varied environmental conditions; also, it included, an intensive study of the morphological, cultural, pathogenic and serological properties of variants.

THE INCIDENCE OF VARIANTS IN NEWLY ISOLATED STRAINS

In order to detect variants in any strain of bacteria it is necessary to determine what constitutes a so-called "normal" or typical strain. The characteristics described by Rettger,[2] and by Rettger and Plastridge[3] were accepted as the criterion for the normal type. On plain meat extract agar (p_H 7.0–7.2) liberally seeded with inoculum, characteristic colonies, when viewed through the low power objective, appear discrete, smooth, homogeneous, entire, and transparent, and vary in form from round to oval, and occasionally more or less angular. On liver infusion agar the growth is much more luxuriant than on meat extract agar, and the colonies are less trans-

---

Received for publication, July 20, 1935.

From the Department of Bacteriology, Yale University.

1. J. Infect. Dis. **47**: 334, 1930.
2. New York M. J. **71**: 803, 1900.
3. Storrs Agric. Exper. Sta., Bull. 178, 1932.

parent (figures 1 and 2). Crowded colonies remain small (1 mm. or less), but well isolated colonies may attain a diameter of from 3 to 4 mm., or more. Surface markings may appear as the colony increases in size and age, but as a rule the colonies on heavily seeded plates change little with age.

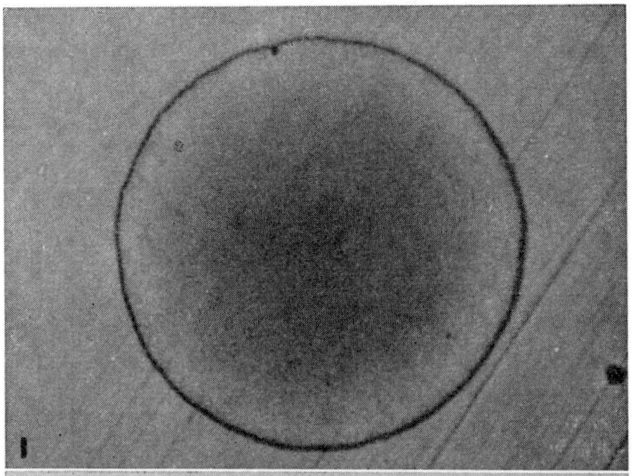

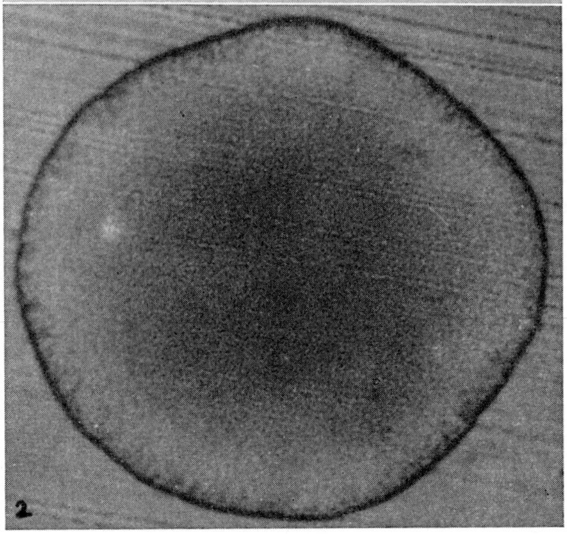

Fig. 1.—Typical S. pullorum colony on meat extract agar. 24 hours incubation. ×125 diameters.

Fig. 2.—Typical S. pullorum colony on liver infusion agar. 24 hours old. ×100 diameters.

The "normal" cell type is a Gram-negative rod (0.4–$0.5\mu \times 1$–2.5μ) with slightly rounded ends, which usually occurs single, and rarely in chains of more than two bacilli. Filamentous forms are observed occasionally. Films prepared from colonies on liver infusion agar often contain cells that vary greatly in size, morphology and staining property.

Freshly isolated S. pullorum strains are identified, further, by the use of fermentable substances (dextrose, lactose, maltose, sucrose and dulcitol) and serological tests. The production of acid and gas in dextrose broth is considered typical of the organism, although occasional strains do not produce visible gas. Lactose, maltose, sucrose and dulcitol are not attacked.

A total of 163 strains, isolated from several different sources, including eggs, chicks and mature fowl, was studied in this investigation. The majority of these were received from the Department of Veterinary Science, Massachusetts State College. Of the 163 strains, 13 did not resemble typical S. pullorum in every respect, when grown on plain meat extract agar plates. Salt-sensitiveness was exhibited by 12 strains, of which one also produced atypical colonies and cells, and grew with difficulty on plain meat extract agar and in sugar broth. One strain manifested only rough colonial forms on primary culture.

The atypical strains were tested on several occasions with positive and negative pullorum serums. It was necessary to reduce the concentration of the salt solution from 0.9 to 0.22 per cent, to increase the stability of the salt-sensitive strains. The atypical strains did not behave alike as antigens, with positive and negative serums, in the presence of 0.9 per cent sodium chloride. With most of these antigens it was difficult to determine whether the cells were actually agglutinated. Stable, well defined clumps of cells were not visible to the naked eye, as one ordinarily observes in typical agglutination with S. pullorum. Some antigens appeared unstable in 0.9 per cent salt solution, while the cells remained in suspension in the presence of negative serum and the same salt concentration. In one instance agglutination occurred in a serum dilution of 1:640, but not in 1:1280. In the higher dilution the cells remained in suspension, but settled out in the antigen control. While in some instances the serum appeared to exert a stabilizing effect in maintaining the cells in suspension, in others the opposite effect was observed.

Antigens may vary to such an extent in their mosaic structure as to react differently when placed under certain uniform conditions. The influence of electrolyte on the stability of the organism was demonstrated by the use of a 0.11 per cent salt solution, which in itself permitted the cells to remain in suspension. In this weak concentration of electrolyte the agglutination titer of the positive serums was not only reduced, but the clumping was less definite. The agglutinin titers of the hosts from which some of the atypical strains were originally isolated showed that the organisms were not entirely devoid of the power to stimulate agglutinin production. However, this observation warrants further substantiation, as will be pointed out later.

VARIATION INDUCED BY ARTIFICIAL METHODS

In this phase of the investigation attention was directed chiefly to deviation from the normal colony type. Colony form was selected, therefore, as a starting point, and changes from the normal related to other characters, namely cellular morphology, biochemical and tinctorial reactions, pathogenicity, antigenicity and agglutinability. Repeated transfer and aging in broth were found to bring about variation in a majority of the strains studied. Other methods employed proved, on the whole, to be less successful.

INFLUENCE OF FREQUENT TRANSFER AND OF AGING IN BEEF INFUSION BROTH

Beef infusion broth having the following composition was used in the first three experiments: fresh infusion of 500 grams of lean beef, 1,000 cc.; peptone (Difco), 10 grams. The reaction was adjusted to p_H 6.8–7.0.

The different strains were grown at 37 C. in 10 cc. of the beef infusion broth and subjected to daily transfer over a period of two weeks. After the last 24 hours' incubation at 37 C., all of the broth cultures were kept at room temperature and streaked on agar plates, after various intervals.

EXPERIMENT 1

The following strains of S. pullorum were employed:

Strain	*Source*
I	Ovary of a carrier hen, 1930.
II	Diseased chick, 1929.
III	Diseased chick, November, 1932.
IV	Ovary of a carrier hen, October, 1932.

Strains I and II were subject to more or less variation, when received, due to earlier treatment to bring about dissociation. They developed smooth and rough colonies on meat extract agar. Strain I produced a distinct flaky sediment and slight general turbidity in the broth, while strain II caused a definite uniform turbidity, with only moderate sedimentation. Strains III and IV resembled typical S. pullorum in all respects, at the outset.

Transfers to agar plates from young broth cultures yielded colonies whose morphology was similar to that observed at the beginning. However, aging of the broth cultures for a period of two months brought about a partial loss of the rough colonial characteristics of strains I and II, while strain IV exhibited some typical smooth colonies and numerous extremely small colonies which appeared very irregular in shape. Transfers made from the small colonies to meat extract broth tubes did not result in as pronounced a growth throughout the medium as is usually observed with typical S. pullorum. The peculiar characteristic of this variant (designated IV-a) to produce very small pin-point colonies which increased but little in size on prolonged incubation was preserved indefinitely. The cells of these colonies were highly pleomorphic, and included both coccoid and filamentous forms.

Attempts to develop larger colony types from IV-a by continued selection were unsuccessful. The process of artificial selection was carried on for a period of two years, at the end of which this variant exhibited characteristics which were essentially the same as at the outset, except that the peculiar irregular colony shape had been almost completely lost. But for their extremely small size, the colonies appeared fairly typical of the species. The cellular morphology had been altered to the extent that the filamentous forms were less numerous.

EXPERIMENT 2

The procedure was similar to that of experiment 1, except that 15 strains of S. pullorum were employed, instead of only 4. The sources of these strains were as follows:

Strain	*Source*
I, II and III	Diseased chicks, 1933.
IV	Carrier hen, 1932. (Same as strain IV, exp. 1.)
V and VI	Diseased chicks, 1933.
VII	Old laboratory strain which fermented maltose.
VIII and IX	Diseased chicks, 1933.
X, XI and XII	Carrier hens, 1933.
XIII	Diseased chick, 1933.
XIV	Young pullet, 1932.
XV	Diseased chick, 1933.

All but two of the strains exhibited the typical characteristics of S. pullorum. Strain VII, when originally isolated and for some time after, was, from all appearances, a maltose non-fermenting strain, but later attacked this sugar. Strain XIV grew with difficulty in the different mediums, settled out in broth, and produced some atypical colonies and cellular forms.

One month after the last set of broth tubes was inoculated all of the broth cultures were streaked on agar plates. While previous transfers to agar had revealed no change from the typical, all strains at this time exhibited some degree of colony variation as a result of the frequent broth to broth transfer and aging in the broth cultures. Through a process of selection of colonies that varied from the normal, and by repeated transfer, three definite variants were obtained from strains VI, VIII and IX. Variants VIII-a and IX-a were cultivated and transferred at frequent intervals on meat extract agar. Both of these exhibited a marked change from the original in their colony form, the new colonial variants being quite stable. The new colonial type variants were more or less alike; they exhibited an irregular shape, effuse periphery, raised and opaque central portion, rough surface and brittle consistency. Colonies were frequently observed to attain from five to seven millimeters in diameter. The cells were slightly pleomorphic. Variant VI-a was cultivated on liver infusion agar, with frequent transfers. It developed colony types that were not strikingly different from the so-called "normal" on liver infusion agar, and never approached the marked roughness and colony size (2 cm.) of variant IX-a, when the latter was subjected to the same treatment. The cells were extremely pleomorphic, long and thick filaments predominating.

Two and one-half months after the last set of infusion broth tubes was inoculated, four of the sets were streaked on agar plates, and the colony characteristics noted. No changes were apparent, but after five and one-half months of holding strains I, II and XV in the same broth cultures exhibited definite variation, when plated out. The variants (I-a and II-a) derived from strains I and II were maintained on liver infusion agar through frequent transfer, whereas the one obtained from strain XV gradually reverted to normal. The colony type of variants I-a and II-a were identical and possessed the following features: raised growth with a crenated edge, a marked convoluted periphery, and a slightly rough, dull and opaque interior. Cellular forms were highly pleomorphic.

Six months after the last set of broth tubes was inoculated three additional variants (from strains XII and XIII) were isolated from the broth cultures. One of these variants (XIII-a) was cultivated on liver infusion agar, one (XII-a) on meat extract agar, and the third (XII-b) on liver infusion agar. Variant XIII-a resembled I-a and II-a, while XII-a exhibited a smooth mound-shaped, opaque, undulated colony (figure 3). Few unusual cell types were present. Variant XII-b produced a dentated colony with a striated convoluted and tenacious periphery, and a raised, dense, faintly convoluted central portion. Cells in the periphery were entirely filamentous, while in the central portion they approached the normal (figures 4, 5, and 6)

EXPERIMENT 3

In this part of the investigation 13 of the 15 strains employed in experiment 2, and three additional strains, were subjected to the same treatment as was applied in the second experiment. The three additional strains (XVI, XVII and XVIII) had been maintained under laboratory cultivation for more than ten years.

Six strains (III, V, X, XV, XVI and XVIII) yielded definite colony variants similar to the types previously described; three colonial types of one strain were observed. In a few instances the changes from the normal were not of sufficient magnitude and stability to receive recognition as types. Immediate reversion to the normal parent type was also observed in a few sub-strains that appeared quite remote from the normal in their colonial features. Such types could not be stabilized by the colony selection method.

EXPERIMENT 4

Liver infusion broth was used in place of the meat infusion medium, since the former is regarded as a more complex and favorable medium for stimulating luxuriant growth, which is often conducive to variation. The composition of the liver infusion broth was as follows: extract of 500 grams of beef liver, 1,000 cc., and Bacto-peptone (Difco), 10 grams.

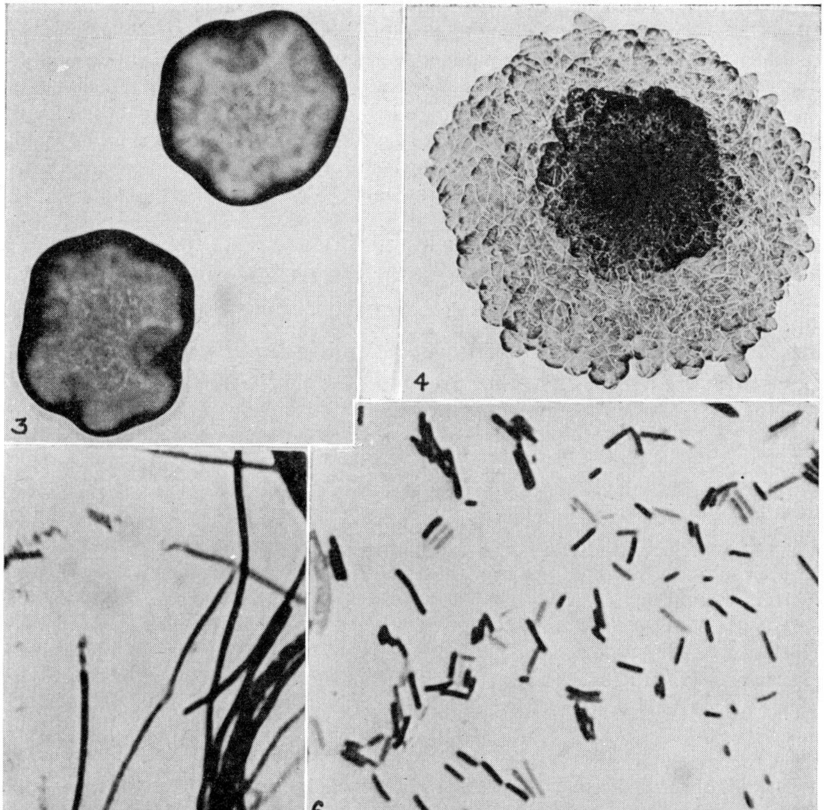

Fig. 3.—Variant XII-a. Two-day-old colonies on meat extract agar. ×50 diameters.

Fig. 4.—Variant XII-b. Three-day-old colony on liver infusion agar. ×10 diameters.

Fig. 5.—Variant XII-b. Filamentous forms in a smear prepared from the peripheral portion of the colony illustrated in figure 4. ×1200 diameters.

Fig. 6.—Variant XII-b. Type of cells in a smear prepared from the central portion of the colony illustrated in figure 4. ×1200 diameters.

Fig. 7.—Variant XVIII-a. Two-day-old colony on meat extract agar. ×25 diameters.

The experimental procedure and bacterial strains were the same as those used in Experiment 2. Variation was not brought about as readily as in the previous studies. The majority of cultures were found to be sterile when examined two months after inoculation. A change from p_H 7.0–7.2 to p_H 4.5–5.8 took place in the H-ion concentration. This pronounced acid production, together with the accumulation of other metabolic products, obviously accounted for the sterility of the cultures. None of the surviving strains produced variants; however, by making frequent transfers on liver infusion agar (liver infusion broth containing 1.5 per cent Difco agar), two definite variants (II-b and X-c) were obtained.

INFLUENCE OF COLONY SELECTION AND FREQUENT TRANSFER ON VARIATION TREND

Selection of marked colonies on solid medium was found to be an important means of deriving variants of S. pullorum. Extreme colonial types may be established by this procedure, particularly when it is continued over long periods of time.

EXPERIMENT 5

Two old strains (I and II employed in experiment 1) which revealed some degree of variation in colony type were selected for this experiment. Both strains produced smooth and rough colonies as well as intermediate types. By means of frequent transfer on meat extract agar, and by selecting the roughest and smoothest types of colonies at each tranfser, it was possible to isolate a rough strain which remained stable and a smooth type which at times would exhibit a certain degree of roughness. The rough variants derived from strains I and II were designated A and B, respectively, while the smooth forms were recorded as A-1 and B-1, respectively. Considerable similarity was observed between the two rough types, both of which resembled the type described for variant VIII-a.

EXPERIMENT 6

The purpose of this experiment was to determine the influence of frequent transfer on variants and on normal S. pullorum strains when cultivated on liver infusion agar. Because liver medium yields a more luxuriant growth than meat extract and infusion mediums, it was regarded as being, perhaps, a favorable factor in producing and stabilizing variants.

The following strains were employed:

I—Same as I in experiment 1.
IV-a—Variant derived from IV in experiment 1.
XII and XIV—Same as XII and XIV in experiment 2.

The same liver infusion agar was used as in Experiment 4. At the beginning the transfers were made at 48-hour intervals, which were later increased to four or five days. The colonial response of strains I, IV-a and XIV was very impressive. A most striking difference was observed between these three strains and the normal strain XII. Strain IV-a did not yield a stable variant on liver agar, even after a second trial, and reversion to the normal colony type occurred after a period of eight months. Strain XIV also produced a type of colony that did not submit to complete stabilization. Variant C, derived from strain I, exhibited characteristics which resembled those of variant IX-b. The two variants (D_1 and D_2) derived from strain IV-a, at the outset produced a very irregular colony possessing numerous projections. The structure was partly or entirely granular and filamentous. The colony appeared dull and could be removed in toto. The cellular forms were thick filaments of various lengths, as well as other bizarre forms. Variant E derived from strain XIV exhibited a very angular colony, and the structure of the projections and interior was markedly striated. The cellular types in the young striated colonies consisted largely of slender filamentous forms, while the older colonies contained cells of various sizes.

Miscellaneous attempts to induce variation by other expedients, such as (a) alternate transfer in liquid and on solid mediums, (b) cultivation in medium with increased concentration of peptone, (c) growing in deep liquid medium, and (d) cultivation in meat extract solution, failed to produce variants of S. pullorum in this investigation.

BEHAVIOR OF VARIANTS IN DIFFERENT ENVIRONMENTS

Numerous investigations, reviewed by Hadley,[4] show that organisms may lose or gain various properties, and that some are more readily altered than others. Colonial and cellular morphology, and pathogenic and serologic characteristics seem to be most susceptible to change, while fermentative and other biochemical properties are more resistant.

In this investigation particular attention was given to the behavior of the variants in (1) broth, (2) NaCl solution, (3) fermentable substances, (4) fresh whole egg (in the shell) and egg yolk, and (5) the natural host. The results are summarized briefly here.

Variants of S. pullorum settled out in broth cultures, but the degree of settling varied among the different sub-strains. Likewise, their stability in NaCl solution varied among different types, and even fluctuated within the same type. The ability to attack different fermentable substances appeared to be changed but little, if any, in all of the variants. The sojourn of the different variants in fresh whole egg and in the natural host (chicks and mature fowl) apparently had little or no influence on their general features.

VIRULENCE AND SEROLOGICAL STUDIES

The virulence of S. pullorum is known to fluctuate greatly. Avirulent strains have been isolated simultaneously with highly virulent types from the same natural disease outbreak. Diminished or complete loss of virulence is frequently associated with change in other properties of micro-organisms, such as colonial and cellular morphology, antigenicity and agglutinability. Virulence study in this investigation included determination of this property in the natural host (chick) and in an alien host (guinea pig). Comparative virulence tests were made of 19 different strains (including variants and their parent strains). Small lots of day-old chicks were employed.

The different groups of chicks within each lot were kept in separate cages. The procedure of infecting the chicks was in general the same throughout the investigation. Saline suspensions of the organism having a turbidity equal to tube 2 of McFarland's nephelometer were prepared from 24 hour agar cultures and inoculated subcutaneously. Previous infection experiments had demonstrated that 0.4 cc. of such suspensions prepared with the so-called normal bacterial strains were fatal, when injected subcutaneously. In order to further insure definite response, the different lots of chicks were chilled immediately after inoculation. Chicks within the same lot were given the same treatment, except in one instance where not all of the chicks were chilled. Clinical manifestations were recorded and all chicks that died were necropsied and examined bacteriologically. Two weeks after the inoculation, the surviving chicks were killed and subjected to the same post-mortem examination.

4. J. Infect. Dis. 40: 1, 1927.

In the eleven lots of inoculated chicks a striking difference in virulence was observed between some of the parent strains and their variants. In a few lots (I, IV and V), the parent strain appeared as nearly avirulent as its derived variant type. As stated earlier, this may be explained in part by the fact that the parent cultures were not typically "normal." In one instance (lot IV) the derived variant (E) exhibited a virulence similar to that of its parent strain (XIV), which at times showed characteristics that were remote from the normal type. These observations confirm those of Plastridge and Rettger,[5] who showed that variants may be extremely virulent. Such types, although apparently rare, are very baffling to the diagnostician and cause considerable difficulty in attempts to establish species identity, especially for one who has not encountered them before.

Variants III-a and VIII-a failed to establish themselves in chicks after five inoculations, but after fourteen inoculations of strain VIII-a positive results were obtained. Relative to the positive isolations, one may question whether strain VIII-a reverted to the normal type, or whether it was a pure variant, and contained a few normal cells which, upon repeated injection gradually established themselves as a so-called typical strain. The latter view seems the more plausible, although this is still a matter of speculation, since it is impossible to follow the cell progeny of a mass culture.

Table 1 gives the comparative results obtained with parent and variant strains, when inoculated into chicks. The differences in the percentages of mortality and positive isolation between the two groups are very significant.

TABLE 1.—*Comparative Virulence of Parent and Variant Strains of S. pullorum*

Treatment	No. of Chicks	Chicks Died		Chicks Yielding S. pullorum	
		No.	Per cent	No.	Per cent
Inoculated with parent strain	120	48	40.00	90	75.00
Inoculated with variant	130	5	3.85	21	16.15
Controls not inoculated	52	2	3.84	0	0.00

A comparative study of the behavior of normal strains and their variants in 46 guinea pigs showed that the variants did not possess the invasive power of their parent strains, which substantiated the general findings recorded in the chick experiments.

Serological investigation of the variants showed that they were different from their parent strains in their antigenic properties. This is in harmony with the observations of Arkwright,[6] De Kruif,[7] Schütze,[8] White,[9] and others, who ascribed peculiar immunizing and agglutinogenic properties to variants.

Several normal strains and their variants were studied. This phase of the investigation bears a direct relationship to the routine serological diagnosis

5. J. Infect. Dis. **47**: 334, 1930; **54**: 23, 1934.
6. J. Path. and Bact. **24**: 36, 1921.
7. J. Exper. Med. **33**: 773, 1921.
8. J. Hyg. **20**: 330, 1921.
9. J. Path. and Bact. **35**: 77, 1932; **36**: 65, 1933.

of pullorum disease, because, as will be pointed out, S. pullorum strains can be altered in their antigenic structure to the extent that they lose their power to produce agglutinins in the host and fail to absorb the specific agglutinins.

Realizing the fact that a salt-sensitive variant cannot be employed as a satisfactory strain for antigen preparation, an effort was made to stabilize such a type and yet maintain optimum conditions for agglutination. From the literature one may gain the impression that the problem of maintaining variants suspended in saline solution is of minor importance. It is possible that the variants reported by others were of a different character from those dealt with here. However, while variant types that are different in their salt-sensitiveness do occur, it is also possible that different interpretations may be made of the behavior of variants in salt solution. In tests conducted with the variants a combination of agglutination and settling of cells occurred in certain instances. Some variants form perceptible clumps in salt solution, while others settle in the salt solutions without perceptible clumping. With either type of variant, the reaction with positive serums may be quite complex and the end result baffling.

White[10] reported that variants can be made stable in salt solution by treating the cells with 95 per cent alcohol, and that the alcoholic extract contains an antigenic substance, which suggests that the variant itself has been deprived of some of its chemical components by the alcohol treatment. To what extent one can proceed in subjecting the organism to extracting agents without depriving the same of its essential constituents for true agglutination remains a question.

To determine the agglutinogenic power of the variants, adult birds which were negative to the macroscopic agglutination test with pullorum antigen, and presumably pullorum disease-free, were inoculated with normal and variant strains of S. pullorum. Their serums were tested at frequent intervals with known pullorum antigen. The results obtained with one series of fowl are reported in table 2. The birds inoculated with the normal strain developed

TABLE 2.—*Behavior of a Parent Normal Strain and its Variant in the Natural Adult Host*

Strain No.	Bird No.	Number of Injections	Agglutinin Titer (Days after first injection) 8	12	19	28	33	40	47	54	69	82	97	124	190	Isolation of S. pullorum
	18950	6	80	1280	2560	—	—	640	—	320	320	160	160	80	20	Positive
VIII	19018	6	320	1280	+5120	—	—	2560	—	640	640	320	320	320	160	Negative
	19050	6	5120	2560	1280	—	—	160	—	40	20	40	20	20	40	Negative
	18882	13	0	0	0	0	20	20	10	0	0	0	0	10	0	Negative
	18989	13	0	0	0	0	20	10	10	0	0	0	0	10	0	Negative
VIII-a	19002	13	0	0	0	0	20	40	10	10	0	10	0	10	20	Negative
	19042	13	0	0	0	0	10	10	10	10	0	10	0	10	20	Negative
	19049	13	0	0	0	0	40	0	10	10	0	0	0	0	10	Negative

a definite titer within eight days after the first inoculation, while those receiving the variant gave no agglutinin response until after a second series of inoculations, which was administered approximately one month after the first inoculation. Furthermore, the agglutinin response observed in the birds receiving the variant was extremely feeble. All birds were necropsied at the

10. Medical Research Council. Special Report Series No. 103, 1926.

end of 190 days. While the titers at necropsy were considerably lower than those observed earlier, the birds may have been infected still, since S. pullorum was recovered from bird 18,950, which yielded a titer of 1:20.

These results showed that the variant VIII-a did not possess the power to stimulate agglutinin production in the living natural host to the extent that its parent strain did. Also, that it failed to establish itself in the natural host.

In the determination of the absorptive capacities of the different parent strains and their variants, five serums which varied in titer were absorbed with 12 original parent strains, 16 variants and 4 miscellaneous strains. It was clearly demonstrated here that variants do not possess the absorptive capacity of their parent strains.

DISCUSSION

It has been shown in this study that S. pullorum variants may occur among freshly isolated strains. Thirteen variants were discovered among 163 strains obtained from infected eggs, chicks and adult fowls. With one exception, they different from the normal type strain in that they exhibited salt-sensitiveness. Peculiarities in colonial and cellular morphology, and atypical behavior in broth, were observed in two instances. No variation in staining and biochemical reactions was detected. Identification of a typical S. pullorum strain requires a study of its various properties. If the colony type had been selected by the authors as the only means of recognizing variants, all of the strains studied, with the exception of two, would have been designated as typical. Likewise, if these strains had been identified only by the Gram-staining method and biochemical reactions, all would have been considered typical. Furthermore, only slight deviations, which may be overlooked by one not familiar with the characteristics of variants, may be observed at times. The property of salt-sensitiveness would in all probability escape detection when the rapid serum agglutination method is employed to determine the agglutinability of a freshly isolated strain.

Strains of S. pullorum placed under different environmental conditions may yield many sub-types. The observations reported in this investigation are in general agreement with those reported for other organisms. The majority of strains studied were susceptible to marked variation, which was induced readily by subjecting the strains to frequent transfer and holding in meat infusion broth. Various so-called normal strains responded differently to the same environment; this was observed particularly when the organisms were grown on liver infusion agar. The liver infusion medium may serve to bring out variation tendencies that otherwise would remain obscure. Differences in colonial and cellular morphology were observed. This was likewise true when the same variant was cultivated on meat extract agar and subsequently placed on liver infusion agar.

Variants were isolated and stabilized on solid mediums by colony selection and frequent transfer. The relation of one colony type to another cannot be explained with any degree of satisfaction. Certain daughter types appeared more remote from the parent strain than others, but this may be applicable only to one or more features such as colony form, virulence, and antigenic structure. To classify all of the different variants according to their order of development or degree of variation is not possible at this time. The realm of variation may possess great latitude, and the border between normal and variant types should not be looked upon as a sharp line of demarcation. A normal type may vary in some of its aspects, but the changes may not be perceptible. The terms "S" and "R" introduced by Arkwright for smooth and rough forms, seem inappropriate, because variants having a smooth surface, but which are far remote from the parent strain in their antigenic structure, may be observed. The correlation between colonial form and antigenic structure is by no means constant. This also applies to other features.

S. pullorum variants may settle out in broth cultures, but the degree of settling varies with the different types. This was likewise true when variants were suspended in sodium chloride solution. The ability of the variants to attack various fermentable substances was practically the same as that of the normal type. Passage through whole fresh egg (in the shell) and through the natural host (chicks and adult fowl) had little or no determining influence on the general features of the different types.

In general, the derived types exhibited a lesser degree of virulence than their parent strains, and in some instances appeared avirulent. Some variants (III-a and VIII-a) that appeared markedly different from the normal type on plain agar seemed to possess no invasive power and induced no gross local tissue response at the site of inoculation. It appeared that the defensive power, as well as the aggressive property, had been lost. However, repeated subcutaneous inoculation of massive doses of the variant yielded an organism of the normal type; this suggests a means of either bringing about reversion of the variant to the normal type, or ascertaining the purity of a given variant. The latter conjecture seems the more plausible in this instance.

Serological investigations showed that the agglutinogenic power and the absorptive capacity of the variants tested were not equal to those of the normal type. These observations appear significant, since they show that stock cultures employed for antigens used in the macroscopic agglutination test may vary in degree of sensitivity, and that the type of agglutination may be greatly influenced by the ratio of the variant to the normal type in a mixed population of cells.

In the selection of antigen strains for the macroscopic agglutination test it is highly important to choose only such as are pure in type, and will, on continued cultivation maintain their agglutinating stability. Furthermore, adopted strains should be tested at frequent intervals, to insure the constancy of their agglutinating properties.

SUMMARY

Among 163 freshly isolated strains of S. pullorum, 13 variants were detected. The behavior of these variants in sodium chloride solution of different concentrations and in the presence of positive and negative serums differed greatly. Other properties, such as colonial and cellular morphology, Gram-staining, and biochemical reactions revealed little or no variation, on the whole.

S. pullorum strains readily underwent variation when subjected to frequent transfer and storage in beef infusion broth.

When variants were cultivated on both meat extract agar and liver infusion agar the colonial and cellular features often appeared markedly different. Some strains that appeared normal on meat extract agar exhibited pleomorphic tendencies when placed on liver infusion agar.

Most variants exhibited a lesser degree of virulence than their parent strains, and in some instances appeared avirulent. The agglutinogenic power and the absorptive capacity of the variants tested were not equal to those of the normal type.

THE BACTERICIDAL EFFECT OF PEROXIDES IN IRRADIATED COD LIVER OIL

FRANKLIN A. STEVENS
NEW YORK

In preceding experiments[1] the observation was made that oil of pine acquired additional bactericidal properties if exposed to ultraviolet light. The following points were emphasized. First, salt solution shaken with certain essential oils retained enough of the oil either in suspension or solution to be bactericidal. Second, the bactericidal action of the salt solution was exhausted if bacteria were repeatedly suspended in the same solution. Third, salt solution shaken with irradiated oil of pine was more bactericidal than salt solution shaken with normal oil. Fourth, peroxides formed in the oil during irradiation were extracted by the salt solution and adhered to bacteria suspended in salt solution containing these peroxides. Since Harris, Bunker and Milas[2] have demonstrated that the bactericidal properties of vapor arising from the surface of animal and vegetable oils which have been exposed to ultraviolet light is proportional to the increase in peroxides in the oils occurring during the period of irradiation, attempts were made to prove that the peroxides formed in oil of pine during exposure to ultraviolet light were responsible for the increased bactericidal effect. The margin between the germicidal effect of normal and irradiated oil of pine was so narrow that experiments in this direction were inconclusive. On the other hand, salt solution shaken with normal cod liver oil is seldom bactericidal. In the following experiments in which the bactericidal action of cod liver oil has been demonstrated, a study of the bactericidal action of peroxides formed in the oil during irradiation with ultraviolet light has been possible. These peroxides are definitely bactericidal.

EXPERIMENTAL

The Bactericidal Action of Irradiated Cod Liver Oil on Hemolytic Streptococcus.—In the preceding paragraph experiments were cited in which it was demonstrated that irradiated oil of pine was more bactericidal than the normal oil. In these experiments hemolytic streptococcus was suspended in salt solutions which had been shaken vigorously with samples of normal and of irradiated oil. Cultures of these suspensions were made at intervals to determine the time limits of the viability of the bacteria in these suspensions. The methods employed in studying the bactericidal properties of irradiated oil of pine on hemolytic streptococcus have been used to study

Received for publication, July 25, 1935.

From the Department of Medicine, College of Physicians and Surgeons, Columbia University, and the Presbyterian Hospital.

1. Stevens, F. A.: J. Lab. & Clin. Med., in press.
2. Indust. & Engin. Chem. **24:** 1181, 1932.

the bactericidal properties of irradiated cod liver oil in the following experiments.

1. *The Bactericidal Action of Irradiated Cod Liver Oil.*—Six strains of hemolytic streptococcus, 273, E 37, NY V, E 38, Si and C 203 were used in this experiment. Twenty cc. of cod liver oil were exposed to the light from an ultraviolet quartz lamp for three hours. A layer of oil 0.5 cm. in depth was exposed to the light in a large flat vessel. This oil was then shaken vigorously with 100 cc. of sterile salt solution in a rubber capped bottle. Twenty cc. of normal oil were shaken with 100 cc. of salt solution for control tests. The bottles were inverted and the salt solutions were withdrawn from beneath the oil after eighteen hours. Nine cc. quantities of 18 hour broth cultures of the strains of hemolytic streptococcus were centrifuged and the bacterial sediment from the centrifuged culture of each strain was suspended in 3 cc. of the salt solution which had been agitated with the irradiated oil. An additional series of tubes containing bacterial sediment from the same quantities of the same cultures of these strains were used for controls. In this control series the sediment was suspended in salt solutions previously shaken with normal oil. The suspensions were cultured at frequent intervals until the bacteria were dead or until it was evident that they would live indefinitely. The results of these tests have been arranged in table 1, to show the death point of the bacteria in terms of hours. The letter D is followed by a numeral indicating the time limit in hours of the viability of the bacteria in each solution. In some instances scant growth with only two or three bacterial colonies on the plated culture is indicated by the letter S followed by the numeral indicating the hours elapsing from the time the bacteria were first suspended in the solution. The letter L indicates that the bacteria were viable and cultures were discontinued at the indicated hour.

TABLE 1.—*The Bactericidal Action of Irradiated Cod Liver Oil on Hemolytic Streptococcus*

Strain	273	E 37	NY V	E 38	Si	C 203
Salt solution shaken with normal oil...	L 80 hrs.	L 80 hrs.	L 80 hrs.	L 80 hrs.	L 80 hrs.	L 80 hrs.
Salt solution shaken with irradiated oil	D 33	S 25 D 33	D 60	S 22 D 25	S 25 D 33	S 33 D 60
Bacteria in physiologic salt solution...	L 80	L 80	L 80	L 80	L 80	L 80

The Bactericidal Action of Peroxides Formed During the Irradiation of Cod Liver Oil.—In previous studies[3] it was observed that both peroxides and aldehydes were formed during the irradiation of mineral oil or of oil of pine. If these oils were tested directly by agitating them with acidified starch potassium iodide mixtures or with Schiff's reagent both tests were positive. Irradiated cod liver oil also gives positive tests when tested directly with these reagents. Furthermore, salt solution shaken with irradiated oil of pine or cod liver oil gives intense reactions for peroxides and weakly positive reactions for aldehydes. In the following experiments neutralized cysteine HCl, neutralized thioglycolic acid and alanine have been added to the bactericidal salt solutions before the bacteria were suspended in them. The two reducing reagents, the cysteine and the thioglycolic acid, destroyed the bactericidal properties while alanine, which is not a reducing reagent, had no effect whatever. The conclusion from these experiments is, that the peroxides are bactericidal, since the addition of reducing reagents prior to the suspension of the bacteria in the solutions destroyed the bactericidal qualities. The final concentration of cysteine, thioglycolic acid and alanine in the solutions in which the bacteria were suspended was .05 per cent. In this concentration none of these reagents affects the intensity of the reaction for aldehydes obtained on the addition of Schiff's reagent, so it is improbable that the cysteine and thioglycolic acid neutralize the bactericidal properties of these solutions through combinations with the traces of aldehydes present.

2. *The Neutralization of the Bactericidal Effect by the Addition of Cysteine*—In this experiment the salt solution and cultures were prepared as in experiment 1. The control of salt solution shaken with unirradiated oil was omitted. Four of the strains previously employed were used. Three tubes containing 9 cc. of the culture of each strain were centrifuged and the

3. Stevens, F. A.: J. Lab. & Clin. Med., in press.

sediment suspended in the following solutions: (1) 3 cc. of salt solution shaken with irradiated cod liver oil, (2) 3 cc. of the same salt solution to which neutralized cysteine hydrochloride was added so that the final concentration of cysteine was .05 per cent, (3) plain salt solution with a concentration of .05 per cent cysteine. These suspensions were cultured as in experiment 1. The results of these tests are arranged in table 2.

TABLE 2.—*The Neutralization of the Bactericidal Effect by the Addition of Cysteine*

Strain	E 38	E 37	Si	273
Salt solution shaken with irradiated oil	S 24 hrs. D 40	S 24 hrs. D 40	S 24 hrs. D 40	S 40 hrs. D 49
Salt solution shaken with irradiated oil +cysteine .05%	L 90	L 90	L 90	L 90
Salt solution +cysteine .05%	L 90	L 90	L 90	L 90

3. *The Comparative Effect of Cysteine and Alanine in Neutralizing the Bactericidal Properties of the Salt Solution.*—The procedure in this experiment was similar to that in experiment 2. The control of cysteine in salt solution has been omitted. An additional suspension of streptococcus in salt solution previously shaken with irradiated cod liver oil has been included. Alanine to the concentration of .05 per cent has been added to this suspension. The results of the cultures are to be found in table 3.

TABLE 3.—*The Neutralizing Effect of Thioglycolic Acid, Cysteine and Alanine on the Bactericidal Properties of the Salt Solution*

Strain of hemolytic streptococcus	Si	C 203	NY V	E 38	273
Suspension of culture in salt solution shaken with irradiated oil	S 6 hrs. D 22	S 22 hrs.	D 22 hrs.	S 6 hrs. D 22	S 22 hrs. D 30
Suspension in salt solution shaken with irradiated oil +.05% alanine	S 6 D 22	D 22	D 22	S 22 D 30	D 22
Suspension in bactericidal salt solution +.05% thioglycolic acid	S 22 D 30	D 46	L 46	D 46	D 46
Suspension in bactericidal salt solution +.05% cysteine	L 54			L 54	S 54

4. *The Neutralization of the Bactericidal Effect by the Addition of Thioglycolic Acid.*—In this experiment the cultures and the salt solution were prepared as in the preceding experiments. The sediment from 9 cc. of culture of each strain was suspended (1) in 3 cc. of salt solution which had been shaken with oil irradiated 3 hours, (2) in 3 cc. of this salt solution to which alanine to the concentration of .05 per cent had been added and (3) in the salt solution to which neutralized thioglycolic acid had been added to the concentration of .05 per cent. The results of this experiment are charted in table 3 together with the results of experiment 3.

The Bactericidal Effect of Peroxides Adsorbed on Bacteria from Salt Solution Shaken with Irradiated Cod Liver Oil.—It was observed in one of the preceding experiments (1) that salt solution shaken with cod liver oil which had previously been exposed to ultraviolet light was bactericidal. When this salt solution was tested for peroxides and aldehydes with potassium iodide, starch and acid and with Schiff's reagent, strong tests for peroxides and weak tests for aldehydes were obtained. In further experiments (2, 3, and 4), in which neutralized cysteine HCl and thioglycolic acid were added to the salt solution before bacteria were suspended in it, the bactericidal effect was destroyed. In experiments with irradiated oil of pine peroxides formed in the oil by irradiation were similarly extractable in salt solution and adhered to bacteria suspended in solutions of salt containing the peroxides. In the following experiments the adsorption of the peroxides in salt solution agitated with cod liver oil has been studied. First, bacteria have been suspended in these solutions and subsequently tested for peroxides after centrifugation. Second, the sediment from cultures has been suspended in the salt solution, centrifuged, and the viability of the bacteria studied after these bacteria previously exposed to peroxides were suspended in normal salt solution. Third, the protective action of cysteine and thioglycolic acid on bacteria exposed previously for short periods to the peroxides has been investigated. The conclusions from these experiments are that peroxides adhere to the bacterial bodies and that reducing agents introduced into the environment of the bacteria subsequent to this reaction afford little if any protection.

5. *The Adherence of Peroxides to Bacteria.*—Cultures of hemolytic streptococcus were grown 24 hours. Two tubes containing 50 cc. of the culture of each of five strains were centrifuged and the sediment washed with salt solution. The sediment from one tube was suspended in 3 cc. of salt solution previously agitated with irradiated cod liver oil. After 18 hours the bacteria in the second tube were centrifuged, washed once in salt solution and resuspended in 3 cc. of fresh salt solution. 0.1 cc. of 2 per cent solution of KI, .5 cc. of 5N, H_2SO_4 and starch indicator were added to all the tubes and the suspensions were allowed to settle overnight. The bacteria exposed to the salt solution agitated with cod liver oil were blue. The controls showed negative tests for peroxides.

6. *The Bactericidal Effect of Peroxides Adherent to Hemolytic Streptococcus.*—In this experiment cultures of three strains, 273, E 38 and Si were employed. Three tubes containing 9 cc. of a culture of each strain were centrifuged and the sediments in these tubes were suspended in salt solution previously agitated with irradiated cod liver oil. One of these tubes was centrifuged after two hours, the second after four hours and the third after six hours. All the three sediments were resuspended in physiologic saline solution and cultures made at intervals to determine the duration of the viability of the bacteria (table 4).

TABLE 4.—*The Bactericidal Effect of Peroxides Adherent to Hemolytic Streptococcus*

Strain	273	E 38	Si
Contact 2 hours	D 28 H	S 2 H D 28 H	S 20 H D 28 H
Contact 4 hours	S 20 H D 28 H	D 20 H	S 20 H D 28 H
Contact 6 hours	S 20 H D 28 H	D 20 H	S 20 H D 28 H

7. *The Bactericidal Effect of Adherent Peroxides in the Presence of Reducing Agents (Thioglycolic Acid and Cysteine).*—In these experiments cultures of hemolytic streptococcus were centrifuged and the sediment from 9 cc. of culture suspended in salt solution previously agitated with irradiated oil. After two hours the bacteria were centrifuged and the sediment resuspended (1) in normal salt solution, (2) in salt solution containing .05 per cent of neutralized thioglycolic acid and (3) in a solution containing .05 per cent cysteine. Cultures were made at intervals on the resuspended bacteria (table 5). In previous experiments the oil was irradiated three hours. In experiment 7 the oil was irradiated six hours.

TABLE 5.—*The Continued Action of Adherent Peroxides in the Presence of Reducing Agents*

Strain	Si	C 203	NY V	E 38	273
Resuspended in saline solution	S 2 H D 18 H	L 2 H D 18 H	L 2 H D 18 H	S 2 H D 18 H	S 2 H D 18 H
Resuspended in saline solution + cysteine	S 18 H D 26 H	L 2 H D 18 H	S 18 H D 26 H	S 2 H D 18 H	L 2 H D 18 H
Resuspended in saline solution + thioglycolic acid	S 2 H D 18 H	L 2 H D 18 H	S 2 H D 18 H	S 18 H D 26 H	S 2 H D 18 H

SUMMARY AND CONCLUSIONS

In the preceding experiments the bactericidal effect of peroxides formed in cod liver oil during irradiation with ultraviolet light has been demonstrated. These peroxides are either soluble in or are miscible with salt solution, and by adding reducing agents such as cysteine or thioglycolic acid the bactericidal effect on hemolytic streptococcus is overcome. Peroxides are taken out of salt solution by the bacteria. Either brief contact is sufficient to injure the bacteria so that they eventually die, or the effect of the peroxides adherent to the cells continues over several hours, because the introduction of reducing agents into the environment of streptococcus previously exposed to the peroxides fails to overcome the bactericidal effect.

THE ANTIGENIC SIMILARITY OF TWO STRAINS OF NON-CAPSULATED, METHEMOGLOBIN-PRODUCING ORGANISMS TO TYPE XXIX PNEUMOCOCCUS

SARAH EYRE

AND

W. D. STOVALL

MADISON, WISCONSIN

Considerable attention has been directed to the antigenic structure of the pneumococcus. It is well established that pneumococcus types I, II, and III are composed of two fractions, one a carbohydrate complex conferring type specificity; the other protein in nature and species specific. The same antigenic structure is assumed for the other types of pneumococci. While very little investigation has been made of the related methemoglobin-producing Streptococcus viridans, Lancefield[1] has demonstrated the presence in this group of antigenic components analogous to the carbohydrate and protein fractions of the pneumococcus. The latter fraction as derived from Streptococcus viridans shows a close relationship to the protein fraction of the pneumococcus. In this paper we wish to present evidence of the similarity of the carbohydrate or type-specific fraction of two strains of methemoglobin-producing, non-capsulated organisms, not pneumococci by the recognized tests, to type XXIX pneumococcus.

SOURCE AND DESCRIPTION OF STRAINS

Strain Br was isolated from a blood culture of a case of bacterial endocarditis. When first obtained, the colonies on 5 per cent rabbit-blood-agar were small, smooth, dome-shaped and opaque. Upon subsequent transfer they became larger, flat, and granular. The growth in broth was diffuse. The organisms were not soluble in a 1:10 or a 50:50 mixture of Bacto ox-bile. They did not agglutinate spontaneously in 0.85 per cent saline. No capsule could be demonstrated. Doses of 0.1 cc. of a 16-hour broth culture caused death of mice in twenty-four hours. Mice survived smaller doses. Fermentation reactions classified the strain as Streptococcus salivarius sub-group 2 (Brown).[2]

Strain L 3 was isolated from nasopharyngeal culture of a normal individual. On 5 per cent rabbit-blood-agar the colonies were opaque, coarsely granular, flattened, with a central elevation and irregular edges. When first isolated the strain grew as a coarse floccular sediment in broth. After several mouse passages a diffuse type of growth was obtained, but the strain tended

Received for publication, July 25, 1935.

From the State Laboratory of Hygiene, University of Wisconsin.

1. J. Exper. Med. 42: 397, 1925
2. Rockefeller Inst. for M. Res., Monograph 9, 1919.

to revert to the aggregate type of growth. The strain was partially soluble in a 50:50 Bacto ox-bile mixture after twenty-four hours exposure at 37 C., but there was no decrease in the number of organisms after the same time in a 1:10 bile mixture. No capsule could be demonstrated. The organisms did not agglutinate spontaneously in 0.85 per cent saline. Virulence for mice was slight, 0.1 cc. of broth culture causing death in 24 hours. Fermentation reactions classified the strain as Streptococcus salivarius sub-group 1 (Brown).[2]

AGGLUTINATION IN PNEUMOCOCCUS ANTISERUM

Sabin[3] slide-agglutination tests were performed with cultures of strains Br and L3 using pneumococcus antiserums for types I to XXXII. It was found that the strains agglutinated slightly in a number of the type-serums, definitely in a few; and markedly in type XXIX antiserum. Tube agglutination tests were then run using those serums which gave the most definite agglutination by the slide method.

Type-specific agglutination of a typical pneumococcus strain, due to the union of the carbohydrate fraction with its antibody, is characterized by "compact" agglutination. The agglutinated organisms are formed into a disc, large flakes, or compact particles which do not break up upon being shaken. Non-specific agglutination, on the other hand, observed with rough pneumococci, and due to the protein antigen-antibody union, is characterized by agglutination into fine particles which are easily shaken apart. The Br and L3 strains agglutinated in type XXIX pneumococcus antiserum in large compact flakes which are not broken up by shaking. The agglutination of these strains in type VI a and b antiserum is also of the type-specific character. The particles are large and do not shake out. Three strains of type XXIX pneumococcus tested agglutinated in low dilutions of type VI a and b antiserum, with the formation of large compact particles.

Agglutination of strains Br and L3 in the other pneumococcus antiserums used was of the fine type, and is due presumably to the similarity in the protein fractions of the methemoglobin-producing group.

AGGLUTINATION TESTS IN ANTISERUMS PREPARED FOR STRAINS BR AND L3

Antiserums were prepared for strains Br and L3 by essentially the same method as is used in our laboratory for preparing pneumococcus antiserums. Intravenous injections of heat-killed (54 C. for one-half hour) organisms from a 16-hour broth culture are given a rabbit on three successive days followed by four days' rest. A total of 15 such injections is given to produce pneumococcus antiserum of required type-specific titer (1:320). It was found that six injections (two series) of strains Br and L3 were sufficient to produce antiserums with a titer of 1:4000. In order to guard against a possible variation in the strain during culture over the period of the injections, sufficient quantity of the heat-killed vaccine was prepared from one culture to last during the course of injections. A required quantity of this stock was centri-

3. Proc. Soc. Exper. Biol. & Med. **26:** 492, 1929.

TABLE 1.—*Agglutination Tests with Type XXIX Pneumococcus, Strains Br and L3*

Test Strain	Antiserum	Antiserum Dilutions 1:5	1:10	1:20	1:40	1:80	1:100	1:200	1:400	1:800	1:1000	1:2000	1:4000	1:8000	Control
Type XXIX	Type XXIX	+++	++++	++++	++++	++++	++++	+++	++	(+)					
	Br (6)	+++	+++	+++											
	Br (9)	++++	(+)												
	L3 (6)	++++	(+)												
	L3 (9)	(+)													
	L3 (15)														
Br	Type XXIX	++	+++	+++	+++	+++	+++	+	±	±	±	(±)			
	Br (6)	++	++	++	++	++	++	++	++	+	+	+	±	±	
	Br (9)	++	+	+	+	+	±	±	±	±	±	±	(±)	(±)	
	L3 (6)	++	+++	+++	(+++)	++	++	++	+	±					
	L3 (9)														
	L3 (15)	+	+	+	±	±	±	±	(±)						
L3	Type XXIX	++*	++*	++*	++*	++*	+†	±							
	Br (6)	++*	++*	++*	++*	++*	++*	+†	+†	±					
	Br (9)	++*	++*	++*	+†	+†	+†	±	(±)						
	L3 (6)	+†	+†	+†	++*	++*	++*	++*	++*	+†	+†	±	±		
	L3 (9)	±	±	±	±	±	±	(±)	(±)						
	L3 (15)	±	±	±	+†	++*	+†	+†	+†	+†	+†	±	±	±	

++++ Compact disc.
+++ Large compact flakes.
++ Large compact particles.
\+ Medium granular agglutination.
± Fine agglutination.
++* Compact floccular.
+† Medium floccular.
( ) Incomplete agglutination.
[ ] No agglutination.

Figures in parentheses after "Antiserum" represent number of injections which rabbit had received at time serum was tested for agglutinins.

fuged, the organisms were taken up in 0.85 per cent saline, and the suspension was reheated for each injection.

For agglutination tests dilutions of the antiserum were made in 0.5 cc. quantities, and an equal volume of broth culture of the test organisms was added. The tests were placed in a water-bath at 54 C. for two hours, then in the icebox until the next morning. Final readings were made after refrigeration.

The results of agglutination tests with antiserums prepared against strains Br and L3 and type XXIX pneumococcus are shown in table 1. It is evident from cross-agglutination that strains Br, L3, and type XXIX contain some similar antigenic fraction. From the type of agglutination observed we believe that this is the carbohydrate or type-specific fraction.

It was found that serum drawn from a rabbit after six injections of the Br strain agglutinated type XXIX pneumococcus in a dilution of 1:20, whereas after nine injections true disc agglutination occurred only in a dilution of 1:5. The tests were performed with the same culture of type XXIX pneumococcus. Likewise, serum from a rabbit receiving only six injections of strain L3 gave disc agglutination of type XXIX in a dilution of 1:5, and coarse particles in a 1:10 dilution. Serum from the same rabbit after nine injections of L3 agglutinated type XXIX in a dilution of 1:5 with the formation of coarse particles. Serum from another rabbit which had received 15 injections of strain L3 failed to agglutinate type XXIX pneumococcus. The difference in titer and type of agglutination of the homologous strain in serum drawn from a rabbit after six injections and again after nine injections of the strain is evident from the tables. It has been recognized by Lancefield[1] and others that the titer of the specific antibodies for certain groups of organisms may decrease as the course of injections is lengthened. This is in contrast to the condition described for pneumococci where a long course of injections is necessary to produce type-specific serum of high titer.

Difference in manner and type of agglutination were marked in the two strains, Br and L3. The L3 strain agglutinated very rapidly and maximum agglutination took place during the two hours in the water-bath. The agglutination in homologous antiserum was floccular and corresponds to the H type of agglutination found in the typhoid group. The Br strain agglutinated more slowly in homologous antiserum, the maximum titer being evident only after refrigeration. The agglutination was more granular than floccular.

ABSORPTION TESTS

Absorption tests with antiserum prepared against strains Br, L3 and type XXIX pneumococcus were performed in the following manner. The growth from a 16 hour broth culture of the strain to be used for absorption was concentrated by centrifuging and a 1:10 dilution of the serum to be absorbed was added in the proportion of 10 parts of diluted serum to one part of packed organisms. The mixture was placed in a water-bath at 45 C. for two hours, stirred frequently, and left in the icebox overnight. A maximum of three such absorptions were done if the antibodies for the test strain were not removed by one or two absorptions. The results may be summarized as follows:

Type XXIX pneumococcus removes its own and the agglutinins for Br and L3 from type XXIX antiserum. It removes its own and the agglutinins for L3 from Br antiserum, and reduces the specific titer for Br organisms. Type XXIX removes its own and Br specific agglutinins from L3 antiserum, and reduces the titer for the homologous organism, L3.

Br organisms remove Br and L3 specific agglutinins from type XXIX serum. After three absorptions the specific titer for type XXIX is reduced from 1:320 to 1:40. Br removes its own and the agglutinins for type XXIX and L3 from Br serum. It removes its own and type XXIX agglutinins from L3 serum, and reduces the L3 specific agglutinins leaving only fine agglutinins above a dilution of 1:200.

L3 strain removes its own agglutinins from type XXIX antiserum, but after three absorptions has no effect on the titer of type XXIX and Br agglutinins specific type. It removes all but a part of the fine agglutinins from homologous antiserum in three absorptions, and for Br in two adsorptions. L3 removes its own agglutinins from Br serum, and reduces the specific agglutinins for Br and for type XXIX after three absorptions.

DISCUSSION

In this paper we have demonstrated a similarity in the antigenic composition of two strains of organisms, which may be classified in the group of Streptococcus viridans, and certain types of pneumococci, particularly type XXIX. While the similarity is made apparent by cross-agglutination and absorption tests, certain dissimilarities are also evident. Thus, strain L3 (streptococcus) reduces the titer of Br (streptococcus) antiserum for the homologous organism, but fails to affect the titer of pneumococcus type XXIX antiserum for its homologous organism; while paradoxically the Br strain reduces the titer of specific agglutinins in type XXIX antiserum from 1:320 to 1:40 for type XXIX organisms. The contradiction here is that while there is clearly demonstrated, by absorption tests, a relation between strains L3 and Br, the failure of L3 to effect a reduction in the titer of type XXIX antiserum for type XXIX pneumococcus is not explained. In other words while there is clearly a specific relation between strains Br and L3, the tests do not show a specific relation between L3 and type XXIX pneumococcus, although there is a suggestion in the fact that type XXIX reduces the specific agglutinins for L3 in homologous antiserum.

From these results it seems possible that in type XXIX pneumococcus and strains Br and L3 there are specific antigens, not identical, but of sufficiently similar chemical structure to give cross-agglutination and some degree of cross-absorption. Such a possibility has been proposed by Avery, Heidelberger and Goebel[4] to explain the similarity of the type specific substance in type II pneumococci and a strain of Friedlander's bacillus.

SUMMARY

The experiments reported in this paper demonstrate the antigenic similarity of two strains of organisms classified as Streptococci viridans and type XXIX pneumococcus. This similarity appears to reside in the type specific carbohydrate fraction.

4. J. Exper. Med. 42: 709, 1925.

THE EFFECT OF BILE ON THE BACTERIOPHAGE PHENOMENON

MARTHA APPLEBAUM

AND

MARJORIE B. PATTERSON

NEW YORK

LITERATURE

The medical literature[1] of recent years pertaining to the bacteriophage phenomenon has repeatedly contained brief statements that bile is inhibitory to the action of the lytic agent. This reiteration has discouraged investigation, although the experiments have remained inconclusive. It seemed probable that an erroneous impression had prevailed due to the emphatic statement by d'Herelle[2] in 1926 that "when added to a bacterium-bacteriophage mixture, substances devoid of action upon the bacteria, have in general, no effect upon the phenomenon. Thus, the process is not modified, for example, by normal serum, ascitic fluid or urine. Bile is unquestionably inhibitory." D'Herelle[3] based this opinion on the work of Hauduroy who found that "in vitro the addition of bile to the medium inhibits bacteriophagy. The bacteriophage protobe is not destroyed, but its action is completely inhibited. In vivo, the bacilli which are found in the gall bladder are thus completely protected against bacteriophagy, and consequently when the infection involves the bladder the administration of bacteriophage can have no effect upon the course of the disease."

D'Herelle's opinions on the lack of phage inhibition by body fluids have not been fully corroborated by later work. It has been shown in our laboratory[4] that serum, blood, and pus definitely inhibit bacteriophagy. Other workers[5] have also found serum to be inhibitory to phage. Colvin,[6] in addition, noted inhibition with ascitic fluid and urine. The purpose of the present investigation was to study the relation of bile to the bacteriophage phenomenon.

Calalb[7] found staphylococcus, coli and dysentery bacteriophages to be

---

Received for publication, July 26, 1935.

From the Department of Pathology and Bacteriology, New York Post-Graduate Medical School and Hospital, Columbia University.

These studies have been aided by a grant from the Josiah Macy, Jr. Foundation

1. Eaton, M. D., and Bayne-Jones, S.: J. A. M. A. **103:** 1771, 1934; Soule, M. H.: J. Michigan M. Soc. **32:** 8, 1933.
2. The Bacteriophage and Its Behavior, Baltimore, Williams and Wilkins, 1926, p. 71.
3. Ibid., p. 552.
4. Applebaum, M., and MacNeal, W. J.: J. Infect. Dis. **49:** 225, 1931; **50:** 269, 1931.
5. Gratia, A., and Mutsaars, W.: Compt. rend. Soc. de biol. **106:** 943, 1931.
6. J. Infect. Dis. **51:** 527, 1932.
7. Compt. rend. Soc. de biol. **92:** 1442, 1925.

completely inhibited by ox bile in dilutions up to approximately 1–20. De Jong and Hauduroy[8] discuss a single case of typhoid fever in which a blood culture was positive for typhoid bacilli when bile was added to a peptone medium but remained negative for this organism when cultured in the absence of bile. It is assumed by these authors that bacteriophage was present in this blood and they attributed the positive blood culture to the inhibitory action of bile upon bacteriophage, as previously reported.[7] They also conclude that typhoid carriers harbor typhoid bacilli in the gall bladder because of the inhibitory action of bile. No proof is given that bacteriophage was involved in the reported cultural results, and it is possible that the added bile enriched the medium, thus stimulating the growth of the typhoid bacilli.[9]

Caublot[10] in 1926 treated a urinary infection due to dysentery bacilli (Flexner group) with a potent specific phage. After the patient was discharged, this phage was diluted with bile (1–2) and stored in sealed ampoules. Five months later, the patient had a recurrence of the same infection and at this time, the phage was retested for potency and found to be fully active against the infecting microbe. In vitro tests showed that lysis took place in bile with phages active against staphylococcus, colon, para-typhoid, and dysentery bacilli. Bile was found to stimulate the growth of certain bacteria but had no appreciable effect upon phage.

Kline[11] in 1927 briefly stated that no inhibition of phage by bile was noted when it was added in 10 per cent and 50 per cent amounts in test tube experiments with colon, typhoid, Shiga and Mt. Desert dysentery phages.

Evans[12] in 1933 reported experiments she performed with one race of streptococcus bacteriophage. A part of the study was devoted to the effect in vitro of ox bile on bacteriophagy. She found ox bile completely inhibitory to phage action in a 1–2 dilution in one test, and partially inhibitory in the same bile dilution in another test. Partial phage inhibition is reported in a 1–5 dilution of bile, and sometimes in a 1–10 dilution. Higher dilutions of bile were usually without effect but occasionally dilutions such as 1–5,000 caused complete inhibition of phage. Evans refers to these findings as examples of the zoning phenomenon which she has also observed in the absence of bile. We have not noted such irregularities in lysis when optimum temperatures, potent phages and truly sensitive bacterial strains were employed.

Few reports of animal experiments with bile and bacteriophage appear in the literature. Kabeshima[13] in 1920 injected ten rabbits intravenously with 1 cc. Shiga phage and was able to recover it in a fully active state in

8. Bull. et mém. Soc. méd. d. hôp. de Paris **49:** 1561, 1925.

9. Besson, A.: Practical Bacteriology, Microbiology and Serum Therapy, London, Longmans, Green and Company, 1913, pp. 372 and 391.

10. Compt. rend. Soc. de biol. **93:** 1583, 1926; abstract in English, J. A. M. A. **86:** 987, 1926.

11. Proc. Soc. Exper. Biol. & Med. **24:** 735, 1927.

12. Pub. Health Rep. **48:** 411, 1933.

13. Compt. rend. Acad. d. sc. **170:** 71, 1920.

the bile in from thirty minutes to sixteen hours later, but rarely after 24 to 48 hours. He next attempted phage therapy in animals with induced biliary infection. Rabbits were injected with dysentery bacilli directly into the biliary vesicle. This was followed seven days later by intravenous injections of bacteriophage in daily doses of from 1 to 5 cc.; the total number of injections varying from two to seven in the different animals. Two sets of 12 rabbits each were treated in this way and all killed 24 to 48 hours after the last phage injection. The first set received bacteria only and of these one had a sterile gall bladder, while the remaining 11 showed Shiga bacilli. The second set received phage treatment after bacteria were injected. Ten of the 12 rabbits in this series had sterile gall bladders.

Doerr and Grüninger,[14] in 1922, were unable to corroborate many of these findings. Ten rabbits received coli phage only, and it was necessary to use large intravenous doses (2 cc. for a 1,700 gram rabbit) of a phage with a titer of 10^{-8} in order to recover it in bile or urine. Phage was present four hours later in low concentration, but not after fourteen hours. When rabbits were injected intravenously with colon bacilli alone, only one out of six showed these bacteria in the gall bladder. When in addition to colon bacilli, phage also was given intravenously, four out of eight had infected gall bladders. Phage therapy was then tried in animals with experimentally induced gall bladder infections. Colon bacilli were injected directly into the gall bladder and phage was given intravenously several days later. It was found that the organisms were not destroyed even when 2 cc. phage was used. In vitro control tests proved bile itself was not inhibitory to the phage.

McKinley[15] treated three patients with pyocyaneus phage for subacute catarrhal cholecystitis with symptomatic relief, followed by recurrence. D'Amato, Pizarro, and Vacarezza[16] of Buenos Aires are the only clinicians reporting the extensive use of bacteriophage in human biliary infections. Best results were obtained when "Bacte-coli-phage" was administered subcutaneously, and "Bacte-intesti-phage" given simultaneously by mouth. Fifty-seven cases of various biliary tract diseases such as hepatalgia, biliary lithiasis, cholangitis, and cholecystitis were treated with bacteriophage. In 36 of these, 8 were reported as cured, 23 improved, and 5 unbenefited. In 21 remaining cases, good general results followed bacteriophage therapy. The authors mention without comment Hauduroy's statement of phage inhibition by bile, but were not deterred by it in attempting phage therapy in biliary infections.

EXPERIMENTAL

In Vitro Tests with Ox Bile.—To determine whether bacteriophage could exert its action in bile, a series of in vitro experiments with ox bile was undertaken. A fresh unopened gall bladder of a steer was obtained from the slaughter house. Before removal from the animal, a ligature was applied close to the gall bladder and the duct was then cut at a distance below this ligature. In the laboratory, the wall was seared and punctured with a sterile Pasteur pipette.

14. Schweiz. med. Wchnschr. **52:** 761, 1922; abstract in English, J. A. M. A. **79:** 1277, 1922.
15. Arch. Int. Med. **32:** 899, 1923.
16. Semana med. **38:** (2) 1809, 1931.

Approximately 250 cc. of sterile ox bile was collected for experimental purposes. This procedure is to be preferred to sterilization of a body fluid by autoclaving or passing it through a Berkefeld filter, as has been reported from other laboratories.[12]

The phages employed were of high titer and were completely active in broth against the strains of bacteria indicated. In each case, they represent a mixture of different races of bacteriophage; the coli phage used contained forty separate phages, the staphylococcus phage was a mixture of five races; there were four races in the streptococcus phage, and two in the typhoid phage.

For each bacterial strain, six tubes were used, three to which phage was added, and three without phage. The first tube in each set of three contained sterile undiluted ox bile; the second, a 1–10 dilution of bile in beef infusion broth of p_H 7.6 and the third contained sterile broth. The medium was apportioned to total 5 cc. in each tube. To the first set of three tubes, 0.1 cc. of phage to be tested was added. All six tubes received 0.05 cc. of a light bacterial suspension (of approximately 1,000 million bacteria per cc.) in saline, made from a 24-hour agar slant culture. Tubes were shaken and incubated at 32 C. After five hours and again after twenty-four hours incubation, tubes were read for growth and lysis. At these periods, one loopful from each tube was spread on a freshly solidified agar plate with a sterile glass spreader. After inoculation, plates were incubated for twenty-four hours at the same temperature and read for growth and lysis.

Undiluted bile is too opaque for macroscopic readings. A 1–10 dilution of bile causes a slight clouding of the medium which does not signify growth but obscures the lysis readings. For this reason, descriptions of tubes are omitted. It is necessary to rely upon the plate findings for accurate results, the records of which are shown in table 1.

TABLE 1.—*Growth on Agar Plates Inoculated from Respective Tubes of Liquid Medium after 5 Hours and after 24 Hours at 32 C.*

	Undiluted ox bile		Ox bile 1:10		Broth	
	5 hours	24 hours	5 hours	24 hours	5 hours	24 hours
Microbe	Tubes with respective bacteriophage					
Staphylococcus C......	300P	400	2	3	0	0
Colon bacillus C.......	0	85P	4P	0	5P	0
Colon bacillus De......	moderate	moderate	1	0	0	0
Streptococcus M.......	moderate	slightP	200	slight	0	30P
Typhoid bacillus.......	very slightP	moderateP	2P	6	0	0
Microbe	Tubes without bacteriophage					
Staphyloccocus C......	confluent	confluent	confluent	confluent	confluent	confluent
Colon bacillus C.......	confluent	heavy	confluent	heavy	confluent	heavy
Colon bacillus De......	heavy	heavy	confluent	confluent	confluent	confluent
Streptotoccus M.......	light	light	confluent	confluent	confluent	confluent
Typhoid bacillus.......	confluent	confluent	confluent	confluent	confluent	confluent

Note: P indicates evidence of lytic phage action seen in colonies which are notched, glassy, transparent, thin or small. The numbers indicate the exact or approximate colony count of the plate. When colony count was not possible, the descriptive terms have been employed.

Plates show definite partial inhibition of all phages tested in undiluted ox bile. No inhibitory influence on phage was noted by a 1–10 dilution of bile, except for the streptococcus bacteriophage. In another experiment, not included in the table, the staphylococcus phage was inhibited also in the 1–10 dilution of ox bile. The slight inhibition when coli phage was used with colon bacillus "C" was not observed upon repetition of the experiment. The amount of inhibition by the same sample of bile varies with different phages and for the same phage with different strains of bacteria.

In Vitro Tests with Bile, Blood and Serum.—In order that the amount of phage inhibition caused by bile might be compared with various body fluids parallel experiments were undertaken with bile, whole blood and blood serum. These three fluids undiluted and diluted 1–10 in broth, were tested for their inhibitory action on bacteriophage, at the same time and under similar conditions. Comparative experiments were undertaken for staphylococcus, streptococcus, colon and typhoid bacteriophage with ox bile, defibrinated rabbit's blood and rabbit serum from the same animal. The ox bile used in this series was a fresh sample different from that previously mentioned. The volume of the fluids in each test amounted to 1 cc. Two series of tubes were set up for each bacteriophage. One set received 0.1 cc. specific bacteriophage. Both sets were inoculated with 0.05 cc. of a weak suspension of the homologous organism. Tubes were shaken, then incubated at 32 C. After five hours incubation and again after 24 hours, the tubes were read for lysis and growth when the transparency of the medium permitted. At these times, a loopful from each tube was streaked on the surface of freshly solidified agar plates which were incubated over night and then read for growth and lysis. The results of the plates only are recorded in the following table.

TABLE 2.—*Growth on Agar Plates Inoculated from Respective Tubes of Liquid Medium after 5 Hours and after 24 Hours at 32 C.*

	Colon bacillus Mg		Staphylococcus 16		Typhoid bacillus B		Streptococcus M	
	5 hrs.	24 hrs.	5 hrs.	24 hrs.	5 hrs.	24 hrs.	5 hrs.	24 hrs.
	Tubes with respective bacteriophage							
Undiluted ox bile.....	0	0	16^{P}	5	0	100^{P}	mod-	mod-
Ox bile 1:10.........	1	0	1	0	0	0	5	0
Rabbit blood........	mod^{P}	100^{P}	mod	mod^{P}	25^{P}	100^{P}	mod	mod
Rabbit blood 1:10....	300^{P}	2	slt	35^{P}	0	35^{P}	0	slt
Rabbit serum........	mod^{P}	65^{P}	mod	mod	0	100^{P}	mod^{P}	mod^{P}
Rabbit serum 1:10...	mod^{P}	1	125	50^{P}	0	150	2	20
Broth..............	10	3	10	0	0	150	0	0
	Tubes without bacteriophage							
Undiluted ox bile	confl	slt	mod	mod	confl	confl	mod	mod
Ox bile 1:10.........	confl	confl	confl	confl	confl	confl	mod	confl

Controls without bacteriophage for undiluted rabbit blood, rabbit blood 1:10, undiluted rabbit serum, rabbit serum 1:10, and broth all gave confluent growth on the plates.

Mod = moderate Slt = slight Confl = confluent

With the strain of staphylococcus and colon bacillus tested, the respective phages were able to exert complete lytic action in ox bile whereas the same phages were distinctly inhibited by rabbit blood and serum. Previously,[4] we have reported similar results on inhibition of staphylococcus and coli phages by blood and serum using other bacterial strains. The typhoid strain "B" recently isolated from a carrier was lysed in the body fluids employed here to about the same degree as in broth. The streptococcus bacteriophage seemed more inhibited by undiluted bile than by blood and serum.

These experiments were repeated using a fresh sample of ox bile, and blood and serum obtained from another rabbit. The results were comparable with those recorded in table 2 with a few exceptions. The new rabbit blood exerted a greater inhibitory effect on the staphylococcus bacteriophage. The streptococcus bacteriophage was not inhibited as much by the ox bile this time, so that lysis was as good or better in bile than in blood and serum.

Identical experiments, employing the same bacteriophages and bacterial strains were carried out using sterile human bile, sterile defibrinated human blood, and sterile human serum. The latter two were obtained from the same normal individual. The bile was obtained by aspirating the contents of a non-infected gall bladder freshly removed at operation. The coli phage was not inhibited by any of the human fluids used. The staphylococcus phage was slightly inhibited by bile but less so than by blood or serum. The streptococcus phage was slightly inhibited in five hours by all three human body fluids to about the same degree, the amount of inhibition becoming more evident in twenty-four hours. The growth of the typhoid bacilli was so greatly inhibited by human blood and serum that it is difficult to record lysis in these mediums. However, in five hours, less growth appeared with phage than without, in all of the body fluids. The twenty-four hour plates were too irregular for comparison. Repetition with another typhoid strain gave similar results.

In general, phage inhibition was either absent in bile or was not as great as that found in blood and serum.[4] This applies to human body fluids as well as those obtained from animals.

In Vivo Experiments.—In vitro studies showed that bile was partially inhibitory to some races of bacteriophage, while others were not affected. Since none of the races of phage were completely inhibited by the presence of bile, it was assumed that some phage action might occur in vivo, and be of therapeutic value in biliary infections. It was necessary to show that phage given by the intravenous route could be recovered from the human gall bladder in sufficient concentration to combat infection. It was possible to study five patients without infection, who were admitted to this hospital for cholecystectomy.

Intravenous injections of bacteriophage in asparagin medium were given before operation. The doses varied from 0.5 cc. to 2 cc. of undiluted phages active against the staphylococcus and the colon bacillus. The time interval elapsing between the last phage injection and operation varied from one hour and 26 minutes to 22 hours and 45 minutes. The gall bladder was sent to the laboratory immediately upon removal, and the bile aseptically collected. Cultures were made of the bile, gall bladder wall and stones if present. Serial filtrations were undertaken to determine if phage was present in the bile. At this time, in vitro tests were made using the bile specimens obtained from the five patients. Two sets of dilutions were made from each bile specimen in nutrient broth of p_H 7.5.

To the first set, phage and bacteria were added; to the second, bacteria only. Controls in plain broth were included. These in vitro tests were made to ascertain the degree of inhibitory action which human bile might exert upon phage. It was found not to inhibit coli phage when a susceptible stock strain "C" was used. Slight inhibition was noted in one case where a recently isolated coli strain "O" was the test strain. In another case, no inhibition of coli phage was noted when a different, freshly isolated strain of colon bacillus "T" was employed. The bile of the fifth patient (A.D.) was found to inhibit phage partially but very definitely even in 1–1,000 bile dilution. In this instance, staphylococcus bacteriophage was used together with a stock susceptible strain "C". This bile was unusual, however, in that a large cholesterol stone almost filled the gall bladder, and was surrounded by a small amount of thick reddish brown bile. From none of these five specimens was it possible to recover the injected bacteriophage.

These patients exhibited no reaction to the phage injections. In no case was it possible to recover the lytic agent from the bile, and in three cases the urine was found negative for phage. The urines of the two remaining patients were not tested for the presence of bacteriophage. In two respects these results were contrary to our previous experience with patients having infections: first, we have generally noted a reaction with the use of coli bacteriophage given intravenously in similar doses, when the colon bacillus was the infecting microbe; second, we have been able to recover the lytic agent from various body fluids after its injection when the doses were no larger. It is possible that if large enough doses of phage were used, it could be recovered even from non-infected patients, but we were unwilling to submit them to the inconvenience of possible reaction. Subsequently, an intravenous injection of 5 cc. of undiluted staphylococcus bacteriophage was administered to a healthy person just after a control specimen of urine had been collected. Following the phage injection, six additional urine specimens were obtained over a period of 22 hours. Each specimen was filtered immediately through a Berkefeld filter. Subsequently serial filtrations were made with a phage-susceptible strain of staphylococcus, "C". No lysis was detected in filtrates of any specimen in 4, 5, or 24 hours incubation at 32 C., in four successive filtrations.

Animal Experiments.—The failure to recover bacteriophage after intravenous injection in the six non-infected individuals just discussed, may have been related to the absence of infection. Experiments with rabbits were therefore undertaken to determine whether phage could be more easily recovered when the homologous bacterium was present.

Rabbit No. 10, weight 3090 grams, received intravenously 2 cc. of a bacterial suspension of colon bacillus "De," (four billion bacteria). One half hour later, the rabbit received intravenously 3 cc. of a 1–10 dilution of asparagin coli phage of titer 10^{-9}. The animal was killed four hours and ten minutes after the phage injection. At autopsy, heart's blood and bile were collected. Both contained colon bacilli, with approximately 80 bacteria per cc. in the blood. Bacteriophage was recovered from both specimens but in an attenuated state, giving complete lysis in four hours incubation at 32 C. but none in 24 hours; nor could the phage be enhanced to its former potency in three successive filtrations.

Rabbit No. 13, weight 3650 grams, received no bacteria but was given 3 cc. of a 1–10 dilution of the same coli phage intravenously. Five hours five minutes later, the animal was killed and autopsied. Heart's blood, bladder urine and a very small quantity of bile were collected. Cultures of all three were negative for bacteria. No phage was detected in any of them in three successive filtrations.

Rabbit No. 2, weight 2820 grams, received 2 cc. of a suspension (four billion bacteria) of colon bacillus "De" intravenously. The animal was killed four hours ten minutes later and autopsied. Cultures of bile and urine were negative for bacteria. The blood contained approximately 97 bacteria per cc. No phage was recovered in bile, urine, or blood in four successive filtrations.

Rabbit No. 9, weight 3050 grams, received 2 cc. of the same suspension, followed one half hour later by 3 cc. of a 1–10 dilution of the same coli phage in asparagin as was used previously. The animal was killed four hours forty-five minutes after phage injection. Bile, a small quantity of urine with thick gray sediment, and heart's blood were collected. Cultures of all three were positive for colon bacilli, with approximately 100 bacteria per cc. blood, and 6 per cc. in the bile. Coli phage was recovered from the bile and blood which was completely active in four hours but showed hardly any lysis in twenty-four hours in each of three successive filtrations. This mysterious diminution of lytic potency challenges further investigation. No phage was recovered from the urine in four successive filtrations.

Rabbit No. 278, weight 3350 grams, received 3 cc. of a 1–10 dilution of coli phage as above. The animal was killed four hours five minutes later. Bile, heart's blood and bladder urine were negative for bacteria and phage. Three serial filtrations were unsuccessful in detecting phage.

These animal experiments showed that a small dose of bacteriophage could be recovered when the homologous organism was present, but not in its absence. This may explain why no phage was recovered in six individuals without infection when doses of from 0.5 cc. to 5 cc. undiluted phage were injected intravenously. It will be shown presently that similar doses were sufficient to permit recovery of phage in two patients with biliary infection. When biliary infection exists, it is highly probable that such doses of potent phage will be sufficient to reach the gall bladder. Further studies on this and allied problems are now in progress.

*Two Typhoid Carriers.**—As a result of the findings in rabbits, an attempt was made to recover injected phage from patients with biliary infection. Accordingly studies were made on two typhoid carriers admitted to this hospital for cholecystectomy.

The first patient, man, 42 years old, a recently detected typhoid carrier, was admitted January 22, 1935 for operation in an attempt to relieve the carrier condition. Several bile drainages had been done previously, all being culturally positive for typhoid bacilli. Upon admission, a voided urine specimen was collected and filtered through a Berkefeld filter. The patient then received intravenous injections of stock typhoid bacteriophage in asparagin medium, (titer 10^{-9}), as follows: 1.0 cc. phage of 1–10 dilution in saline at 3:10 P.M.; 2.0 cc. of 1–10 dilution in saline at 4:00 P.M.; 4.0 cc. of 1–10 dilution in saline at 4:45 P.M.; 7.0 cc. of 1–10 dilution in saline at 5:30 P.M.; 1.0 cc. of undiluted phage at 6:30 P.M. At 8:30 P.M., two hours after the fifth injection, the patient chilled for ten minutes, the temperature rising to 102.4 F. On the following morning, January 23, a second voided urine was collected and filtered. At 9:30 A.M. the sixth and last injection, 5 cc. of a 1–10 dilution of bacteriophage was given. A third urine was taken later that morning and filtered at 12:15 P.M. Operation took place on the afternoon of January 23. After incision of abdomen the surgeon aspirated the contents of the gall bladder.

The bile collected in this manner was sent to the laboratory for study, in addition to gall stones and a portion of gall bladder wall. Typhoid bacilli in abundance were cultured from bile, stones and wall. The organism was found to be susceptible to lysis by the injected phage. The urines were negative for typhoid bacilli and no bacteriophage was detected in filtrates of any of the three urine specimens. Filtered broth cultures of bile and gall bladder wall yielded typhoid

---

* The study of human material was made possible by the coöperation of Dr. R. Franklin Carter and the Gall Bladder Clinic of the New York Post-Graduate Hospital.

phage in successive filtrates when tested with a stock phage-susceptible strain. A more potent bacteriophage was isolated from the gall bladder wall than from the bile. These results suggest that phage will reach the infected gall bladder by the intravenous route. It may be recovered after injection more readily when the homologous susceptible organism is present. On February 2, ten days after operation, the patient's stool was negative for typhoid bacilli. Bile drainage specimens taken February 20, 27 and March 6 were negative for typhoid bacilli. The unusually rapid cure of this typhoid carrier by cholecystectomy may have been aided by the injected bacteriophage. In vitro experiments undertaken with the patient's bile indicate that undiluted bile greatly inhibits the action of typhoid phage with this carrier strain "W." Lysis was slightly inhibited also in 1–2 and 1–5 dilutions of bile in broth, but not in 1–10 dilution.

In vitro tests performed with sterile ox bile indicated that partial inhibition of typhoid bacteriophage occurred when bile was undiluted or diluted 1–2. Inhibition of phage was greater with the above described freshly isolated typhoid strain "W" than with an old stock strain of typhoid bacillus. Inhibition of lysis by ox bile with typhoid strain "W" was comparable to that found for staphylococcus bacteriophage when a strain of staphylococcus "M" was employed.

Experiments were carried out with the carrier strain of typhoid bacillus and a bacteriophage active against it using human bile and human plasma. Inhibition of phage by plasma was much greater than by human bile after five hours incubation. In 24 hours, the amount of inhibition of phage by both of these body fluids was similar. The protocols of these experiments are omitted.

Another typhoid carrier, age 45, was admitted for cholecystectomy on April 22, 1935. Bile drainage specimens taken in the gall bladder clinic during March had been positive for typhoid bacilli. One of these was tested for presence of bacteriophage but none was detected. A specific bacteriophage active against the causative organism was prepared in an asparagin medium. On April 23, the day following admission, a voided urine specimen was collected and filtered through a Berkefeld filter. Fifteen minutes later, intravenous injections of specific bacteriophage were begun: 1.0 cc. of 1–10 dilution of specific bacteriophage at 3:30 P.M.; 2.0 cc. of 1–10 dilution of specific bacteriophage at 4:10 P.M.; 4.0 cc. of 1–10 dilution of specific bacteriophage at 4:50 P.M.

The patient complained of malaise and chilliness after having received only 3 cc. of bacteriophage diluted 1–10. At 5:30 P.M. the temperature had risen to 101.4 F. and by 8 P.M. that evening, it had reached 104 F. On the morning of April 24, a second voided urine was collected and filtered. The patient received a fourth and last injection of 2 cc. of a 1–10 dilution of phage at 8:15 A.M. About one hour later the patient had a slight chill lasting seven minutes with a rise in temperature to 101.2 F. Cholecystectomy took place 11:05 to 11:34 A.M. on April 24. Bile was removed approximately three hours after the last injection of bacteriophage. The lytic agent was recovered in this operative bile, lymph node, and gall bladder wall, where typhoid bacilli were also found. Phage was obtained in this case also in greatest concentration in the gall bladder wall. A control of a previous bile specimen from drainage was negative for bacteriophage, showing that the recovered phage was not native. Further, no bacteriophage was isolated from either of two urine specimens which were also negative for typhoid bacilli. The first urine, serving as a control, was collected just before phage was given, the second four hours before operation after a total of 7 cc. 1–10 dilution of phage had been injected. Bile collected from this pathological gall bladder was insufficient for in vitro tests of phage inhibition by bile itself. In all other respects, this corroborates the findings on the first patient.

Further work with typhoid carriers and patients with biliary infection is in progress. An attempt is being made to study the therapeutic value of bacteriophage in these conditions.

COMMENT

These experiments indicate that the lytic action of bacteriophage is to some extent interfered with by the presence of bile, particularly when undiluted. However, the amount of such inhibition is distinctly less than that encountered with blood, blood serum, and purulent exudate as previously reported. Partial lysis can usually be demonstrated in vitro in body fluids. Evidently when given the assistance of bacteriophage in combating the infecting microbe, the body is sometimes able to destroy it completely by calling into use its own defense mechanisms. In spite of inhibition of phage by blood, intravenous bacteriophage therapy has yielded gratifying results.[17] In bile, where the amount of phage inhibition is definitely less than in blood, a measure of success may be expected with the use of phage. It seems fairly certain that the usual intravenous doses of phage will be sufficient to reach the gall bladder of patients with biliary infection. It might be advantageous to attempt phage therapy when a biliary infection due to a susceptible colon or typhoid bacillus is present. If phage should fail, one may later resort to cholecystectomy.

CONCLUSIONS

Ox bile interferes in varying degrees with the lytic action of some races of bacteriophage. Human bile exerts a similar interfering action, even in dilution, with some bacteria-bacteriophage combinations, while it has no effect upon others. The amount of phage inhibition by bile is, in general, less than that exerted by blood or serum.

Bacteriophages active against colon and typhoid bacilli are less inhibited by body fluids than the bacteriophages for staphylococcus and streptococcus.

Following intravenous injection, we did not recover bacteriophage from the bile or urine of patients without biliary infection.

In five rabbits injected intravenously, coli phage was recovered in blood and bile of two animals when the colon bacillus had previously been injected. In two others receiving no bacteria but similar doses of injected phage, the phage could not be recovered. No phage was obtained from bile or blood in a fifth animal receiving bacteria only.

In two typhoid carriers submitting to cholecystectomy, it was possible to recover intravenously injected bacteriophage in the bile and gall bladder wall removed at operation. Typhoid bacilli were isolated from both situations. In urines of these patients which were negative for typhoid bacilli, none of the injected phage could be recovered.

---

17. MacNeal, W. J., and Frisbee, Frances C.: Am. J. M. Sc., in press.

THE EFFECTS OF OZONE UPON CERTAIN BACTERIA AND THEIR RESPECTIVE PHAGES

STUDIES IN BACTERIAL METABOLISM, CV

ARTHUR ISAAC KENDALL

AND

ARTHUR WILLIAM WALKER

CHICAGO

Certain investigators[1] have reported that staphylococcus phage is destroyed after brief exposure to sunlight in presence of methylene blue. B. coli phage, similarly treated, appears to be unaffected.[2] This difference in behaviour of the two respective phages may be due either to a quantitative lack of resistance of the staphylococcus phage to mild oxidization, or, possibly, to a qualitative fundamental distinction involving deep seated individual characteristics. This is not merely an academic problem: it involves reactions to physical agents which, rightly understood, may throw considerable light upon the controversial nature of phage itself, regarded by some as an enzyme, and by others as an ubiquitous slayer of microbes. Staphylococci are usually found to be distinctly more tolerant of chemical and physical agents than colon bacilli, hence it is instructive to find that the staphylococcus phage is less resistant to inactivation by mild oxidization than colon phage.

The experiments which are presented herewith illustrate the effect of a powerful oxidizing agent-ozone- upon the same strains of bacteria referred to above-B. coli and Staphylococcus-, upon their respective phages, their "induced lysogenic" variants, and upon their respective filterable forms. The "induced lysogenic" variants were obtained by cultivating the respective bacteria in presence of dilute phage. The resulting strains, themselves apparently undissolved by phage, were "carriers" of phage. It was shown in a previous communication[2] that staphylococci in the nonfilterable state could be recovered from staphylococcus phage which had been inactivated by methylene blue in presence of sunlight. It was also shown that coli phage was not only unaffected perceptibly by exposure to this mild oxidizing system, but also that attempts to recover bacteria in the nonfilterable state were unsuccessful from coli phage thus treated. With these differences in response to slight oxidization in mind, the much more powerful oxidizant, ozone, was tried.

The effects of ozone upon phage do not seem to have been reported possibly because suitable ozone generating apparatus is not generally available. Therefore, a brief discription of the procedure followed will be made, together

Received for publication, August 1, 1935.

From the Departments of Bacteriology, Northwestern University Medical School.

1. Clifton: Proc. Soc. Exper. Biol. & Med. **28:** 745, 1931.
2. Kendall and Walker: J. Infect. Dis. **53:** 355, 1933.

with a discussion of certain precautions which must be taken to insure reasonably consistent results. The more important precautions are: first, to maintain a uniform flow of air containing ozone through the test solution; second, to use a constant volume of test solution; third, to keep the composition of the test solution with reference to soluble organic substances as nearly uniform as possible. The apparatus employed was loaned by the Ozone Corporation. Throughout the experiments a uniform volume of 20 cc. was observed, unless otherwise indicated. Plain, nutrient broth was used both for the production of phage, and as a diluent for the phage, unless otherwise specified. Inasmuch as rubber is rapidly disintegrated by ozone, all tubing through which ozonized air passed was either aluminum or glass. Wide mouth bottles, holding 100 cc. and of 4 cm. internal diameter were found to be convenient. Bottles with lesser internal diameters were unsatisfactory because of frothing of the contents, and those of greater diameter did not give the requisite depth of solution, a factor of some importance because ozone is but slightly soluble in water. The delivery tube for the introduction of ozonized air into the test solution was of glass, approximately 6 mm. in internal diameter, and having a crown of 6 minute, equally spaced openings at the delivery end to insure an effective distribution of ozone within the test solution. A glass mantle originating on the ozone delivery tube above the bottle holding the test solution, and fitting loosely over the bottle, downward for a distance of some 6 cm. kept out dust and air contaminants without interfering with the escape of spent air from the bottle itself. The glass mantle was wiped off with $HgCl_2$ solution immediately before using, to reduce further the possibility of aerial contamination. All glass ware coming into contact with the test solution was sterilized.

The first series of experiments was designed to show the effect of soluble organic substances (the ingredients of plain, nutritive broth), upon the resistance of phage to ozone. In each experiment, 2 cc. of phage were diluted with 18 cc. of broth, giving thereby a total volume of 20 cc. and a dilution of 1:10 of phage. The details of a single experiment will indicate the procedure followed:

Two cc. of coli phage diluted with 18 cc. of broth were placed in one of the wide mouth bottles described above. The mantle was adjusted, the delivery tube was connected with the ozonizer, and so arranged that the delivery end just touched the bottom of the bottle. The ozonized air was turned on, rapidly enough so that the bubbles coming from the orifices of the delivery tube formed a continuous stream. Time was taken from the appearance of the first bubbles. At appropriate intervals samples of 1 cc. each were removed with sterile precautions and placed at once in 9 cc. of sterile broth. This gave a dilution of 1:10 of the ozonized phage, but 1:100 of the original phage: it will be recalled that the phage was diluted 1:10 at the start of the experiment. At the end of the experiment, all the samples thus removed were diluted in decreasing multiples of 10 to the original limit of activity of the phage. Usually the original titer of the phages used was 1×10^{-10}. It was noticed that within the first minute, the broth-phage mixture darkened: after 10 minutes the broth became much lighter in color, and after 20 minutes the color was nearly gone. Upon standing, however, the color reappeared, and was considerably darker than that of unozonized broth. Broth without any bacteriophage underwent a similar series of color changes.

Titration of B. coli II phage, diluted with broth (2 cc. phage, 18 cc. of plain broth) after various exposures to ozonized air.

Start titer 10^{-10}
after 5 minutes' exposure to ozone titer 10^{-10}
after 10 minutes' exposure to ozone titer 10^{-10}
after 15 minutes' exposure to ozone titer 10^{-4}
after 20 minutes' exposure to ozone titer 10^{-2}
after 25 minutes' exposure to ozone titer 10^{-1} (doubtful)
after 30 minutes' exposure to ozone titer nil: phage completely gone.

Hence B. coli II phage was completely inactivated by 30 minutes' exposure to ozonized air.

Titration of Staphylococcus (lyt.) phage, diluted with broth (2 cc. phage, 18 cc. of plain broth) after various exposures to ozonized air.

Start titer 10^{-10}
after 5 minutes' exposure to ozone titer 10^{-5}
after 10 minutes' exposure to ozone titer 10^{-3}
after 15 minutes' exposure to ozone titer 10^{-1}
after 20 minutes' exposure to ozone titer nil: phage completely gone.

Hence Staph. lyt. phage was completely inactivated by 20 minutes' exposure to ozonized air.

It would appear from these experiments that Staph. lyt. phage is distinctly less resistant to ozonized air than B. coli II phage: this is in accord with the observations referred to above, where, it will be remembered, Staph. lyt. phage was inactivated by brief exposure to sunlight in presence of methylene blue, and B. coli phage was not noticeably affected.

Next, the effects of the soluble organic constituents of nutrient broth upon the resistance of phage were studied. This was achieved by decreasing the amount of broth, substituting therefore distilled water. For brevity of presentation, the results only are recorded: the experiments were carried out precisely as those in the previous tabulation, with the exception that the broth was decreased progressively, and the volume (20 cc.) was kept constant by the addition of sterile, distilled water.

B. coli II phage 2 cc.,	broth 18 cc.,	water 0 cc.,	phage inactivated in 30 minutes
B. coli II phage 2 cc.,	broth 9 cc.,	water 9 cc.,	phage inactivated in 20 minutes
B. coli II phage 2 cc.,	broth 4.5 cc.,	water 13.5 cc.,	phage inactivated in 15 minutes
B. coli II phage 2 cc.,	broth 0 cc.,	water 18 cc.,	phage inactivated in 10 minutes.

Therefore, decreasing the soluble organic constituents of broth, and substituting therefore distilled water, led to a progressively decreased inactivating time of the phage of B. coli II.

Coli II phage was next generated in an ammonium lactate-asparagin medium (a socalled "protein free" medium). Its resistance to ozonized air was next tested.

Start titer 10^{-10}
after 5 minutes' exposure to ozone titer 10^{-3}
after 10 minutes' exposure to ozone titer 10^{-1}
after 15 minutes' exposure to ozone titer nil: phage completely gone.

From which it would appear that B. coli II phage, generated in a socalled "protein free" medium had about the same resistance to ozonized air as a corresponding phage, of like potency, in a 10 per cent broth medium: that is, a medium containing 2 cc. of phage, generated in broth, and diluted 10 times with distilled water. The question is very properly raised: would Staph. lyt. phage react similarly to ozone, in mediums where the soluble organic constituents are reduced in like manner. The following tabulation contains the results of this experiment. The details are similar to those for the corresponding coli II phage,

Staph. lyt. phage 2 cc.,	broth 18 cc.,	water 0 cc.,	phage inactivated in 20 minutes
Staph. lyt. phage 2 cc.,	broth 9 cc.,	water 9 cc.,	phage inactivated in 20 minutes
Staph. lyt. phage 2 cc.,	broth 4.5 cc.,	water 13.5 cc.,	phage inactivated in 10 minutes
Staph. lyt. phage 2 cc.,	broth 0 cc.,	water 18 cc.,	phage inactivated in 3 minutes.

Therefore, it appears that Staph. lyt. phage is less resistant to the ozone oxidization than B. coli II phage, and, also, decreasing the broth constituents decreases the inactivation time. One iregularity appeared, namely, that decreasing the broth constituents 50 per cent had no appreciable effect upon activation: this was repeated twice, with the same general result. This was not noticed with B. coli II phage. Comment: reference has been made to the "induced lysogenic" strains of B. coli II and Staphylococcus lyt.: these organisms are "carriers" of phage, without themselves being noticeably dissolved by the phage. Phage is readily obtained from these "lysogenic" strains by the simple expedient of cultivating them in plain, nutrient broth over night in the incubator. The next morning the bacteria are filtered off, leaving the phage in the clear filtrate. This "lysogenic" phage will dissolve the corresponding "lytic" strains in characteristic manner. "Lysogenic" phages for B. coli II and Staphylococcus lyt. were prepared, and tested for their resistance to ozonized air. Inasmuch as their resistance was almost exactly that of the corresponding "lytic" phages, the fact is hereby mentioned, without tabulating the details of the experiments. B. coli II "lysogenic" phage resisted ozonized air for 30 minutes, and Staphylococcus "lysogenic" phage resisted ozonized air for 20 minutes. Here again, the coli phage is distinctly more resistant than the staphylococcus phage, to the powerful oxidizing agent ozone.

It was deemed important to determine the time required for ozonized air to either kill, or to so injure B. coli II and Staphylococcus lyt. they would no longer grow in nutritive broth. Many experiments are recorded in the literature upon this point, and for many bacteria, but such experiments are difficult to compare one with another. Very many factors influence the results: the strain of organism, the age and condition of the culture, the absolute amount of ozone, the concentration of the ozone in the ozonized air, the composition of the suspending medium, and the after care of the cultures. The purposes of this investigation were served by exposing B. coli II and Staphylococcus, respectively, to ozone under the same conditions as those obtaining for the exposure of their various phages. The procedure was single: 3 loops of an 18 hour agar slant culture of the required organism were thoroughly emulsified in broth, or whatever medium was selected, and samples of 1 cc. removed at the intervals stated, and placed at once in 10 cc. of plain, nutrient broth. The table shows only the length of exposure to ozonized air necessary to kill, or prevent the growth of the particular microbe. Otherwise the tabulations are self explanatory.

B. coli II, 3 loops. broth 20 cc., 50 minutes' exposure to ozone killed
B. coli II, 3 loops. broth 10 cc., distilled water, 10 cc., killed in 30 minutes
B. coli II, 3 loops. broth 2 cc., distilled water, 18 cc., killed in 15 minutes
B. coli II, 3 loops. broth 0 cc., distilled water, 20 cc., killed in 3 minutes.

It should be stated that control cultures in distilled water were not affected by a 2 hour exposure: evidently the water alone was without noteworthy effect. This same control was made for Staphylococcus lyt. with the same negligible effect.

Staph. lyt. 3 loops. broth 20 cc., 50 minutes' exposure to ozone killed
Staph. lyt. 3 loops. broth 10 cc., distilled water, 10 cc., killed in 40 minutes
Staph. lyt. 3 loops. broth 2 cc., distilled water, 18 cc., killed in 20 minutes
Staph. lyt. 3 loops. broth 0 cc., distilled water, 20 cc., killed in 5 minutes.

These experiments indicate that Staphylococcus lyt., is distinctly more resistant to ozonized air than B. coli II: this is in harmony with the generally accepted experience that staphylococci are among the most resistant of non-spore forming bacteria, and also the experiments are significant in that the phages of the two bacteria are inversely resistant to ozone in comparison with the organisms themselves. No adequate explanation for this difference between phage resistance and microbe resistance to ozone presents itself at this time.

It was reported in a preceding communication (2) that staphylococci in the nonfilterable state could be recovered from staphylococcus phage, if the phage, diluted nearly to its limit of potency, was allowed to stand in the incubator in contact with a heavy suspension of homologous killed (autoclaved) bacteria. The technic followed was single: first, the phage was diluted in multiples of 10 to its limit of potency. Then to each tube of diluted phage, 1 cc. of a heavy suspension of killed bacteria was added. At stated intervals, cultures were made from each of these tubes, upon agar plates, together with suitable controls, of course. If the experiment was successful, growth would occur in one, rarely two, of the tubes, the remainder being sterile. Almost always, growth occurred only in one of the higher dilutions, the higher concentrations remaining sterile. The organisms recoverable by this procedure may or may not agree in cultural characteristics with the original culture from which they came. Often two strains of bacteria could be isolated from the same tube, differing the one with the other in respect to fermentation reactions. A tentative explanation was advanced to account for these several phenomena. It was as follows: phage liberates filterable forms of bacteria from the nonfilterable forms. These filterable forms may, and often do, remain viable in the phage for weeks or months. These filterable forms are ordinarily constrained from growing up into nonfilterable forms, partly at least, by the presence of the phage itself, which originally made them filterable. Absorbing the phage upon killed, homologous bacteria tends to reduce the lytic power of the phage. Also, possibly, the killed culture adds something to the medium which tends to facilitate growth from the filterable to the nonfilterable state. In this connection, it is not without significance that successful recovery of nonfilterable forms from phage is almost always achieved in the higher dilutions of the phage, where the amount of phage is less, and where the anchorage of the small amount of phage is probably more nearly complete upon the dead organisms. Perhaps it should be added that phage, diluted as above outlined, but without added killed bacteria never yielded cultures of bacteria.

The inactivation of B. coli II phage by ozone in 30 minutes, whereas 50 minutes of ozonization was required to sterilize the homologous broth cultures of the organism, obviously offered a possibility of testing the resistance of the filterable forms of B. coli II to ozone. This possibility of testing the resistance of the filterable forms is based upon the assumption that the filterable forms (produced by action of the phage upon the homologous bacteria, and existing in the phage freed from residual, unlysed bacteria by filtration) are more resistant to ozone than the phage itself. To test this assumption, phage prepared from a "lysogenic" culture of B. coli II was obtained in the usual manner, namely, by cultivating the "lysogenic" culture in nutrient broth in the incubator over night, then filtering the culture to remove all nonlysed bacteria. It should be stated that this "lysogenic" culture had been under observation several weeks before and after this experiment, indicating clearly that its phage "carrying" power was unimpaired during the time this study was made. The titer of the "lysogenic" phage was 10^{-10}. One cc. of the phage was diluted with 9 cc. of mutrient broth, and subjected to ozonized air for 30 minutes. A test for phage potency made at this time showed that the phage was inactivated completely. It should be stated that the "lysogenic" culture itself required 50 minutes' exposure to ozonized air for complete sterilization.

The "lysogenic" phage, thus ozonized was diluted with nutrient broth in the usual manner, in multiples of 10 to 10^{-10}, making ten dilutions, therefore, in the series. To each of these 10 several dilutions there was added 1 cc. of a heavy, autoclaved suspension of B. coli II. Then, with proper controls for phage and suspension sterility, the entire set of tubes was incubated for several days. The controls remained sterile for 10 days; then they were discarded. Each day, for 5 days, agar slants were inoculated from each tube, respectively. A loopful was used in each instance. Also, daily, fresh controls were made, both from the autoclaved suspension, and from some of the ozonized, undiluted phage to which no bacteria had been added. These, also remained sterile for 10 days, indicating that neither phage alone, nor killed culture alone had any cultivable bacteria or contaminants. The agar slants made the first and second days remained sterile. Those made the third, fourth and fifth days were also sterile, except those made from the third dilution (10^{-3}): from this dilution, after 48 hours of incubation, a considerable number of small, clear, transparent colonies appeared in the agar slant cultures of the third, fourth and fifth days, respectively. These colonies upon longer incubation increased somewhat in size, but did not exceed about ½ millimeter. Several of these colonies, well separated the one from another, were transferred to agar slants, and incubated. Then their fermentation reactions were tried in soft agar, using dextrose, lactose, saccharose and mannitol. Readings were made in 24 and 48 hours: after that time no changes took place. They were as follows:

		Dextrose	Lactose	Saccharose	Mannitol
B. coli II (original)	24 hrs.	ag	ag	ag	ag
	48 hrs.	ag	ag	ag	ag
B. coli II (lysogenic)	24 hrs.	ag	0	0	0
	48 hrs.	ag	0	0	0
Colony, type 1.	24 hrs.	g	g	g	g
	48 hrs.	ag	ag	ag	ag
Colony, type 2.	24 hrs.	ag	ag	ag	ag
	48 hrs.	ag	ag	ag	ag
Colony, type 3.	24 hrs.	a	0	0	0
	48 hrs.	ag	ag	0	ag
Colony, type 4.	24 hrs.	a	0	0	0
	48 hrs.	a	a	a	a

Legend: a = acid: g = gas: O = growth, no acid formed.

Several features brought out in this tabulation deserve specific mention. The "lysogenic" culture (that is "phage carrying" culture) of B. coli II was obtained directly from a 1:10 dilution of coli phage acting upon a culture of B. coli II. After 48 hours, a slight clouding appeared, which upon isolation on agar, yielded this "lysogenic" culture. Twenty-four hour broth cultures of this organism have not yet failed to yield a potent phage, lysing the parent culture, B. coli II, in high dilution. The potency has been quite uniformly 10^{-10}. This lysogenic culture, unlike the parent strain, ferments only dextrose, from which it produces acid and gas. It is not uncommon to find that "lysogenic" cultures differ culturally and antigenically from the parent strains. This has been commented upon by Hadley[3] and by d'Herelle[4] and many others. This loss of fermentative power for lactose, saccharose and mannitol has persisted to the present time (July, 1935). Of the four types of organisms emerging from the filterable state to the nonfilterable state, type 2, fermening dextrose, lactose, saccharose and mannitol, was found to be identical with the parent culture, B. coli II, not only in its action upon sugars, but also in that it was lytic. This seems to be significant. It indicates clearly two hitherto unmen-

3. J. Infect. Dis. **42:** 263–1928.

4. The Bacteriophage and Its Behavior, Williams and Williams Company, Baltimore, 1926.

tioned phenomena of phage action, namely, that phage made from "lysogenic" cultures contains viable organisms in the filterable state, and, also, that among these organisms in the filterable state there may be, and in this instance, was, one that became lytic upon recovery, although derived from a "lysogenic" culture. Type 1 culture, fermenting dextrose, lactose, saccharose and mannitol, but more slowly than type 2 culture, was neutral: that is, it neither was a phage "carrier" (a "lysogenic" culture) nor did it lyse with either the B. coli II phage, or the "lysogenic" B. coli II phage. Thus far it has been impossible either to make it a "carrier" of phage, or to be lysed by phage. Types 3 and 4 departed somewhat more widely from the parent strain, especially the one designated as type 4. Neither of these cultures was lytic, "lysogenic" nor reminiscent of either B. coli II or "lysogenic" B. coli II. One of their most outstanding characteristics was their inability to grow in either plain or dextrose broth. Both of these organisms produced yellowish, thin, shiny films upon agar slants. The fact should not be overlooked that all of these variants were isolated from the same tube of ozonized phage-killed bacteria: all of the remaining tubes of the series remained sterile. The cultural reactions of these several types of bacteria remained constant for several weeks, at the end of which time they were discarded.

The "lysogenic" coli culture was plated directly upon mannitol Andrade agar plates, several times. Three principal types of cultures were obtained, of which the following were illustrative, insofar as their fermentation reactions are concerned:

	Dextrose	Saccharose	Lactose	Mannitol	
Type 1.	ag	0	0	0	"lysogenic"
Type 2.	ag	ag	0	0	neutral
Type 3.	ag	ag	ag	ag	neutral

Legend: a = acid: g = gas: 0 = growth, no acid formed.

Type 3 is a replica of B. coli II, but it neither "carried" phage, nor was the organism lysed by B. coli II phage. It was neutral in other words. Type 1 agreed with the reactions of B. coli II "lysogenic": it carried phage. Type 2 was neutral, and agreed with none of the other strains in its fermentative reactions. By direct plating of a "lysogenic" culture of B. coli II, therefore, bacteria were readily isolated, apparently in pure state, which differ in their fermentative reactions, among themselves, the "lysogenic" culture, and the parent culture, B. coli II. It is, therefore, perhaps not surprising to find a number of variants among those recovered in the nonfilterable state from the "lysogenic" phage.

Having thus recovered a typical, lytic culture of B. coli II from phage generated by this "lysogenic" culture, after inactivating the phage with ozonized air, a similar study was made of a culture of "lysogenic" staphylococcus, to see if it also contained staphylococci in the filterable state. The organism selected was a typical S. aureus (Staph. lyt.), which had been kept in culture in the laboratory for several years. This was the culture from which filterable bacteria were recovered in the nonfilterable state in some previous studies (2). The phage for this Staph. lyt. was built up in the usual manner from sewage.

It had a titer of 10^{-10}. A consistent peculiarity of this phage, not noticed in previous experiments, was noted: in every test for potency, the first dilution of this phage in broth (10^{-1}) showed a slight, but distinct turbidity, not manifested in the succeeding dilutions. For want of a better name, this slight turbidity was referred to as a "prezone." This "prezone" was reminiscent of the "prezone" occasionally met with among agglutinating serums. It is not to be assumed, however, that this phage "prezone" implies any essential relationship with the agglutination "prezone." From this "prezone" a "lysogenic" culture of Staph. lyt. was readily cultured upon agar, and this "lysogenic" culture, grown in broth over night, then filtered to remove bacteria, always yielded a potent phage, whose titer was uniformly 10^{-10}: that is, it would lyse the original, lytic culture in a dilution of 10^{-10}. Furthermore, this "lysogenic" phage always exhibited the "prezone" phenomenon, a detail of some interest inasmuch as it agreed in this respect, as in all others, with the phages prepared for the lytic strain, as above noted.

Growth from 3–20 hour agar slants of Staph. "lysogenic" were washed off with 15 cc. of sterile, physiological salt solution. After vigorous shaking to break up clumps, the bacterial suspension was centrifuged until all the organisms were sedimented. The clear, supernatant solution was filtered through a Berkefeld N filter. The clear, faintly yellowish, filtrate about 10 cc. in volume, was divided into three parts, which were tested as follows: a— a few drops were added to broth, and also spread upon agar, to determine sterility in the usual manner. b— dilutions were tested for phage activity. None was found. This is somewhat uncommon, because experience with other "lysogenic" cultures washed from agar slants, as above indicated, usually have phage activity. c— dilutions of the phage were made in broth, in multiples of 10, in the usual manner. To each of these several dilutions, 1 cc. of a killed (autoclaved) culture of Staph. lyt. was added. These several tubes, together with controls for sterility of the killed culture, and of phage, without added, killed bacteria, were incubated for several days. The controls, both those mentioned in a (filtered phage) and the killed organisms, remained sterile for two weeks. Then they were discarded. Plates were made from each of the several tubes, after 1, 2, and 3 days incubation. Those made on the first and second days remained without growth. Those of the third day, except from tube 2 (10^{-2}) also remained sterile. From the tube 2 cultures of the third day, incubated for 48 hours, small, clear, colorless colonies appeared. They were numerous: it was estimated that about 50 colonies eventually appeared. Three types of organisms, as shown by fermentation reactions, were detected. These reactions, upon the common sugars, dextrose, lactose, saccharose, and mannitol, in soft agar were as follows:

	Dextrose	Lactose	Saccharose	Mannitol	Remarks
Type 1.	a	0	a	a	neutral
Type 2.	a	a	0	0	neutral
Type 3	a	a	a	a	lytic
S. lyt.	a	a	a	a	parent culture
S. "lysogenic"	a	0	±	0	

Legend: a = acid: 0 = growth, no acid produced: ± = slight acid.

DISCUSSION

The ozone generator used in these experiments was said, by the manufacturers to produce 8 grams of ozone per hour, with the voltage and air pressure employed. No attempt was made to check the amount, however. The primary objective of the experiments was satisfied by comparative results, utilizing ozone merely as a convenient reagent, to determine the resistance of certain phages to strong oxidization, and also to make certain observations upon "lysogenic" bacteria, from which titratable phage was inactivated by ozone. Interest, in other words, centered upon the bacteria and their respective phages rather than upon the ozone.

The principal facts brought out through ozonization of phage in presence of nutrient broth are fairly simple and direct: under the conditions of the experiments, Staph. lyt. phage was found to be distinctly less resistant to ozonization (oxidization) than B. coli II phage. The same holds true for the corresponding "lysogenic" phages of these microbes. This is in accord with the results of mild oxidization induced by methylene blue and sunlight, where it will be remembered, Staph. phage was inactivated, whereas B. coli phage was apparently not weakened. On the other hand, Staph. lyt. organisms were found to be distinctly more resistant to ozone than B. coli II organisms. Decreasing progressively the amount of soluble organic substances in solution other than phage, conveniently achieved by substituting distilled water for broth as a diluent of phage, resulted in a porportionate and relative decrease, both of phage resistance and organism resistance to ozone, but always the relation between the phages and their respective bacteria remained parallel. The results seem to indicate that the protective action of soluble constituents of broth, while increasing the time required for inactivation of phage, or killing of bacteria, tempered the reaction, and thereby increased the chances of successful differentiation. From this, it is inferred that ozone provides a simple and direct means of inactivating phage in presence of certain bacteria, and also, of inactivating the phage of "lysogenic" cultures without destroying the organisms. Of some interest, also, is the recovery of bacteria in the nonfilterable state from certain lytic and "lysogenic" phages (those of Staph. lyt., Staph. "lysogenic," Coli II lyt. and Coli II "lysogenic") after these respective phages had been inactivated by ozone. Details of the experiments with the "lysogenic" phages only were described, but the procedure was equally successful with the lytic phages. The facts to be learned from the study of these particular filterable forms of bacteria, and their isolation are two, namely, first: that the filterable forms of Staph. lyt. and B. coli II are more resistant to ozone than the phages from which they were isolated. Whether these filterable forms are more resistant to ozone than their corresponding nonfilterable forms was not determined, and secondly, that phages made from these specified "lysogenic" cultures of Staph. lyt. and B. coli II respectively, freed from nonfilterable bacteria by filtration, yielded filterable forms of bacteria which, upon recovery in the nonfilterable state were found to be fully lytic. Thus far it has not been possible to obtain lytic strains from "lysogenic" strains by direct plating, and selection of colonies in this laboratory, using these specific cultures. And inasmuch as there has been considerable literary controversy upon this point, these definite recoveries of lytic bacteria from phage made from the "lysogenic" strains would seem to justify the statement that "lysogenic" cultures may, and these did, actually contain lytic bacteria. In addition to these lytic forms, recoverable from "lysogenic" phages, atypical strains also were recovered in the nonfilterable state, cultures which were neither lytic, lysogenic nor, indeed, replicas of either the lytic or the "lysogenic" strains, from which they were derived. These variants, morphologically resembling the parent cultures, ran the gamut of fermentation reactions. Several of these retained their peculiar sugar reactions with great tenacity for considerable periods of time: others were rather transitory, and upon artificial cultivation soon exhibited unmistakable tendencies to revert to type. Just what value and significance is to be attached to these disturbing variants depends upon the view point of the commentator.

SUMMARY AND CONCLUSIONS

Lytic and "lysogenic" phages were prepared for a particular strain of Staphylococcus and B. coli respectively, and their resistance to ozone was studied.

The lytic and "lysogenic" phages of the Staphylococcus were distinctly less resistant to ozone than the corresponding phages for B. coli.

The staphylococci on the contrary were more resistant to ozone than the colon bacilli.

The bacteria (Staphylococcus and B. coli), were more resistant to ozone than their respective phages.

Certain soluble organic substances materially increase the resistance of phage and of bacteria to ozone.

Typical lytic bacteria in the nonfilterable state were isolated respectively from "lysogenic" and lytic phages, both of B. coli and of Staphylococcus.

OBSERVATIONS UPON THE "PREZONE" OF CERTAIN BACTERIOPHAGES

STUDIES IN BACTERIAL METABOLISM, CVI

ARTHUR ISAAC KENDALL

AND

ARTHUR WILLIAM WALKER

CHICAGO

It is a matter of not uncommon observation that certain phages, but by no means all, exhibit a peculiarity, when they are tested by the dilution method in broth upon their respective homologous bacteria, which has no adequate explanation. This peculiarity consists in a clouding, or lack of clearing, in the highest concentrations of the phage, the lesser concentrations being clear up to the limit of potency of the phage. This clouding, or lack of clearing, which in absence of a better term, will be referred to as "prezone" is due to the presence of unlysed bacteria, which may be identified either by examination of direct smears, or by direct cultivation upon agar. The bacteria recoverable upon agar are almost always "lysogenic" that is, they are "carriers" of phage. Phage prepared from these lysogenic strains, thus recovered, also usually show this "prezone" phenomenon when they are tested upon their specifically homologous organisms. It should be emphasized that this "prezone" phenomenon (clouding), in point of time is different from the secondary clouding that may appear in any or all tubes of a phage titration in broth, in that the former—the "prezone" clouding appears during the first hours of incubation, whereas the latter, the secondary clouding—develops only after prolonged incubation. Phage recovered from the filtration of a "prezone" tube is as potent as that of any tube not showing "prezone" in the series. Also, phage thus prepared from a "prezone" tube exhibits a "prezone." Two other pecularities of this "prezone" phenomenon deserve mention. First, "prezone" is, or may be elicited only when the phage lyses its specifically homologous organism. Other lysable, but not specifically homologous bacteria may fail to produce it, even though they dissolve in "prezone" phage of very great potency. Yet phage generated by the action of a "prezone" phage upon alien, but lysable bacteria not itself manifesting "prezone" may, and apparently often does, revert to the "prezone" type when it is tested against its original, specifically homologous strain of organism. In other words, a phage exhibiting "prezone" for one lysable strain, may not exhibit "prezone" when it lyses another strain: but the phage generated by this mismating may, and certainly occasionally does, carry the "prezone stamina" which is remanifested when the phage and its specifically homogeneous strain of microbe are

---

Received for publication, August 1, 1935.

From the Laboratories of Bacteriology, Northwestern University Medical School.

brought together. Notwithstanding the obvious fact that this phenomenon, tentatively designated "prezone" has been observed many times, very little seems to have been done in the way of specifically studying it: indeed, the only reference thus far encountered is that of Zaytzeff-Jern and Meleney[1] who noticed that a certain phage, exhibiting apparently the "prezone" phenomenon would fail to show this initial clouding if the number of bacteria added were increased from some 25 million to 250 million, using otherwise the same concentration of phage. "More potent phages are obtained by using large inoculations of bacteria (150–250 million per cc.) and small inoculations of phage, 0.1 to 0.01 cc. (approximately 1 to 10 million phage corpuscles) in 10 cc. of medium than with smaller quantities of bacteria and larger amounts of phage." This observation does not bear directly upon the phenomena about to be described, however.

The experiments recorded here were made with two phages, Staph. lyt. and Staph. 1038, together with their respective, specifically homologous organisms Staph. lyt. and Staph. 1038. Staph. lyt. was isolated from a case of impetigo some years ago. It is a typical Staphylococcus aureus. A phage was built up for it from sewage at the time of its isolation. Staph. 1038 and its specific phage were obtained from outside sources about two years ago. It happens that either phage will lyse either organism in high dilution, (10^{-10}) when measured in the usual manner in broth. The potencies of these two phages have remained unchanged for several months before and after these experiments were made. It was noticed that the phage for Staph. lyt., from the start, produced a "prezone" consistently, whenever it was tested against its specifically homologous organism (S. lyt.): It does not produce a "prezone" against Staph. 1038. The phage for Staph. 1038 does not produce a "prezone" either against Staph. lyt. or against Staph. 1038.

EXPERIMENTAL

The following tabulation shows the essential details of the "prezone" phenomenon which led to a more extended examination of this peculiar clouding, which occurs in the highest concentrations of phage (10^{-1}) in a series of dilutions in broth, extending to the limit of potency, (10^{-10}) of Staph. lyt. phage for its specifically homologous organism.

Staph. lyt. phage + Staph. lyt. = "prezone," 10^{-1}: dilutions 10^{-2} to 10^{-10} clear.
Staph. lyt. phage + Staph. 1038 = no "prezone": dilutions 10^{-1} to 10^{-10} clear.
Staph. 1038 phage + Staph. lyt. = no "prezone": dilutions 10^{-1} to 10^{-10} clear.
Staph. 1038 phage + Staph. 1038 = no "prezone": dilutions 10^{-1} to 10^{-10} clear.

The clouding, or "prezone" in dilution 10^{-1} of Staph. lyt. phage and Staph. lyt. remains unchanged for at least 48 hours, the remaining tubes being entirely clear.

From this, it appears that the "prezone" in this series appears only when Staph. lyt. phage lyses its specifically homologous organism, Staph. lyt. This experiment has been repeated many times with the same results. Next, the clouding in tube 1 (10^{-1}) was subcultured on agar. After 24 hours a fairly luxuriant growth of typical staphylococci resulted. The organisms were found

1. J. Lab. and Clin. Med. **20:** 862, 1935.

to be "lysogenic" that is, "carriers" of phage. Phage made from this "lysogenic" culture was found to have a "prezone" for the homologous organism, but not for the heterologous organism, thus:

Staph. lyt. "prezone" phage+Staph. lyt.="prezone," 10^{-1}: remaining tubes clear.
Staph. lyt. "prezone" phage+Staph. 1038=no "prezone" all tubes clear.

The potency of this Staph. lyt. "prezone" phage was found to be 10^{-10} for each organism. It appears from these experiments that the clouding or "prezone" manifested by Staph. lyt. phage is due to unlysed bacteria, and that these unlysed bacteria become "carriers," but only when the phage acts upon its homologous organism. When the phage acts upon the heterologous organism, (1038) no clouding appears, and all the organisms dissolve. Also, phage made from the Staph. lyt. "prezone" tube are carriers of phage which has the same peculiarity, namely, that it produces "prezone" acting upon Staph. lyt. but not when acting upon Staph. 1038.

It might be assumed, and the possibility is freely admitted, that the "prezone" lysogenic phage produces a prezone when lysing Staph. 1038, but that this prezone is too little in amount to detect in the lowest dilution used, 10^{-1}. But in any event, no detectable prezone was noticed under any circumstances not involving Staph. lyt. and its phage, or its "lysogenic" variant. And this raises the interesting question: is the transmission of this "prezone" through the phage itself, or through its specific organism, Staph. lyt. An attempt was made to obtain information upon this point through the following set up:

A. Staph. lyt. phage+Staph. lyt., were allowed to act over night in the usual manner, than filtered. The ninth tube of the series (10^{-9}) which was clear and showed no evidence of "prezone" ("prezone" was observed in tube one, however) will be referred to as Phage A for brevity. B. In like manner Staph. lyt. phage was allowed to act upon Staph. 1038, using the customary set of dilutions in broth (10^{-1} to 10^{-10}). No "prezone" was observed. Tube 9 (10^{-9}) of this series was filtered, and will be referred to as Phage B. Phages A and B were tested respectively against Staph. lyt. and Staph. 1038. The results elicited were as follows:

Phage A+Staph. lyt.: tube 10^{-1} had a "prezone" tubes 10^{-2} to 10^{-10} were clear.
Phage A+Staph. 1038: no "prezone" tubes 10^{-1} to 10^{-10} were clear.
Phage B+Staph. lyt.: tube 10^{-1} had a "prezone": tubes 10^{2}, to 10^{-10} were clear.
Phage B+Staph. 1038: no "prezone": tubes 10^{-1} to 10^{-10} were clear.

COMMENT

The ninth dilutions (10^{-9}) were used in preference to others of the same series for two reasons: first because there was no clouding, or "prezone" and secondly because these dilutions approached the limits of potency of the phages, which were found to be 10^{-10}, as previously stated, The suggestive feature of this experiment is found in the phage obtained through the lysis of Staph. 1038 by the Staph. lyt. phage. This phage (B) has, so to speak, a mixed ancestry in that it was not specifically developed originally for the organism it happened to lyse. Yet this phage, resulting from the lysis of the alien strain, retested upon its specifically homologous organism. Staph. lyt. manifested the initial clouding, or "prezone" in quite as definite manner as it did when generated upon its own specific strain. From this it was inferred that the capacity for "prezone" formation resides in the phage rather than in its homologous organism, and also that this peculiar phenomenon of "prezone" formation or production was not lost by passage of the phage through the alien strain. To elicit the "prezone" phenomenon, however, it is apparently essential to have the homologous strain. Whether other phages exhibiting the "prezone" phenomenon would exhibit the same entailability cannot be answered at this time.

Other combinations involving a "prezone" phage and alien organisms readily present themselves, but they were passed by in order to study somewhat more in detail just what the nature of the "prezone" really is.

A fully satisfactory explanation of the "prezone" phenomenon, in addition to the fundamental, antecedent problem of the nature of phage itself, should be prepared to answer the following questions: 1—why do some, but by no means all, phages have a "prezone": 2—how is, or how may, "prezone" be produced: 3—how may "prezone" be accentuated: and 4—how may "prezone" be temporarily or permanently be lost or destroyed? The experiments hereby described, admitting failure, frankly in answering most of these queries, are cited to show how the "prezone" phenomenon was apparently very definitely increased in one phage—that for Staph. lyt., described above. One very definite objective was rigorously adhered to in this extension of the "prezone" phenomenon, namely, that the titre of the phage should not be materially lessened coincidently with the "prezone" increment. It was assumed that advancing the "prezone" by experimental measures, the phage meanwhile remaining unchanged in its titre, would be indicative, or at least suggestive, of quantitative interference with the action of the phage, without thereby lessening its ultimate capacity of inducing lysis, as measured by the smallest concentration that would dissolve its homologous organism. A mere extension of "prezone" concomitant with a marked diminution of its potency to lyse, on the other hand, could be construed, very properly, as essentially a linear destruction of the phage, with concomitant supplemental effects. A number of procedures, involving the use of chemicals, were tried, unsuccessfully, before the method herein described was arrived at. These numerous failures are passed by in favor of that one which seems to be reasonably effective for the phage studied. Attention is directed here to the notorious variations different phages exhibit under presumably comparable conditions, which suggest that the study of "prezone" among different phages may require considerable variation in procedure to achieve the desired results.

EXPERIMENTAL

It has long been known that certain soluble nitrates, in moderate concentration, stimulate the growth of bacteria, due probably to the availability of oxygen in the nitrate molecule. Having in mind the inactivation of Staph. phage by mild oxidization, induced by methylene blue and sunlight, Staphylococcus phage (Staph. lyt. phage, having a natural "prezone") was set up in the following manner: Staph. lyt. phage, 1 cc., M/1 $NaNO_3$ 1 cc., broth, 8 cc. The mixture was inoculated with Staph. lyt., and incubated over night. The following morning it was filtered through a Berkefeld N filter, and, together with a control to ensure sterility, was diluted in broth in the usual manner, to test its potency, using the homologous organism, Staph. lyt., for this purpose. After 18 hours of incubation, all the tubes were cloudy, some more so than others, as appears in the tabulation below. For purposes of comparison, the relative degrees of clouding, or turbidity, are designated by numerals, 4 indicating maximal; 3, 2, and 1 progressively less: 0 indicates complete clearing, or, in other words, complete lysis.

Tube	1	2	3	4	5	6	7	8	9	10	Control (culture)
"Nitrate" phage	3	3	3	3	2	1	2	2	2	2	3
Control phage	2	1	0	0	0	0	0	0	0	0	3

At first sight, it might appear that the "nitrate" phage had been almost completely inactivated. However, tubes 3 and 9 of the "nitrate" phage were filtered, and tested for phage activity, using the homologous organism for this purpose. The results, set forth below, indicate very clearly that there is phage in all the tubes, unimpaired in strength, and showing the "natural prezone" in tubes 1 and 2, like that of the unnitrated phage,

Dilution	1	2	3	4	5	6	7	8	9	10	Control (culture)
Tube 3	3	1	0	0	0	0	0	0	0	1	3
Tube 9	2	1	0	0	0	0	0	0	0	2	3

From which it would appear that both tubes 3 and 9, showing originally little evidence of phage, in reality had phage of initial potency, (10^{-10}). Such an experiment is not particularly convincing, however, and the procedure was modified by using an alien organism to effect the "prezone" formation, by oxidizing the phage in presence of nitrate. B. coli II, a typical B. coli, was used for this purpose. The Staph. phage used was, as before, Staph. lyt. phage. The initial set up was as follows: Staph. lyt. phage, 1 cc., M/1 $NaNO_3$, 1 cc., broth, 8 cc., B. coli II inoculum. Incubation was practiced for 18 hours, at the end of which time the cloudy culture was filtered through a Berkefeld N filter, and the filtrate set up in the usual manner in broth for the testing of phage potency. Proper controls were made, to insure the sterility of the filtrate. Staph. lyt. was used to test the potency of this coli-nitrate-phage.

Dilution	1	2	3	4	5	6	7	8	9	10	Control (culture)
Coli-nitrate phage	4	4	4	2	4	0	0	0	0	2	3

Tubes 1, 2, 3, and 5, (1:10, 1:100, 1:1,000, 1:100,000) were distinctly more turbid than the control culture. Tube 4 (dilution 1:10,000), although turbid, was somewhat less turbid than the control, an irregularity often observed in experiments of this kind. Tubes 6 to 9 inclusive, were perfectly clear, indicating complete lysis of the organisms. In this experiment, therefore, clouding, or "prezone" was marked in the first 5 dilutions, without any detectable impairment of the potency of the phage, which cleared the homologous organism through the ninth dilution. To be certain that the cloudy tubes really contained phage, and that the highest dilution also contained phage, tubes

2 and 9 were filtered, and tested in the usual manner against the homologous organism, Staph. lyt. with the following results:

Dilution	1	2	3	4	5	6	7	8	9	10	Control (culture)
Tube 2	3	1	0	0	0	0	0	0	0	0	3
Tube 9	2	1	0	0	0	0	0	0	0	2	3

Two facts stand out, first, that the potency of the phage was not perceptibly altered as a result of the nitrate-coli growth, and secondly, that the "prezone" artificially developed as a result of the coil-nitrate action upon the Staph. lyt. phage, manifested by turbidities in the first 5 dilutions of the main experiment, was completely lost in the second generation of phage, as shown by the titration of tubes 2 and 9. The "natural prezone" however, characteristic of the Staph. lyt. phage, remained without detectable change. It would appear, therefore, that an artificial "prezone," or at least an extension of a "natural prezone" had been brought about by the use of an alien organism, B. coli II, acting in presence of sodium nitrate, upon Staph. lyt. phage. That the alien organism had no appreciable effect upon the potency of the phage is evidenced by the high titre (10^{-10}): and that an "artificial prezone" had been created, or greatly extended, seems to be shown by the marked clouding induced in tubes 1 to 5 inclusive.

Inasmuch as $NaNO_3$ is the reagent involved in the production of "prezone" in these experiments, the next series of observations was made upon the effect of varying the concentration of this reagent. The details of the set up are as follows:

Staph. lyt. phage, 1 cc., 5M $NaNO_3$, 1 cc., broth, 8 cc. inoculum, B. coli II
Staph. lyt. phage, 1 cc., M/1 $NaNO_3$, 1 cc., broth, 8 cc. inoculum, B. coli II
Staph. lyt. phage, 1 cc., M/10 $NaNO_3$, 1 cc., broth, 8 cc. inoculum, B. coli II
Staph. lyt. phage, 1 cc., M/20 $NaNO_3$, 1 cc., broth, 8 cc. inoculum, B. coli II

The series of cultures was incubated over night, and then filtered through Berkefeld N filters. The clear filtrates were diluted in broth in the usual manner, and tested for "prezone" and for potency, using Staph. lyt. as the test organism.

Dilution	1	2	3	4	5	6	7	8	9	10	Control (culture)
5M $NaNO_3$ phage	3	3	2	2	1	0	0	0	1	1	3
M/1 $NaNO_3$ phage	4	4	3	2	1	0	0	0	0	1	3
M/10 $NaNO_3$ phage	3	2	1	1	1	0	0	0	0	1	3
M/20 $NaNO_3$ phage	2	1	2	0	0	0	0	0	0	1	3
Control: no $NaNO_3$	0	0	0	0	0	0	0	0	0	0	3

The results indicate that molar $NaNO_3$ is on the whole the most effective concentration of this reagent to use for the induction of "prezone" in this particular phage (Staph. lyt. phage). Next, the effect of molar $NaNO_3$ was studied upon undiluted Staph. lyt. phage. For comparison, phage diluted one half, and 10 times was included in the set up, which was initially as follows:

Staph. lyt. phage, 9 cc., broth 0 cc., $NaNO_3$, M/1, 1 cc., inoculum B. coli II
Staph. lyt. phage, 5 cc., broth 4 cc., $NaNO_3$, M/1, 1 cc., inoculum B. coli II
Staph. lyt. phage, 1 cc., broth 8 cc., $NaNO_3$, M/1, 1 cc., inoculum B. coli II

After incubation for 18 hours, the turbid cultures were filtered through Berkefeld N filters, set up in the usual manner in broth dilutions, and tested with Staph. lyt. for "prezone" formation and potency. The results appear in the following table, in the order presented above:

Dilution	1	2	3	4	5	6	7	8	9	10	Control (culture)
Concentrated phage	4	3	3	3	3	0	0	0	0	2	3
Phage 1:5	4	3	4	2	2	0	0	0	1	3	3
Phage 1:10	4	2	3	3	0	0	0	0	2	3	3

From which it would appear that molar $NaNO_3$ is as effective in inducing "prezone" in undiluted phage, without impairment of potency, as it was found to be in broth diluted 10 times.

One more type of experiment, illustrating the effect of crossing "nitrated" Staph. lyt. phage, which it will be recalled, had a persistent natural "prezone," with an alien, but lysable organism, Staph. 1038, deserves mention. The plan of this experiment was very simple: Staph. lyt. phage and Staph. 1038 phage, respectively were subjected to mild oxidization through the action of B. coli II and $NaNO_3$. The oxidized phages thus obtained were tested by the broth dilution method upon their respective organisms, both for potency and for "prezone" extension. The details were as follows:

A. Staph. lyt. phage, 1 cc., M/1 $NaNO_3$, 1 cc., broth, 8 cc., inoculum B. coli II
B. Staph. 1038 phage, 1 cc., M/1 $NaNO_3$, 1 cc., broth, 8 cc., inoculum B. coli II

After 28 hours incubation, A and B were filtered, and the clear filtrates were tested against both Staph. lyt. and Staph. 1038, respectively. For controls, the respective, unnitrated phages were tested against their homologous organisms

Dilution	1	2	3	4	5	6	7	8	9	10	Control (culture)
Phage A+Staph. lyt.	4	4	4	0	3	3	0	0	0	2	3
Phage A+Staph. 1038	4	4	4	4	4	0	0	0	3	3	3
Phage B+Staph. lyt.	0	0	0	0	0	0	0	0	0	3	3
Phage B+Staph. 1038	0	0	0	0	0	0	0	0	0	1	3
Control, Staph. lyt. phage	2	0	0	0	0	0	0	0	0	3	3
Control, Staph. 1038 phage	0	0	0	0	0	0	0	0	0	1	3

Legend: turbidities are expressed, as before, numerically: 4 being the most turbid, 1 the least but perceptible, turbidity. 0 = clear, and complete lysis.

DISCUSSION

The table shows quite clearly that a very considerable extension of "prezone" was induced in Staph. lyt. phage in presence of molar $NaNO_3$ by B. coli II, without materially impairing the initial potency of the phage itself. In this particular experiment, the "prezone" phenomenon extended to the sixth tube, of the dilution series, whereas in the control, unoxidized phage, the prezone was detectable only in the first dilution. Tube 4 was clear: this irregularity not infrequently occurs. The extension of "prezone" in the Staph. lyt. phage tested against Staph. 1038 is significant: it seems to corroborate in unequivocal fashion the effect of mild oxidization of Staph. lyt. phage upon the extension of the "prezone" phenomenon. This particular experiment was repeated with essentially similar results. The tubes showing clouding were examined microscopically; in each instance the clouding was found to be due to large numbers of typical staphylococci. Phage 1038 was apparently unaffected by the nitration in presence of B. coli II. No "prezone" was created but the potency of the phage was unchanged. The controls show the "normal prezone" in Phage Staph. lyt., and the absence of "prezone" in Phage Staph. 1038. The third tubes of Phage A were filtered, and tested for phage potency and "prezone": for this purpose, the homogeneous organisms were used, as appears in the table. For brevity, Phage A, tube 3, Staph. lyt. will be designated Phage X: Phage A, tube 3, Staph. 1038 will be designated Phage Y.

Dilution	1	2	3	4	5	6	7	8	9	10	Control (organism)
Phage X, Staph. lyt.	2	1	0	0	0	0	0	0	0	2	3
Phage X, Staph. 1038	0	0	0	0	0	0	0	0	0	3	3
Phage Y, Staph. lyt.	0	0	0	0	0	0	0	0	0	3	3
Phage Y, Staph. 1038	0	0	0	0	0	0	0	0	0	3	3

Legend: turbidities recorded as before: 4 the most turbid, 1 the least turbid. 0 = clear, complete lysis.

From which it follows that the very turbid tubes (number 3), which exhibited the "prezone" phenomenon generated in Staph. lyt. by B. coli, in presence of $NaNO_3$, contained phage of practically undiminished potency, but no "prezone" beyond that found in unaltered Phage Staph. lyt., when it was regenerated under the conditions of this experiment. Here again, therefore, the extension of "prezone": observable in the nitrated Staph. lyt. phage, does not reappear in the filtrate of this cloudy phage, retested upon its homologous organism. This would suggest that the artificially extended "prezone" is a direct, but unentailable result of mild oxidization rather than a permanent modification of the phage. Attempts to create a "prezone" in Staph. 1038 phage, which never had a natural "prezone" have thus far been unsuccessful, as has also a similar attempt to create "prezone" in two distinct phages for B. coli. Whether this lack of success is to be construed as indicating a highly specific peculiarity of Staph. lyt. phage, or whether a "natural prezone" is a prerequisite for prezone extension is left an entirely open problem at this time. The experimental data thus far elicited may be summarized as follows:

The "prezone" phenomenon is a peculiarity of some, but by no means all. phages.

The "prezone" may be a temporary, or a permanent quality.

"Prezone" when present, is manifested by a clouding in the highest concentration, or concentrations, of phage, when it is tested against its specifically homologous organism.

"Prezone" often is not manifested when the phage is tested against an alien, but lysable strain.

Thus far, phages not having a "natural prezone" have been refractory to the creation of prezone.

In one specific phage, Staph. lyt. phage (which had a persistent "natural prezone"), this "prezone" was extended by mild oxidization to such a degree it was clearly discernible in a dilution of 1:1,000,000. The potency of this phage was not perceptibly diminished by this mild oxidization. Unlike the naturally occurring "prezone," this artificially extended "prezone" was detectable when it was tested with an alien, but lysable strain of organism.

The "prezone" phenomenon, originally a peculiarity of a specific phage, may still manifest this peculiarity after the phage has been passed through an alien, lysable strain, and then retested against its specifically homogeneous strain. There is no perceptible loss of potency by this passage.

The mechanism of "prezone" extension deserves brief discussion: in these experiments, the extension of the prezone from its original level, to its artificial level (1:10 to 1:1,000,000, as determined by broth titration) was brought about by mild oxidization. The oxidizing agent was molar $NaNO_3$, and the organism inducing the oxidization was B. coli II. The result of this peculiar, mild oxidization is to so alter the phage that it, still possessing its combining power (specificity) for its homologous organism, has lost to a considerable degree that (hypothetical) property in virtue of which it actually effects lysis. Not all of the phage is thus altered, as is clearly indicated both by the presence of active phage in the cloudy tubes, and, also, by the unaltered potency of the phage, which, in the instance cited was 10^{-10} in spite of the induced "prezone." Upon this theory, the clouding in the higher concentration of phage that has been thus oxidized is due to bacteria which are saturated with the partly changed phage-phage which still combines, but no longer lyses-whereas in the highest dilutions, there is little or no partly changed phage, and lysis proceeds to clearing in the usual manner.

The closest biological analogy (which is mentioned here for purposes of illustration, without necessarily inferring any definite parallelism) is to be found in the much criticised, but still useful Ehrlich concept of toxin and toxoid as constituents of a specific toxin. Labelling the "prezone" for purposes of discussion, "phagoid," meaning merely that "phagoid" is a possible constituent of phage which, retaining its specific combining power for its homologous organism, has lost (still retaining the Ehrlich symbolism) its ergophore group, it is tentatively postulated that the experiments cited above, may be explained on this basis. By mild oxidization, of specific character, some phage is changed to "phagoid," manifested by a noteworthy increase in the number of tubes, or dilutions in broth, in which the "prezone" phenomenon is clearly apparent. However, this induced or extended "prezone" is a temporary change; for two reasons. When the tubes containing artificially extended "prezone" are further incubated, they often clear completely, indicating that the saturation with "phagoid," protecting those bacteria so saturated, does not protect the descendants of these bacteria, which, it will be remembered are in presence of active phage, even if it is masked by the "prezone." Secondly, the clear filtrates of cloudy tubes, retested upon the homologous bacteria, phage in the usual manner, with the limited, "natural, prezone, but not the induced, extended, prezone being discernible. It might be objected that this extended "prezone" is due to $NaNO_3$, carried over from dilution to dilution. This is apparently not so for two reasons: experiments with M/20 $NaNO_3$ in place of M/$NaNO_3$, it will be recalled, showed a very decided reduction in oxidization effect, and secondly, it is a simple matter of calculation to find that in the 5th dilution tube, where the effect was still marked, the $NaNO_3$ concentration is but 0.00085 milligrams. Also, experiments with the Staph. 1038 phage were unsuccessful in the creation of prezone, although there was no appreciable diminution in phage potency through the use of this reagent. From this it is inferred that $NaNO_3$ per se is not the effective agent in extending "prezone."

This tentative hypothesis fails to explain certain important details of "prezone," however.

It fails to afford an explanation of failure to create "prezone" in the few phages thus far studied, which had at the start no natural prezone.

It fails to explain why the "prezone" phenomenon is observed in phage generated by passage of a "prezone" phage through an alien, but lysable strain, incapable of itself generating "prezone."

It fails to explain why "prezone" is, or may be, detectable only when the specifically homologous strain is lysed, whereas lysis of an alien strain may fail to create "prezone."

It may well be that the "prezone" phage described in some detail above is an unusual phage, and therefore, the phenomena are chance ones, not to be met with very often. But the fact remains, that whatever the explanation may be, and whatever may be the rarity of its occurrence, the possibility of artificially extending "prezone" is a very real one. And as a biological phenomenon, it should be taken into account in a searching discussion of the origin, nature and mode of operation of phage.

SUMMARY AND CONCLUSIONS

"Prezone" formation is a peculiarity of some, but by no means all, phages.

A method of chemically augmenting "prezone" is described for one specific phage.

Certain characteristics of this "augmented prezone" are described.

A very tentative hypothesis is advanced in explanation of the phenomena observed.

FERMENTATIVE VARIETIES OF SALMONELLA AERTRYCKE

PHILIP R. EDWARDS
LEXINGTON, KENTUCKY

The problem of distinguishing different strains of bacilli within a single bacterial species has occupied the attention of bacteriologists for a number of years. In 1901 Jensen observed that certain cultures of E. typhi fermented xylose while other cultures did not. Kristensen and Henricksen[1] observed that the fermentation of xylose by E. typhi possessed epidemiologic significance and that in a given epidemic all the cultures isolated were identical in their action on xylose. Schiff[2] confirmed the observations of Kristensen and Henricksen.

Kristensen and Bojlen[3] examined 1019 cultures of S. schottmülleri from 414 patients in a number of epidemics. They found pronounced differences in the time required for certain strains to ferment rhamnose, dulcitol and inositol. By dividing the cultures into groups based on the rapidity of their action on inositol and rhamnose and their reaction in the rhamnose test of Bitter, Weigmann and Habs,[4] these workers were able to show that all the cultures derived from an epidemic belonged to the same type. Kristensen and Bojlen found that these types were remarkably constant and were of the opinion that the differences on which the types were based were of genetic origin.

Warren and Iredale[5] confirmed the observations of Kristensen and Bojlen and reached the same conclusions concerning the origin of the different types. Vogelsang[6] also confirmed the statements of Kristensen and Bojlen regarding S. schottmülleri.

The literature concerning the existence of different types among S. aertrycke cultures is extremely limited. Moltke[7] in the study of 13 cultures from 6 outbreaks of food poisoning found that 8 cultures from 3 outbreaks failed to ferment inositol in 14 days. The remainder of the strains produced acid and gas from inositol in 24 hours. All the cultures from any one outbreak were the same in their behavior toward inositol. Moltke suggested that this observation might be of value in studying the epidemiology of S. aertrycke infection. Kristensen and Bojlen[3] studied the action of several S. aertrycke

---

Received for publication, August 1, 1935.
From the Department of Animal Pathology, Kentucky Agricultural Experiment Station.
1. Acta path. et microbiol. Scandinav. **2:** 289, 1926.
2. Centralbl. f. Bakteriol. (Abt. 1) **110:** 90, 1929.
3. Centralbl. f. Bakteriol. (Abt. 1) **114:** 86, 1929.
4. München med. Wchnschr. **73:** 940, 1926.
5. J. Hyg. **34:** 203, 1934.
6. J. Infect. Dis. **55:** 276, 1934.
7. Acta path. et microbiol. Scandinav. **3:** 711, 1926.

cultures in the same way they examined S. schottmülleri. They noted no distinctive difference in the reaction of the different strains. Warren and Iredale[5] stated "A number of aertrycke or ? aertrycke strains which we tested gave quite different fermentative typing, but actually many of the strains had not been definitely typed serologically." No further reference to S. aertrycke is found in their paper. Edwards and Rettger[8] noted that certain cultures of S. aertrycke produced acid from xylose quite slowly, whereas other cultures fermented the sugar vigorously. The full significance of this observation was not realized at that time.

The purpose of the present paper is to point out the possibility of dividing cultures of S. aertrycke from animal diseases into types based upon their rate of action on various fermentable substances, and to demonstrate that these types possess epizoötic significance. The methods used here closely resemble those used by Kristensen and Bojlen[3] in their study of S. schottmülleri.

MATERIAL AND METHODS

The cultures used in the study were all typical S. aertrycke cultures which had been fully examined serologically. With one exception, cultures were included only when two or more strains from the same outbreak of disease were available. The cultures employed were as follows:

A. Two cultures (C8 and C9) isolated from ducks in Connecticut. See Rettger and Scoville.[9]

B. Two cultures (OW and CW) isolated from ducks in Massachusetts. See Rettger and Scoville.[9]

C. One culture (M22) isolated from a duck on Long Island. See Edwards and Rettger.[8]

D. Two cultures (Cy I and Cy III) isolated from canary birds in New Jersey. See Beaudette and Edwards.[10]

E. Thirteen cultures (17666–17671, TeB, TeF, Du, RD, Af, Ma, TwB) isolated from foals in Kentucky. See Edwards.[11]

F. Six cultures (NMI, NM2, 19170M1, 19170M2, 19176M1, M19187) isolated from mice recently shipped into Kentucky from Pennsylvania.

G. Eleven cultures (19176GPA, 19176GPB, 19187GPA, NGPI-NGP8) isolated from guinea pigs recently shipped into Kentucky from Missouri.

Each group of cultures represents an outbreak of animal disease and since in each instance the animals were from widely separated communities there can be no reasonable doubt that the outbreaks were etiologically distinct.

Methods.—Two methods were used to examine the rate of acid production from the fermentable substance. First the organisms were inoculated into meat extract-peptone broth. This medium, which had an initial reaction of p_H 7.6, contained .0016 per cent of bromthymol blue and 0.5 per cent of the fermentable substance to be tested. The inoculum consisted of a 3 mm.

8. J. Bact. **13:** 13, 1927.
9. J. Infect. Dis. **26:** 217, 1920.
10. J. Bact. **12:** 51, 1926.
11. J. Infect. **54:** 85, 1934.

loopful of a 24 hour broth culture. The cultures were incubated at 37 C and examined at frequent intervals to determine the length of time necessary for complete decolorization of the dye.

The second method used was the substitution of various fermentable substances in the rhamnose test of Bitter, Weigmann and Habs.[5] The basic medium had the following composition:

Dipotassium phosphate	0.5 gr.
Ammonium sulphate	1.0 gr.
Sodium citrate	2.0 gr.
Sodium chloride	5.0 gr.
Bacto peptone	0.05 gr.
Distilled water	1000 cc.

The medium was tubed in amounts of 2 cc. in small tubes and a sufficient amount of the fermentable substance to be tested was added to make a final concentration of 0.5 per cent. The tubes were inoculated with a 3 mm. loopful of a 24 hour broth culture and incubated at 37 C for 15 hours. One drop of a 0.5 per cent alcoholic solution of methyl red was added to each tube. A yellow color was recorded as a negative test, a red color as a positive test. Tubes which developed an orange color were recorded as doubtful.

Using these two methods the organisms were tested for their action on xylose, rhamnose, arabinose, trehalose, maltose, dulcitol, sorbitol, mannitol, inositol, glycerol and dextrin.

RESULTS

The only substances that yielded significant results were xylose, rhamnose and maltose. In extract broth containing xylose the cultures from outbreaks A, E, and F completely decolorized bromthymol blue in 10 to 12 hours, whereas the cultures from outbreaks B, C, D, and F did not attain a full acid reaction until after 36 to 48 hours incubation. In rhamnose broth all cultures decolorized the dye in 12 hours. In maltose broth, cultures from outbreaks A, D, E and F produced a full acid reaction in 7 hours while cultures from outbreaks B and C required 12 hours to fully decolorize the dye.

With the exception of the results obtained with xylose-bromthymol blue broth the tests detailed above were of no differential value. However, when xylose, rhamnose and maltose were used in the peptone-salt medium definite groups were established. The results of these tests are givin in table 1. It is evident that four groups were defined by these tests and that the groups coincide with the sources of the cultures. The first group gave positive tests with all three substances and is composed of strains from epizoötics A and E. The second group gave negative tests with maltose and xylose and positive results with rhamnose. It is composed of strains from outbreaks B and C. The third group gave positive tests with maltose and rhamnose and negative tests with xylose. Strains from epizoötics D and G comprise this group. Cultures from outbreak F gave positive tests with maltose and xylose and negative or doubtful tests with rhamnose.

DISCUSSION

The groups established can be accepted as having epizoötic significance only after their constancy and permanence are established. The tests tabulated above were repeated and constant results obtained. The only variance observed was a change from a negative to a doubtful reaction in rhamnose medium by two of the cultures in outbreak F. A change from a negative to a positive reaction has not been observed.

TABLE 1.—*Reaction of Cultures of S. Aertrycke in Peptone—Salt Medium*

Outbreak	Culture	Maltose	Xylose	Rhamnose
A	C8	+	+	+
	C9	+	+	+
B	OW	0	0	+
	CW	0	0	+
C	M22	0	0	+
D	CyI	+	0	+
	CyIII	+	0	+
E	17666	+	+	+
	17667	+	+	+
	17668	+	+	+
	17669	+	+	+
	17670	+	+	+
	17671	+	+	+
	TeB	+	+	+
	TeF	+	+	+
	Du	+	+	+
	RD	+	+	+
	Af	+	+	+
	Ma	+	+	+
	TwB	+	+	+
F	NMI	+	+	±
	NM2	+	+	0
	19170M1	+	+	0
	19170M2	+	+	0
	19176M1	+	+	±
	M19187	+	+	0
G	19176GPA	+	0	+
	19176GPB	+	0	+
	19187GPA	+	0	+
	NGP1	+	0	+
	NGP2	+	0	+
	NGP3	+	0	+
	NGP4	+	0	+
	NGP5	+	0	+
	NGP6	+	0	+
	NGP7	+	0	+
	NGP8	+	0	+

The only statement that can be made in regard to the permanence of the types over long periods is in regard to the action of certain of the cultures on xylose. Cultures from outbreaks A, B, C and D have been in the writers possession for 12 years. Eleven years ago it was observed that cultures from epizoötic A fermented xylose rapidly, whereas cultures from outbreaks B, C and D fermented xylose slowly. These characters have been retained. The two cultures in outbreak D represent a group originally composed of 9 cultures received from Dr. F. R. Beaudette. All 9 cultures acted slowly upon xylose, as do the two remaining strains. The single culture from outbreak C is one of 3 cultures isolated by Dr. L. F. Rettger from ducks on Long Island. When first tested by the writer these three strains fermented xylose slowly, as does the one remaining culture today. The thirteen cultures from epizoötic E were isolated 3 years previously. At the time of isolation these cultures fermented xylose rapidly, as they now do.

As stated above the cultures from outbreak F give negative tests in the rhamnose medium, that is they are Bitter negative. This is unusual in that the Bitter test has been rather widely used by European workers to differentiate S. aertrycke (Bitter positive) from S. schottmülleri (Bitter negative). It must be remembered, however, that Kristensen and Bojlen[3] isolated 27 cultures of S. schottmülleri which were consistently Bitter positive. Therefore it is not surprising that certain cultures of S. aertrycke should be Bitter negative.

If the groups defined above are accepted as significant, their value in the study of epizoötic and epidemic disease can be perceived easily. A practical illustration of the value of the tests is contained in the cultures from outbreaks F and G. A group of mice and a group of guinea pigs were received at the laboratory at the same time. They came from widely separated points. At the time they were received one mouse was dead. This animal was not examined. Within a few days both lots of animals began to die and from them S. aertrycke was isolated. The question arose as to whether the animals were infected when received and whether the infection had spread from one lot to the other. Closer examination of the cultures isolated revealed the differences given in table 1. The obvious conclusion is that both the guinea pigs and mice were infected with S. aertrycke when they were received. This conclusion is supported by the absence of paratyphoid infection in other animals in the laboratory.

It is probable that the examination of cultures from a number of outbreaks will reveal the presence of still other fermentative varieties of S. aertrycke and that they will be of value in tracing the origin of paratyphoid infection.

SUMMARY

Cultures of S. aertrycke can be divided into groups by their reaction toward rhamnose, maltose and xylose in the peptone—salt medium of Bitter, Weigmann and Habs. These groups coincide with the sources of the strains and apparently are of epizoötic significance.

THE RELATIONSHIP OF STRAINS OF GREEN STREPTOCOCCI TO THE CLINICAL CHARACTER OF SUBACUTE BACTERIAL ENDOCARDITIS

HERBERT FOX
PHILADELPHIA

There is perhaps no more acute problem in the realm of medical bacteriology than the relationship between clinical medicine and the bacteria that can be isolated from a given case. Among the most serious problems of today is the understanding of subacute bacterial endocarditis, its causation, and treatment. To this end this laboratory has been engaged in a variety of studies as have many other places. During the past five years 42 isolations of the viridans group have been made during life and in 22 thereof this was confirmed by autopsy. Twenty-six of the isolations have been followed for varying lengths of time and from 10 of these, adequate data have accumulated for analysis and comparison and for an attempt to show the relationship between the biology of streptococci and the condition of the patient. The remaining 16 could not be or were not followed with sufficient completeness to permit conclusions; some strains died, some would not live on the medium for sufficient length of time to make the comparisons. These organisms were isolated on 7.4 p_H plain and glucose brain broth and after isolation were carried in the ice box on chocolate agar. Throughout this entire work 1 per cent human defibrinated blood agar at 7.4 p_H has been used. Sugar mediums corresponded to the formula of Holman save for the use of serum. Determinations were made primarily by the Holman scale, confirmed by the Brown criteria and established as to type by the biologic standards of Lancefield; precipitation methods were not used.

The organisms were grown on sealed plates in the second or third generation from isolation. After 3 days' incubation, isolations were made from S and R colonies as they appeared. Further study at the end of 10 days showed if true dissociation had occurred and pickings were repeated.

The 10 strains now reported, from 11 to 96 generations, have been cultivated for 10 months to 2 years; 6 of the remaining 16 have had similar treatment but are not reported upon because of the absence of complete bacteriological or clinical data. Incomplete data from them are consistent with those upon which these comments are made.

The plates were sealed, incubated at 37 C. and observed at 3 to 5 day intervals for 5 weeks. Determinations were made at the end of 3 and 10 days according to the biological scales mentioned above. The observations were made three times over eight months.

Analysis of this ten permits no final conclusions but affords a confirmation of the irregularity of bacteriological findings in subacute bacterial endo-

---

Submitted for publication, August 13, 1935.
From the Pepper Laboratory of Clinical Medicine, University of Pennsylvania.

carditis, suggests a certain difference between the clinical types and reveals a somewhat definite relationship between colonial type and clinical features.

The clinical cases were divided into 4 groups. The first consisted of 4 cases that were rapid, stormy, and complicated in course, leading to death in a few months from the earliest record that could be established as the beginning of subacute bacterial endocarditis. The second group was slow in course but ended with an episode that lead to death. The third group was likewise slow but progressive with marked anemia and cachexia so that the patient died without flagrant episodes. The next group gave a history that demanded their separation as truly recurrent cases. One of these is now well for at least 8 months and may be a truly recovered case or one with an intermission of considerable length; this shall be the subject of publication at a later time.

Group 1, the rapid, stormy cases, were due to the salivarius and equinus streptococci corresponding to Lancefield's human group. One of these gave smooth and rough colonies from the start yet the two were biologically identic; it therefore might be called a mixed isolation. Its characters were repeated by autopsy culture. The next case though human, was truly rough originally and its character was repeated at autopsy. Cases 3 and 4 were originally smooth but became rough. Cases 2 and 4 were pathogenic for mice.

It is therefore, noticeable that we have human types which, while partly smooth, were predominantly rough, either originally or by dissociation under laboratory cultivation. Three of these were confirmed by autopsy and 2 were pathogenic for mice.

Only one case, number 5, was slowly progressive and sudden in end. It was due to a human form of a rough and G type of Streptococcus non-hemolyticus No. 1; this was also found at autopsy.

Two slowly progressive cachectic cases gave Streptococcus ignavus in one and Streptococcus non-hemolyticus No. 1 in the other, the former being of the human type, the latter being of the non-human type. The human type was smooth, the non-human type rough. The human type was isolated at autopsy and was found pathogenic for mice. The original culture taken during life, was not pathogenic for mice.

The three recurrent cases were due to Streptococcus faecalis twice and salivarius once. The faecalis type was not human although it was smooth and without dissociation. Unfortunately no autopsy has been had in this recurrent group and two of the three isolations were not pathogenic for mice.

It can be seen from the foregoing that all of the serious and rather rapid cases were of the human type according to Lancefield and that every one thereof had a dissociation to rough or were originally rough. The slowly progressive cases were twice human and twice rough. Two of the three recurrent cases were not human and were smooth. The living recurrent case, while human biologically, was rough.

It would appear then that the possibility of dissociation to rough was associated with the maintained pathogenetic power of the organisms even though they may have begun as smooth.

If one were to divide these cases into rapid and stormy, and slow with a serious episode on the one hand, against the slowly progressive cachectic and recurrent cases on the other, it is easy to see that the human type of organisms with the smooth-rough combination and rough dominant was associated with the more virulent attacks. The slower cases have a dominance of the smooth type.

The pathogenic possibilities of isolated strains are not high but it would appear from these meager data that the more pathogenic strains were associated with the more stormy clinical course.

The same relativity between clinical activity and colony formation was followed partly in 2 flagrant cases and 3 cachectic cases, the bacteriological data of which could not be completed. We have also one partial record of a recurrent case of a year and a half due to Streptococcus faecalis that was constantly human-smooth from two isolations three months apart but the organisms died in all mediums after the tenth day.

Colonial types of these streptococci were constant in their behavior over the five weeks incubations as described and over the eight months observation. Smooth remained smooth with the exception of faint daughter colonies at the end of three weeks in two of the strains. They showed pearl-necklace appearance in hanging drop and stained preparations.

The R colonies when they occurred, appeared after the third day in every one of the strains, developing to their full recognizable and describable form at the end of ten days. There was no true relationship between the type of roughness and the number of rough colonies, whether or not the strain was originally rough or whether it developed from smooth by dissociation. Two types of R colonies could be detected. One had a coarse granular edge with a flat or crateriform center; the other was centrally coarse or granular, the edges becoming petaloid. The diameter of the first seldom reached 2 mm.; the diameter of the second rose on a few occasions to 3 mm. One constant rough form gave homogeneous broth growth of a pearl necklace type of chain and was pathogenic for mice.

In one case only, No. 1, did there seem to be on the original cultivation the development of both S and R colonies on the blood plate.

S colonies and S broth retained throughout, the pearl necklace chains of varying length. The R colonies, whether original or dissociated, were found to be diplococci, pneumococcoid, very short chains or bacillary.

Two strains of established Rs, one human No. 5, one not human No. 7 and one smooth No. 8, were cultivated anaerobically on plates for twelve days. All remained pure and without dissociation, which would seem to indicate that anaerobic growth had no influence upon their colonial differentiation. After anaerobic growth they bred true to type in the Holman scale but were not run out by the Lancefield method.

DISCUSSION

The data presented seem to suggest that there is a relationship between the clinical character of subacute bacterial endocarditis and the biological criteria accepted by Lancefield[1] as indicative of the human origin of certain

1. J. Exper. Med. **57**: 571, 1933.

streptococci. They would also indicate that there is a direct relationship of the rough character of colonies on the mediums used in this study to the violence of the morbid process. They would suggest that the slower cases of subacute bacterial endocarditis are associated with non-human streptococci and are relatively more often smooth originally or throughout. It would seem to indicate that pathogenicity for mice may be found more often than is customarily reported.

This study fits in with the work of Tunnicliff and Woolsey[2] and complements their work by adding the thought of the degree of relativity of clinical and bacteriological findings. It adds to some extent to the assumption of Rosenow discussed in the reference just given which would credit considerable value to rough colonies. Finally it appears to assign to roughs, which are usually accredited with a degree of invasiveness less than that of smooths, a special value perhaps high enough to be considered of sufficient importance for the bacteriologist to report them to the clinician and for the latter to evaluate them as significant in the interpretation of his clinical case.

2. J. Infect. Dis. **56**: 116, 1935.

QUANTITATIVE DETERMINATIONS OF CARBOHYDRATE UTILIZATION BY BACTERIA

COMPARISON WITH ACID-INDICATOR METHODS

A. G. WEDUM

CHICAGO

Fermentation reactions are an important tool in the study of bacterial classification, variation, and metabolism. The usual system for determining fermentation reactions consists of a medium, the carbohydrate in question, and an acid-indicator. Although there are other methods they ordinarily have the common fault like the acid-indicator system of dependence for their reliability upon the production of certain expected end products. If the end products are unorthodox or less in amount than the limit of accuracy of the method, then the conclusions may be erroneous in regard to whether the carbohydrate is utilized. The literature contains many such instances.

Lately there has been an increasing realization of this weakness of the acid-indicator method. The present tendency is to report reactions merely as acid or alkaline instead of reporting an alkaline reaction as a failure to utilize the carbohydrate in question. Such a report is commendable for its accuracy but not for its thoroughness. Surely the utilization of a carbohydrate is a more fundamental characteristic than the rapidity with which it is utilized or the nature of the mechanism or end products. In this regard the work of Karstrom[1] and of Vaughan and Hubbard[2] upon adaptive and constitutive enzymes is a step in the right direction. These workers found that some resting bacteria fermented certain sugars immediately even if grown on and harvested from plain agar. Such carbohydrases were called "constitutive." Other sugars were not fermented unless the organisms were harvested from specific carbohydrate agar. Such carbohydrases were designated as "adaptive." Experienced bacteriologists know only too well that bacterial production of acid from carbohydrates is a somewhat variable property so that sometimes the results of today are difficult to duplicate after a year's interval, particularly where questionable fermentations are involved.

The method which really gets to the root of the matter is one which involves the quantitative determination of the amount of carbohydrate remaining in a bacterial culture after a prolonged period of incubation. There are several of these methods[3] which have been employed in various types of studies by an increasing number of investigators in recent years. Many of

Received for publication, August 14, 1935.

From the Department of Bacteriology, Northwestern University Medical School.

1. Über die Enzymbildung in Bakterien. Helsingfors, Akademische Buchhandlung, 1930.
2. Proc. Soc. Exper. Biol. & Med. **30:** 405, 1932.
3. Schmidt, C. F.: J. Bact. **22:** 31, 1931.
   Smith, M. L.: Biochem. J. **26:** 1459, 1932.

these workers have incidentally demonstrated that the lack of evident acid in a bacterial culture in a carbohydrate medium is no conclusive indication of lack of utilization of the carbohydrate.[4] Many micro-organisms utilize carbohydrate but either produce no acid or else produce so little that it is neutralized by the buffer qualities of the medium or by concomitantly produced alkali. For that reason the practice of reporting carbohydrate reactions without specifying the period of incubation and the medium in which they were obtained must be condemned.

Some three years ago the present study was begun with the object of determining just how accurate the usual acid-indicator method is in reflecting the true state of the carbohydrate reactions of a number of common bacteria when compared with the results obtained by quantitative analysis. Also, amid the welter of work on bacterial variation, it would be interesting to know just how much stability of biochemical characteristics one might expect from a bacterial culture incubated in a carbohydrate medium for weeks and months. This study further gives one an idea of what might be found by careful study of the carbohydrate reactions of any large group of stock cultures.

METHODS

The basic procedure has been briefly described.[4 f, l] This procedure was to examine by quantitative analyses all carbohydrate reactions which appeared to be negative according to the usual acid-indicator methods. First, all organisms were tested at least in duplicate for acid formation by incubation 4 days in carbohydrate beef heart infusion peptone soft agar acid-indicator medium. However, soft agars were often less satisfactory than fluid mediums and the latter had to be used in many instances. Then repeated quantitative carbohydrate analyses[5] were made of cultures of all bacteria in all carbohydrates in which abundant acid was not produced. The minimum number of cultures analyzed before a conclusion was reached that a carbohydrate was not utilized by any one strain of organism was 4. These 4 comprised at least 3 experiments and at least 2 mediums: carbohydrate beef heart infusion peptone broth, and carbohydrate 2 per cent peptone 0.5 per cent sodium chloride, with or without an acid-indicator (usually Andrade). These mediums will hereafter be referred to as broth medium and peptone medium. All carbohydrates were sterilized in 10 per cent solutions by Berkefeld filtration and added separately without being subjected to heating to make concentrations of about 0.5 per cent for monosaccharides and 0.8 per cent for disaccharides. The initial p_H was 6.8–7.4. The mediums were dispensed in tubes 15 to 20 mm.×150 mm., 8–10 cc. per tube. Incubation was practiced at 37 C. for from 14 days to 21 months, the usual time being 14 days. In all doubtful cases additional tubes were incubated for 14 days, 3 months, or 21 months.

All bacteria showing fermentation by analysis but not by indicator were then inoculated in

4. (a) Fred, E. B., Peterson, W. H., and Anderson, J. A.: J. Bact. **8:** 277, 1923.
   (b) De Bord, G. G.: J. Bact. **8:** 7, 1923.
   (c) Merrill, M. H.: J. Bact. **20:** 235, 1930.
   (d) Jones, F. S., Orcutt, M., and Little, R. B.: J. Bact. **23:** 267, 1932.
   (e) Goresline, H. E.: J. Bact. **26:** 435, 1933.
   (f) Wedum, A. G., and Sorkin, S. S.: Proc. Soc. Exper. Biol. & Med. **30:** 1132, 1933.
   (g) Reynolds, H., McCleskey, C. S., and Werkman, C. H.: J. Infect. Dis. **55:** 207, 1934.
   (h) Goddard, D. R.: J. Infect. Dis. **54:** 149, 1934.
   (i) Conn, H. J., and Darrow, M. A.: J. Bact. **27:** 51, 1934.
   (j) Roberts, J. L.: J. Bact. **29:** 229, 1935.
   (k) Lamb, J. H., and Lamb, M. L.: J. Infect. Dis. **56:** 8, 1935.
   (l) Wedum, A. G., and Walker, A. W.: J. Infect. Dis. **57:** 160, 1935.
5. Stiles, H. R., Peterson, W. H., and Fred, E. B.: J. Bact. **12:** 427, 1926.

fresh mediums. Colorimetric p_H determinations were made with a LaMotte Hydrogen Ion Testing Set every 1–2 days and quantitative analyses at suitable intervals up to 14 days. Ample growth was present in all instances. Purity of the cultures was assured by gross examination of the tubes, terminal plating out of the cultures on specific carbohydrate indicator nutrient agar, and the consistency of results from cultures inoculated in different batches of medium at different times.

No attempt was made to control evaporation in cultures incubated for 14 days—the sugar content of the culture tubes was simply compared with that of 2 or more control uninoculated tubes and with that of cultures of non-fermenting bacteria such as B. alcaligenes. Evaporation in tubes incubated more than 2 weeks was minimized by the use in each tube (in addition to the usual cotton plug, cut short and singed) of a sterile one hole rubber stopper containing a short piece of 1 mm. bore glass tubing.

Supplementary variations and additions to the procedure are indicated in the following pages as far as is practicable. It is quite impossible to record all of the 6,000 or more quantitative analyses in detail.

The inoculums were from standard laboratory strains which had been carried for years on 0.1 per cent dextrose agar slants. The date of receipt and source of most of those organisms which were not isolated at Northwestern University Medical School is given as follows: 1912 Staph. epidermis albus, Harvard; 1913 M. tetragenus, Dr. Winslow, NY.; 1909 B. Dys. Flexner I, Boston Floating Hospital; 1914 B. Dys. Flexner II, Parke Davis & Co.; 1913 B. paratyphosus A, Schottmüller culture Dr. T. Smith, Harvard; B. paratyphosus A No. 9 and No. 219, U. of Chicago; 1913 B. paratyphosus B I (Dr. Burton, Boston Board of Health 1903) (Am. Museum Nat. Hist. 1912) U. of Chicago; 1913 B. paratyphosus B II, Schottmüller culture Dr. T. Smith, Harvard; 1912 B. cholerae suis, Dr. T. Smith, Harvard; 1913 B. enteritidis (Gaertner) (Dr. Dunham, Cambridge, England 1900) Dr. Jordan, U. of Chicago; B. icteroides, Hygienic Lab. U. S. Marine Hospital Service; B. morgani (No. 1?), Dr. Morgan, Lister Institute; 1913 B. avisepticus (Colorado State Agri. College 1910) Dr. Jordan, U. of Chicago; B. diphtheriae (Park 8) Dr. Park, NY.; B. hofmanni, American Type culture Collection; 1917 B. anthracis 28, American Museum of Natural History; 1929 B. anthracis (Dr. Pryor, Detroit Board of Health 1928) U. of Michigan; 1929 B. anthracis (Dr. Koch, Germany) (Dr. Novy 1888) U. of Michigan; 1919 Streptococcus No. 20, Dr. Hektoen, Chicago; 1912 B typhosus I, Dr. Arms, Boston Board of Health; 1923 B. typhosus III, Chicago Health Department; 1927 B. typhosus Hopkins, Chicago Health Dept.; 1917 B. dysenteriae Shiga I and II, Rockefeller Institute; B. proteus vulgaris, Dr. T. Smith, Harvard; B. Proteus No. 3, Dr. Clark, U. S. Bureau of Animal Industry; B. phlei III, Hygienic Lab. U. S. Marine Hospital Service; 1916 B. subtilis (Cohn), American Museum of Natural History; B. leprae, Dr. Hardy, Hygienic Lab. U. S. Marine Hospital Service; 1914 B. leprae No. 86, Dr. Winslow, NY.; 1913 B. smegmatis, Dr. Winslow, NY.

RESULTS

Table 1 presents those micro-organisms with which the findings of non-utilization of sugars were in agreement by both acid-indicator and quantitative analysis methods. In this group, fermentation was accompanied by acid which was clearly evident by p_H or acid-indicator in carbohydrate soft nutrient agar or carbohydrate fluid mediums or both. It is gratifying to note in such a representative collection that the use of acid-indicator methods was quite trustworthy.

Table 2 presents those organisms which within two weeks time in broth, peptone, or soft agar carbohydrate mediums produced clearly evident acid in the presence of some sugars but in other sugars even though quantitatively the sugar was fermented no evident acid was formed. When such cultures showing sugar utilization by analysis but not by indicator were plated out on corresponding carbohydrate Andrade nutrient agar, no acid colonies appeared in 1–10 days. Quantitative analyses after 3–5 days incubation were usually inconclusive as to the sugar utilization.

In a minimum buffer synthetic medium* acid was evident within 10 days whenever the sugar was utilized, except that in lactose the action of B. mesentericus and B. subtilis was irregular and when a slight acidity was produced, it was delayed 4–10 days.

TABLE 1.—*Bacteria Showing Parallel Carbohydrate Non-Utilization by Both Acid-Indicator and Quantitative Analysis Methods*

Organism	Number of Strains	Dextrose	Mannose	Fructose	Galactose	Xylose	Arabinose	Lactose	Maltose
Staphylococcus	5	+	+	+	+	0_3	0	+	+
Staph. citreus	1	0	0	0	0	0_3	0	0	0
M. tetragenus	1	+	+	+	+	0_3	0	+	+
M. catarrhalis	1	0	0	0	0_3	0_3	0	0_3	0
B. alcaligenes	1	0_3	0_3	0	0_3	0_3	0_3	0_3	0
B. dysenteriae Flexner	2	+	+	+	+	0_3	+	0_3	+
B. paratyphosus alpha	4	+	+	+	+	0_3	+	0_3	+
B. paratyphosus beta	2	+	+	+	+	+	+	0_3	+
B. cholerae suis	1	+	+	+	+	+	+	0_3	+
B. enteritidis	1	+	+	+	+	+	+	0_3	+
B. icteroides	1	+	+	+	+	+	+	0_3	+
B. morgani	1	+	+	+	+	0_3	0	0_3	0
B. avisepticus	1	+	+	+	+	+	+	0_3	+
B. diphtheriae	2	+	+	+	+	0_3	0	0	+
B. diphtheriae (Park 8)	1	0	0	0	0	0_3	0	0	0
B. hofmanni	1	0	0	0	0	0	0	0	0
B. anthracis	3	+	0_3	+	0_3	0_3	0_3	0_3	+

+ = clearly evident acid accompanying utilization.
0 = no evidence of utilization according to quantitative analysis, acid-indicator, or p_H.
3 = three months (or more) incubation in addition to the usual 2 weeks tests.

TABLE 2.—*Bacteria Which Produced Abundant Evident Acid in Some Sugars and Yet Utilized Other Sugars Without Evident Acid*

Organism	Number of Strains	Dextrose	Mannose	Fructose	Galactose	Xylose	Arabinose	Lactose	Maltose
B. phlei	2	+	+	+	+	C_p	C_p	+	+
B. mesentericus	1	+	C_p	+	B_p	B_p	C_p	B	0
B. subtilis (Cohn)	1	+	+	+	$+_d$	C_p	+	V	+

+ = clearly evident acid accompanying utilization.
0 = no evidence of utilization according to quantitative analysis, acid-indicator, or p_H.
B = 20–50% sugar utilized in 2 weeks without evident acid.
C = 50–100% sugar utilized in 2 weeks without evident acid.
p = daily p_H determinations for 2 weeks showed increasing alkalinity.
d = utilization delayed 4–6 days.[6]
V = variable.

B. subtilis was a weak irregular lactose fermenter producing moderate acidity after 13–17 days in lactose broth or peptone mediums and utilizing 20–50 per cent of the available lactose.

Quantitative analyses by Merrill[4c] of cultures of one strain of B. phlei demonstrated utilization of dextrose, fructose, galactose, and arabinose, but

* Society of American Bacteriologists. Manual of Methods for Pure Culture Study of Bacteria, ed. 5, Geneva, N. Y., 1933, leaflet 2, p. 12. 0.1 per cent $NH_4H_2PO_4$, 0.02 per cent KCl, 0.02 per cent $MgSO_4$. During this investigation, Andrade was found to be a more delicate indicator than brom cresol purple, providing the medium was adjusted to about p_H 7.5, Berkefeld-feltered, and sterile Andrade and sterile carbohydrate added, tubed, and incubated 3 days to insure sterility.

6. Wedum, A. G.: Proc. Soc. Exper. Biol. & Med. 30: 693, 1933.

no use of lactose. His strain produced no acid in carbohydrate broth and the acid reaction in carbohydrate minimum buffer synthetic medium could be accounted for by the removal of ammonia.[7] The metabolism of the two strains of B. phlei herein reported is evidently different, in that clearly evident acid was present in all carbohydrate broths except xylose and arabinose. In these 2 sugars the method of attack may be the same as that described by Merrill.

Study[4a] of the fermentation of xylose by B. mesentericus vulgatus has determined that the end products are chiefly acetone, ethyl alcohol, and carbon dioxide, thus accounting for the lack of evident acidity.

Table 3 presents those organisms which utilized several sugars and yet produced no evident acid in any broth, peptone, or soft agar carbohydrate medium. With 2 exceptions no acid was evident when the cultures quantitatively showing sugar use were plated on corresponding carbohydrate Andrade nutrient agar and incubated 1–10 days. Occasionally Sarcina lutea would show some acid on maltose and B. pyocyaneus on xylose plates. Massive inoculums according to the procedure of Lewis[8] or incubation in minimum buffer synthetic medium for 15 days gave indications of acid formation accompanying fermentation in about one half the cases. The following were particularly reluctant to produce any evident acid during fermentation or produced none under all conditions under which they were examined: Sarcina lutea in fructose, xylose; B. pyocyaneus in fructose, maltose; B. leprae in all sugars; B. smegmatis in fructose and galactose. Merrill[9] also found that the acid-indicator reactions or presence of growth in a synthetic medium were inadequate compared to quantitative analysis in determining whether a sugar was utilized.

TABLE 3.—*Bacteria Which Utilized Sugars and Yet Produced No Evident Acid in Any Broth or Peptone Carbohydrate Medium*

Organism	Number of Strains	Dextrose	Mannose	Fructose	Galactose	Xylose	Arabinose	Lactose	Maltose
Sarcina lutea	1	C_3#	C_3#	C_3#	0#	A_p	O_3#	O_3#	A_p
B. pyocyaneus	2	C_p	C#	C_p	C#	C_3	C#	0_3#	A_p
B. leprae	2	B_p	B_p	B_p	0_3#	C_p	A_p	O_3#	0#
B. smegmatis	1	B_p	C_p	C_p	C_p	C_p	C_p	0_3#	0#

0 = no evidence of utilization according to quantitative analysis, acid-indicator, or minimum buffer synthetic medium.
A = 10–20% sugar utilized in 2 weeks without evident acid.
B = 20–50% sugar utilized in 2 weeks without evident acid.
C = 50–100% sugar utilized in 2 weeks without evident acid.
3 = A, B, C, with a 3 attached here indicate the sugar utilization after 3 months incubation whereas at 2 weeks the results were inconclusive.
p = daily p_H determinations for 2 weeks showed increasing alkalinity.
# = phosphate buffer mediums were also employed because they seemed to increase carbohydrate utilization.

Table 3 illustrates even better than table 2 the value of quantitative analyses among certain types of bacteria because acid-indicator methods were entirely incompetent to detect certain of the fermentations. The text book descriptions of the carbohydrate metabolism of these four bacteria

7. Merrill, M. H.: J. Bact. **21:** 375, 1931.
8. J. Bact. **28:** 619, 1934.
9. J. Bact. **21:** 361, 1931.

when mentioned at all are incomplete and need revision. This has been emphasized by Sears and Gourley[10] as regards B. pyocyaneus. The present results confirm theirs and add arabinose to the list of sugars fermented. Their failure to find xylose fermentation in all strains may have been due to an insufficient period of incubation because here 3 months time was required to secure decisive results. In their medium of low nitrogen content, acid could be demonstrated only with dextrose whereas in the present study acid was evident in the minimum buffer synthetic medium in all sugars except fructose and maltose.

TABLE 4.—*Comparison of 2 Strains of B. Subtilis*

Strains	Dextrose	Mannose	Fructose	Galactose	Xylose	Arabinose	Lactose	Maltose	Sucrose	Mannitol	Gelatin Liquefaction	Nitrate Reduction	Indole
Michigan.....	+	0	+	0_3	0_3	0	0_3	+	0	0	+	0	0
Am. Museum Nat. Hist....	+	+	+	$+_d$	C_p	+	V	+	+	+	+	+	0

+ =clearly evident acid accompanying utilization. Gelatin liquefaction.
0 =no evidence of utilization of carbohydrate. No nitrate reduction or no indole formation.
3 =three months (or more) incubation in addition to the usual 2 weeks tests.
C =50–100% sugar utilized in 2 weeks without evident acid.
p =daily p_H determination for 2 weeks showed increasing alkalinity.
d =utilization delayed 4–6 days.[6]
V =variable.

TABLE 5.—*Bacteria Which Gave Various Unusual Reactions*

Organism	Number of Strains	Dextrose	Mannose	Fructose	Galactose	Xylose	Arabinose	Lactose	Maltose
Streptococcus..............	1	+	+	+	+	*	0_3	*	+
B. typhosus................	3	+	+	+	+	+	*	0_3	+
B. typhosus Rawlins.........	1	+	+	+	+	+	*	0_3	*
B. pullorum.................	1	+	+	+	+	+	+	0_3	*
B. dysenteriae Shiga.........	2	+	+	+	+	0_3	0_3	*	*
B. proteus..................	6	+	0_3	+*	+	+	0_3	0_3	+
B. proteus (#226)............	1	+	0_3	+	+	+	0_3	0_3	*

+ =clearly evident acid accompanying utilization.
0 =no evidence of utilization according to quantitative analysis, acid-indicator, or p_H.
3 =three months (or more) incubation in addition to the usual 2 weeks tests.
* =unusual reaction.

The reactions of B. leprae and B. smegmatis confirm the quantitative findings of Merrill[4c] and add the reactions in mannose, xylose, maltose. One of his strains of B. leprae was galactose negative, two weakly positive and three decidedly positive. Reactions of other Mycobacteria in galactose were also variable.

In view of the recent discussion[11] in regard to the identity of B. subtilis, the Michigan strain furnished by Dr. Soule has been compared in its biochemical characteristics in table 4 with the present strain which was obtained from the Museum of Natural History in 1916 and is probably of the Marburg type. The study of the reactions is incomplete insofar as quantitative determinations were not made for the Michigan strain in mannose,

10. J. Bact. **15**: 357, 1928.
11. Conn, H. J.: J. Infect. Dis. **46**: 341, 1930.
Soule, M. H.: J. Infect. Dis. **51**: 191, 1932.

arabinose, and sucrose. Nevertheless the results emphasize the divergence of these 2 strains.

Table 5 presents those organisms which gave various unusual reactions, according to the generally known and accepted information.

The streptococcus after a latent period of 10 days, during which time no demonstrable utilization of xylose occurred, suddenly utilized this sugar as evidenced by acid production and quantitative analysis.[6] Xylose positive and xylose negative forms were isolated but no complete study of the variation was made. There were also indications of both lactose positive and lactose negative forms.

B. TYPHOSUS

All four strains of B. typhosus, normally negative in arabinose, after 10–60 days incubation in arabinose fluid medium produced arabinose positive variants with accompanying evident acid. Both positive and negative types were isolated from 2 strains. After 13 days in acid-indicator fluid mediums containing the sugars in table 5 (also sucrose) the reactions of all types were similar with the exception of the reactions in arabinose. It was not determined whether the newly isolated arabinose negative forms would produce positive forms upon further prolonged incubation. Colony morphology remained essentially smooth. This latent capacity to ferment arabinose has been noticed before.[12] Since these 4 strains represented an entirely random selection it seems not at all improbable that most if not all B. typhosus strains have this property as an adaptive enzyme.

The Rawlins strain of B. typhosus gave no indication of fermentation of maltose by evident acid production when incubated as long as 9 days on maltose Andrade nutrient agar plates even when plated from cultures quantitatively showing use of the sugar. Nor was there indication of maltose fermentation when the strain was incubated in maltose broth or maltose peptone acid-indicator mediums 60 days, nor when the p_H was determined every 1–2 days for 14 days, but in these 18 tubes (6 experiments) quantitative analyses showed utilization of variable amounts of maltose. In minimum buffer synthetic medium acid was evident in 2–21 days in only 3 out of 23 tubes. One might well conclude (despite table 1) that in dealing with intestinal pathogens any atypical negative carbohydrate reaction must be subjected to quantitative analysis.

Xylose utilization was delayed 2–3 days.[6] The Rawlins strain has been found atypical in other respects.[13]

B. PULLORUM

B. pullorum gave rise to maltose fermenting forms which were isolated and will be reported in a separate paper. As shown by quantitative analysis

12. (a) Krumwiede, C., and Kohn, L. A.: J. Med. Res. **36**: 509, 1917.
(b) Meyer, K. F., and Neilson, N. M.: J. Bact. **27**: 46, 1920.
(c) A System of Bacteriology in Relation to Medicine, Med. Res. Council **4**: 24, 1929.
(d) Bohdanowicz, S., and Lawrynowicz, A.: Zentralbl. f. Bakt. (Abt. 1) **128**: 43, 1933.
13. Grinnell, F. B.: J. Exper. Med. **56**: 907, 1932.

this variation occurred in 50 per cent of 102 tubes in 10 experiments in 3 different mediums. The variation was evident in 6–60 days, was with or without production of acid evident by p_H or acid-indicator, and with or without the development of maltose positive forms evident when the cultures were plated out on maltose Andrade nutrient agar. Changes in colony morphology were slight and the acid-indicator reactions of the variants in the 8 other sugars (including sucrose) were the same as those of the maltose negative form.

The stock strain was typical in that it was non-motile, reduced nitrates, did not form indol, produced acid and gas from dextrose, fermented mannitol, did not ferment dulcitol, dextrin, sucrose, salicin, or inulin in 21 days in acid-indicator mediums. Reports in the literature on nitrate reduction are not uniform.[14]

The question of the fermentation of maltose by B. pullorum has been much discussed.[12a,14b,15] Undoubtedly there is some alteration of the maltose in alkaline mediums.[15f] However this is insufficient to cause other organisms to attack the maltose in its original or altered form (tables 1, 2, 3). It would seem from the present work that the phenomena of variation offer a likely explanation of the irregular late acidity in this sugar.

B. DYSENTERIAE SHIGA

Two strains of B. dysenteriae Shiga (I and II) fermented as much as 60 per cent of the available lactose with a reduction of p_H from 6.8 to as low as 5.4 if incubated 3 months. In two weeks the p_H would drop to about 6.2 with utilization of 10–20 per cent. Eight of 30 cultures (10 experiments) showed no p_H drop or appreciable quantitative fermentation. No acid colonies appeared when the acid cultures were plated on Andrade lactose nutrient agar although colonial variation was evident. Further study is being made of this variation.

Both of these B. dys. Shiga and also a standard strain (No. 0.01339, supplied by Parke Davis & Co.) produced acid in maltose Andrade broth after a delay of 8 days. Preliminary experiments indicate that maltose positive and maltose negative forms may be isolated. Only the Parke Davis strain produced acid in sucrose after 3–8 days but it formed no acid from lactose in 60 days. Otherwise these strains were quite typical in that they were non-motile, agglutinated in high titer with commercial Shiga antiserum,

---

14. (a) Mallmann, W. L.: Michigan State Col. Agri. Expt. Sta. Tech. Bull. 68, 1925.
(b) Bushnell, L. D., Hinshaw, W. R., and Payne, L. F.: Kansas Agri. Expt. Sta. Tech. Bull. 21, 1926.
(c) Rettger, L. F., and Plastridge, W. N.: Storrs Agri. Expt. Sta. Bull. 178, 1932.
15. (a) Mulsow, F. W.: J. Infect. Dis. **25**: 135, 1919.
(b) Spray, R. S., and Doyle, L. P.: J. Infect. Dis. **28**: 43, 1921.
(c) Edington, J. W.: J. Path. & Bact. **27**: 427, 1924.
(d) May, H. G., and Goodner, K.: J. Bact. **13**: 129, 1927.
(e) Hendrickson, J. M.: J. Am. Vet. M. A. **70**: 629, 1927.
(f) Edwards, P. R.: J. Bact. **15**: 235, 1928.
(g) Cernainau, C., and Popovici, I.: Comp. rend. Soc. de Biol. **105**: 84, 1930.
(h) Gunther, K.: Zentralbl. f. Bakt. (Abt. 1) **128**: 197, 1933.

did not produce acid in xylose, arabinose, mannitol, dulcitol, salicin Andrade broths in 21 days, were indol, Voges-Proskauer, catalase negative, and did not liquefy gelatin in 21 days.

Dudgeon[16] in 1929 expressed the following opinion: "Cultures of the Shiga bacillus isolated from cases of dysentery in various parts of the world and stock laboratory cultures all give the same carbohydrate reactions." "Mannitol, saccharose, lactose, maltose, and dulcitol are unaffected."

In the light of more recent work, the matter cannot be so dogmatically stated either in regard to old laboratory cultures or freshly isolated strains. Fermentation of maltose has been frequently reported,[17] and also a bewildering array of other changes.[17g,18] The conclusion is inescapable that a single strain of B. dys. Shiga is capable of developing extensive variation in biochemical and serological properties.

B. PROTEUS

In the fructose broth or fructose peptone mediums, 5 of the 7 strains of B. proteus produced abundant evident acid. Two strains slowly but consistently utilized 50–75 per cent of the sugar in about 9 days but in 32 cultures (7 experiments) daily p_H determinations showed an average maximum (at 6–9 days) drop of only 0.69 with restored alkalinity at about 12 days. Production of evident acid on fructose Andrade plates by these 2 strains was variable. Quantitative analysis, or at least use of a minimum buffer synthetic medium, is therefore indicated before any B. proteus strain is reported as not fermenting fructose. Although this reaction usually is positive,[19] it has been reported as delayed,[19a] or negative[20] with acid-indicator methods.

---

16. A System of Bacteriology in Relation to Medicine, Med. Res. Council, **4**: 184, 1929.
17. (a) Hiss, P. H.: J. Med. Res. **13**: 1, 1904.
    (b) Davison, W. C.: Medicine **1**: 389, 1922.
    (c) Loffler, E., and Rigler, R.: Zentralbl. f. Bakt. (Abt. 1) **99**: 1, 1926.
    (d) de Assis, A.: Inst. Vital Brasil **13**: 3, 1930. In Biol. Absts. **5**(8–9) No. 20859, 1931.
    (e) Hadley, P., Delves, E., and Klimek, J. W.: J. Infect. Dis. **48**: 1, 1931.
    (f) Isabolinski, M., Judenitsch, W., and Simonow, P.: Ztschr. f. Immunitätsforsch. u. exper. Therap. **77**: 12, 1932.
    (g) Rutschko, I. E.: Ztschr. f. Immunitätsforsch. u. exper. Therap. **74**: 468 and 500, 1932.
    (h) Castellani, A.: Zentralbl. f. Bakt. (Abt. 1) **125**: 37, 1932.
18. Truschina, E. F., and Korolewa, E. G.: Zentralbl. f. Bakt. (Abt. 1) **117**: 506, 1930.
    Nosotti, N.: Soc. Internaz. Microbiol., Boll. Sez. Ital. **4**(10): 391, 1932.
19. (a) Moltke, O.: Zentralbl. f. Bakt. (Abt. 1) **113**: 301, 1929.
    (b) Seligmann, M.: Zentralbl. f. Bakt. (Abt. 1) **115**: 346, 1930.
    (c) Bergey. Manual of Determinative Bacteriology, 1930.
    (d) Yacob, M.: Indian J. Med. Res. **19**: 787, 1932.
20. (a) Berthelot, A.: Ann. Inst. Pasteur **28**: 839, 1914.
    (b) Bach, F. W.: Zentralbl. f. Bakt. **85**: 305, 1921.
    (c) Kendall, A. I., Bly, R., and Haner, R. C.: J. Infect. Dis. **32**: 377, 1923.
    (d) Kendall, A. I., and Yoshida, S.: J. Infect. Dis. **32**: 369, 1923.
    (e) Rochaix, A., and Sarda, H.: Comp. rend. Soc. de biol. **95**: 841, 1926.
    (f) A System of Bacteriology in Relation to Medicine, Med. Res. Council **4**: 308, 1929.
    (g) Kendall, A. I., and Gross, C. E.: J. Infect. Dis. **47**: 249, 1930.

Valle Miranda[21] mentions a strain which utilized fructose without evident acid production. Slow and rapid fructose fermenting variants have been noted.[22]

Maltose is commonly employed with acid-indicators to differentiate Proteus vulgaris, the X_{19}, and X_2 strains (maltose positive) and P. mirabilis, OX Kingsbury (OXK), and HX Kingsbury (HXK) strains (maltose negative).[19c,20f,23] One of the present strains (No. 226) in broth and peptone mediums in 6 experiments (17 cultures) quantitatively showed no utilization of available maltose in 8 cultures, 10–20 per cent utilization in 6, and 20–50 per cent utilization in 3, without production of any acid evident by indicator or by daily p_H determinations. No acid appeared in 11 days when these cultures were plated on Andrade maltose nor in 15 days in the minimum buffer synthetic medium. This strain was indole, mannitol, salicin negative, sucrose, gelatin positive, motile, and would therefore be considered as P. mirabilis. The other 6 strains would qualify as P. vulgaris and were indole, maltose positive and otherwise typical except an old X_{19} which was salicin positive and gelatin negative. There are several recent examples of loss of the power to liquefy gelatin.[19d,24]

Further study was made of the maltose reaction by using 2 indole negative strains which were maltose negative according to the acid-indicator method.* The usual mediums were employed. Daily p_H determinations for 2 weeks showed a gradual rise to at least 8.4. Quantitative analyses revealed no maltose utilization in 16 tubes, 10–20 per cent utilization of available maltose in one HXK and one OXK tube, 20–50 per cent in four HXK and two OXK tubes. Uninoculated mediums and non-maltose fermenting cultures of B. alcaligenes, B. morgani, and B. mesentericus served as controls. Plating to maltose Andrade showed no evident acid or contaminations in 10 days. Variant colony forms were evident but no maltose positive forms have been isolated. The same strains were examined after 30 days in maltose Andrade broth, maltose Andrade 1 per cent peptone, m. A. phosphate buffer broth, m. A. phosphate buffer 1 per cent peptone. Quantitative analysis showed no maltose utilization in 27 tubes, and 10–20 per cent utilization of available maltose in three HXK and two OXK tubes. No acid had appeared during this time except in 3 of 8 B. pullorum cultures which were included to demonstrate indirectly that the acid was not caused by fermentation of maltose degradation products. If the acid had been caused by fermentation of maltose

21. Valle Miranda, F. G.: Comp. rend. Acad. Sci. **166**: 184, 1918.

22. Moltke, O.: Contributions to the Characterization and systematic classification of Bac. Proteus Vulgaris (Hauser). Copenhagen. Levin & Munksgaard. 1927.

23. Topley, W. W. C., and Wilson, G. S.: The Principles of Bacteriology and Immunity **1**: 408, 1929.

de Assis, A.: J.A.M.A. **99**: 238, 1932.

24. (a) Meisel, H., and Mikulasek, E.: Comp. rend. Soc. de biol. **114**: 361, 1933

(b) Welch, H., and Poole, A. K.: J. Bact. **28**: 523, 1934.

(c) Welch, H., Mickle, F. L., and Borman, E. K.: Am. J. Pub. Health **24**: 1157, 1934.

* OX Kingsbury and HX Kingsbury, supplied by Dr. Welch and previously studied in detail by him.[24c]

degradation products, then it might be expected that some of the B. proteus cultures also would have shown evident acid.

The suggestion of Seligmann[19b] that the difference in maltose fermentation between the indole positive (P. indologenes[25]—typically P. vulgaris) and the indole negative (P. anindologenes—typically P. mirabilis) strains is quantitative and not qualitative, is therefore corroborated. Although the indole reaction is generally regarded as unsatisfactory for the subdivision of the genus Proteus, the percentage correlation between maltose fermentation and indole production is high. Nevertheless evident acid production from maltose by indole negative strains occurs[19a,b,24,26] and there are instances of maltose negative indole positive strains.[19d,26d,27] The ability to form indole may be lost or gained.[20a]

The question remains whether P. vulgaris and P. mirabilis are variants in which the adaptive enzyme maltase is closely linked with an adaptive sucrase and less closely to the property of forming indole. Recent studies[24a,b] on the X strains make this seem not unlikely.

Lactose fermentation by B. proteus is rare but has been reported for an old laboratory strain,[24c] for a variant,[24b] after long growth in synthetic mediums,[19b] under anaerobic conditions,[28] and under apparently normal conditions.[20b,21,27b,29] Moltke[22] has questioned the validity of several of these reported lactose fermentations.

In a preliminary paper[4f] the fermentation of a small amount of lactose was indicated for the present strains. Further study fails to extend this finding. Decrease in the p_H of fluid mediums has never been observed nor production of acid on lactose nutrient agar Andrade plates. In three experiments (totaling 7 cultures for each of the 7 strains) use of the minimum buffer acid-indicator lactose synthetic medium inoculated with one loop of culture or with the entire growth from a 48 hour agar slant, observed daily for 2 weeks, gave no indication of acid formation. Over 100 analyses on cultures in lactose broth or peptone mediums incubated 2 weeks, 3 months, 9 months, and 21 months, with and without phosphate buffer, have failed to establish a clear cut utilization. In 3 experiments, incubation for 3 weeks in pyrogallol or phosphorus anaerobe jars followed by incubation in air for 7 days gave only irregular and inconclusive evidence of slight utilization regardless of whether the inoculum was one loopful or the entire growth from a 24 hour agar slant. A brief experiment with Seligmann's synthetic medium[19b] was unsuccessful. Whether or not a minimal amount of lactose is utilized still remains in doubt

25. van Loghem, J. J., and van Loghem-Pouw, J. C. W.: Zentralbl. f. Bakt. **66**: 19, 1912.
26. (a) Horowitz, A.: Ann. Inst. Pasteur **30**: 307, 1916.
    (b) Stewart, M. J.: J. Hygiene **16**: 291, 1917.
    (c) Shaeffer, H.: Zentralbl. f. Bakt. **83**: 430, 1919.
    (d) Bengtson, I. A.: J. Infect. Dis. **24**: 428, 1919.
27. (a) Wilson, W. J., and Blair, E. M. McV.: J. Hygiene **26**: 374, 1927.
    (b) v. Gara, P., and Stickl, O.: Arch. Hyg. **102**: 37, 1929.
28. Glenn, T. H.: Zentralbl. f. Bakt. **58**: 481, 1911.
29. (a) Weil, E., and Felix, A.: Wien. klin. Wchnschr. **29**: 33, 1916.
    (b) Wolf, C. G. L.: J. Path. & Bact. **22**: 289, 1918.

although for all practical purposes there was no fermentation by the 7 strains studied.

Inspection of tables 1 and 5 will show that B. proteus and B. anthracis are the only bacteria which ferment dextrose and fructose, yet fail to ferment mannose. The keto-enol relationships of these three sugars have been frequently emphasized. Critical scrutiny must be made of any report that one or two and not all three of these sugars are fermented. Quantitative analyses are always indicated in such cases, as may be seen from the action of B. mesentericus which fermented mannose without evident acid formation (table 2). Therefore additional experiments were performed with B. anthracis and B. proteus in mannose mediums. These included (1) the Lewis method[8] of massive inoculums in nitrogen poor medium* (from 24 hour cultures on 2 per cent mannose nutrient agar slants), (2) growth of B. proteus for 2 weeks in mannose broth medium and mannose peptone medium, both buffered with phosphates, (3) incubation for 5 months in the usual mediums. All these experiments showed no utilization of mannose by B. proteus or B. anthracis.

Various unsuccessful attempts were made to induce B. alcaligenes to use dextrose or other sugars. These included daily or bi-monthly transfer in dextrose broth, use of starvation medium, massive inoculums in both shake and streak plates of synthetic medium according to the method of Lewis, incubation with radioactive thorium dioxide, and incubation for 2 weeks, 3 months, and 21 months.

SUMMARY

Quantitative studies were made of the carbohydrate reactions of a representative series of common bacteria and compared with the reactions obtained by the use of acid-indicators. Dextrose, mannose, fructose, galactose, xylose, arabinose, lactose, and maltose were employed. Cultures were incubated from 2 weeks to 21 months, usually for 2 weeks.

The results indicate that for most aerobic bacteria of medical importance the use of acid-indicators gives a trustworthy picture of the carbohydrate fermentations. In most instances prolonged incubation did not induce the utilization of ordinarily non-fermentable sugars.

The delayed fermentation reaction was investigated in the case of a streptococcus in xylose, B. typhosus in arabinose, B. pullorum in maltose, and B. dys. Shiga in maltose, and was found to be caused by the appearance of variant forms. It is suggested that variation is the usual mechanism operating in such delayed reactions in which, after a latent period, there is a marked production of evident acid.

The difference in the fermentation of maltose by Proteus vulgaris, X_{19}, strains and P. mirabilis, OX Kingsbury, HX Kingsbury strains was found to be quantitative, not qualitative. The latter utilize the maltose so slowly that evident acid does not appear.

Organisms which utilized one or more sugars without the appearance of evident acid in broth or peptone mediums included B. typhosus Rawlins,

* For these organisms, 1 per cent broth was added to the medium recommended by Lewis.

B. proteus, B. phlei, B. mesentericus, B. subtilis, Sarcina lutea, B. pyocyaneus, B. leprae, and B. smegmatis. In most, but not all of these instances, acid was evident with an acid-indicator when a minimum buffer synthetic medium was employed.

It is concluded that one cannot be certain that the characterization of any species of bacteria is complete in regard to its carbohydrases until some method which is independent of the action of acid-indicators is employed and then often only after prolonged incubation. Whereas in organic mediums with an acid-indicator a positive reaction is definite, a negative reaction should be checked by quantitative analysis.

DISSOCIATION OF TWO UNUSUAL ACIDFAST ORGANISMS ISOLATED FROM HUMAN SOURCES

W. STEENKEN, JR.

AND

A. LANDAU*

TRUDEAU, NEW YORK

Recently many workers have renewed their interest in the study of atypical "tubercle bacilli" isolated from human sources. Some interesting reports on these lines have appeared in the literature from time to time. Thus Beaven and Bayne-Jones[1] described a case of a child suffering from extensive pulmonary disease resembling tuberculosis, from which they isolated an acidfast organism possessing all the cardinal tinctorial characteristics of true tubercle bacilli, but exhibiting no pathogenicity for chickens, rabbits, frogs and guinea pigs. These authors dissociated the isolated strain and obtained two variants, "R" and "S," which possessed distinct topographical differences, but neither were pathogenic. Rabinowitsch-Kempner[2] isolated a non-pathogenic acidfast bacillus from a case of empyema, and another from a case of recurrent dermatomyositis, and Sweaney[3] found non-pathogenic acidfast organisms in a case of lymphogranulomatosis. Branch[4] called attention to a number of acidfast organisms not of mammalian type isolated from human sources, some of which resembled the avian type. He considered them to be new strains of pathogenic acidfast organisms. Pinner[5] collected and studied several strains of non-pathogenic acidfast bacilli isolated from human sputum and urine. Some of these strains he found to be chromogenic while others were not. He also noticed a number of variants developing from single strains.

Lyle Cummins and Williams[6] recently isolated an acidfast organism other than Koch's bacillus, called the "M" strain, from the sputum of a girl suffering from a chronic pulmonary illness. We are about to describe a similar organism, called by us the "I.P." strain, isolated from the sputum of a patient seen by Dr. Baldwin, the patient presenting an almost identical clinical picture to that of Lyle Cummins' case.

The object of the studies about to be reported was to determine whether we could dissociate the "I.P." and "M" strains, and to compare the behavior of the variants on artificial mediums; and whether they possessed any patho-

Received for publication, August 15, 1935.

From the Research and Clinical Laboratory, Trudeau Sanatorium.

* Dorothy Temple Cross Research Fellow in Tuberculosis.

1. J. Infect. Dis. **49**: 399, 1931.
2. Am. Rev. Tuberc. **15**: 225, 1927.
3. Tr. Chicago Path. Soc. **13**: 66, 1928.
4. Tubercle **14**: 337, 1932–33.
5. Soc. Exper. Biol. & Med. **30**: 214, 1932–33.
6. Tubercle **15**: 49, 1933–34; Griffith, A. S.: Ibid., 53.

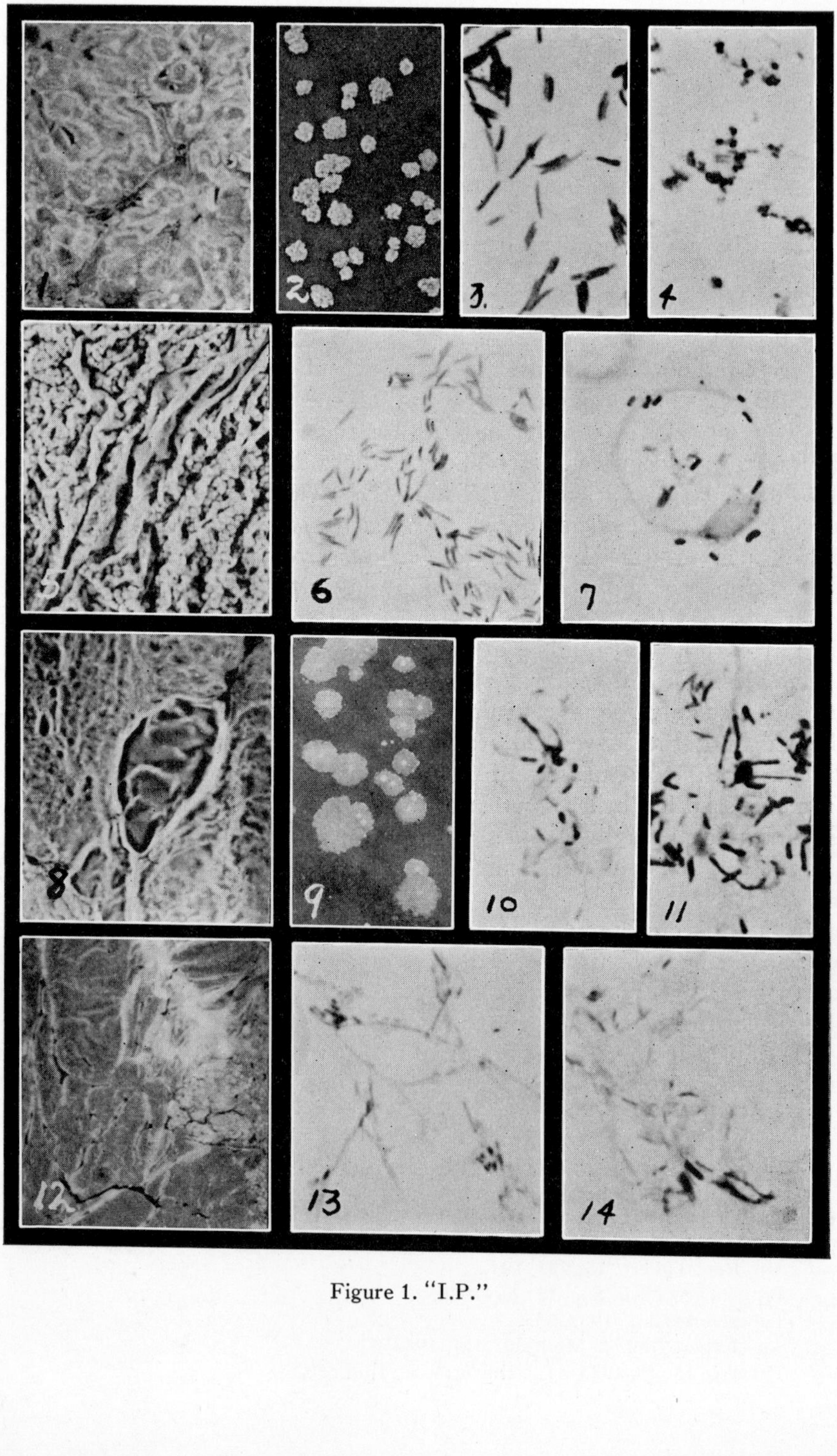

Figure 1. "I.P."

genicity for laboratory animals. We have included in this study a third strain of non-pathogenic acidfast organism isolated by one of us (W.S.) from a BCG culture brought to us by Dr. Frappier from Dr. Birkhaug's laboratory, University of Rochester.

MYCOBACTERIUM "I.P."

This strain was isolated from the sputum of a patient seen by Dr. Baldwin. The patient, a young girl aged 24 years, had been suffering from a chronic pulmonary illness associated with much loss of weight and strength, fever, and a concomitant condition of cardiospasm. Any sputum raised, and that only by vomiting, was on direct microscopic examination persistently negative for acidfast bacilli. X-ray and physical examination of the lungs revealed the presence of an acute pneumonic consolidation, tuberculous in type. After the patient had been ill for several months, a fresh specimen of sputum was obtained and studied. After digestion and sedimentation smears were negative for acidfast organisms. A portion of the sediment was inoculated on Petroff gentian violet egg plates by Mr. Donald Cummings of the Saranac Laboratory, and after a weeks' incubation a few colonies appeared, which revealed acidfast organisms. On subculturing, the organisms developed very rapidly on all the usual mediums used for the cultivation of tubercle bacilli, and the growth that appeared was similar to that of the avian type. It was this strain of organism ("I.P.") that formed the basis of the present bacteriological study.

During the course of the patient's illness intracutaneous tuberculin tests were performed on several occasions, using human O.T., avian, and M. phlei tuberculin, with negative results. However, later the patient gave a mild reaction to human O.T., 0.00025 cc., and a considerably stronger reaction to a tuberculin of the same concentration prepared from the "I.P." culture

DISSOCIATION OF "I.P." STRAIN

The original undissociated culture was on a glycerol agar slant, and immediate transplants were made on glycerol egg and other laboratory mediums. Morphological study revealed acidfast organisms, with an occasional non-acidfast rod. The dissociation method described elsewhere[7] was employed to separate the various colonies. A suspension of undissociated culture was prepared in the usual method, and inoculated on the surface of Petroff gentian violet egg flasks, and incubated at 37.5 C. On the fifth day two types of colonies with distinct topographical characteristics appeared. (a) Variant I, measuring from 2 to 4 mm., raised, coarse, rough and dry, composed of many coils and with clear-cut periphery (figure 1, 2). (b) Variant II, measuring 6 to 12 mm. in diameter, flat, smooth, spreading, with nippled center (figure 1, 9).

At the fifth day of incubation no chromogenicity developed in either variant. However,

---

Figure 1. "I.P."

1. Variant I—17 days on glycerol tomato broth. ×2.
2. Variant I—18 days on gentian violet. ×2.
3. Variant I—48 hours on plain egg medium Ziehl Neelsen. ×865.
4. Variant I—10 days on plain beef agar, Ziehl Neelsen. ×865.
5. Variant I—17 days on Proskauer and Beck's synthetic medium. ×2.
6. Variant I—48 hours on plain agar, Ziehl Neelsen. ×865.
7. Variant I—48 hours on litmus milk, Ziehl Neelsen. ×865.
8. Variant II—17 days on glycerol tomato broth. ×2.
9. Variant II—18 days on gentian violet medium. ×2.
10. Variant I—48 hours on Loeffler's medium, Ziehl Neelsen. ×865.
11. Variant II—48 hours on litmus milk, Ziehl Neelsen. ×865.
12. Variant II—17 days on Proskauer and Beck's synthetic medium. ×2.
13. Variant II—48 hours on Loeffler's medium, Ziehl Neelsen. ×865.
14. Variant II—18 days on Loeffler's medium, Ziehl Neelsen. ×865.

---

7. Petroff, S. A., and Steenken, W., Jr.: J. Exper. Med. **51**: 831, 1930.

after allowing the plates to remain at room temperature for a few weeks, definite chromogenicity developed, but much more pronounced in variant II. This very likely is due to a photochemical reaction in which oxidation probably plays no small part. This reaction occurred only in living cultures. Plates which were sterilized with formaldehyde and left at room temperature for some period of time did not develop chromogenicity.

Variant I on glycerol tomato broth at 17 days was veil-like, tenacious and had a tendency to creep up the sides of the flask (figure 1, 1) whereas variant II was wrinkled, brittle, with no tendency to creep up the sides of flasks (figure 1, 8). Chromogenicity developed in both after 5 days at room temperature. Cultures of variant I on Proskauer and Beck's synthetic medium at 17 days presented a wrinkled growth, with small raised islands with veil-like strands connecting these, also tenacious (figure 1, 5), whereas variant II was dense, smooth and brittle (figure 1, 12). These did not develop chromogenicity at room temperature as readily as those grown on glycerol tomato broth.

Coagulated pleural fluid medium (Loeffler)—Moderate moist growth occurred, variant I being more chromogenic than variant II.

Egg medium—Growth was profuse and chromogenic in both types.

Glycerol agar medium—The two variants developed a profuse chromogenic growth.

Plain agar (no glycerol)—Profuse growth and no chromogenicity in both types.

Pleural fluid broth—The two variants developed a moderate growth which was dry and wrinkled, with slight chromogenicity.

Litmus milk medium—Moderate growth developed on the bottom of the tubes in the two variants, with the development of a slight alkalinity.

Glycerol potato medium—Profuse, wrinkled growth, with more chromogenicity in variant I than in variant II.

MORPHOLOGY AND TINCTORIAL CHARACTERISTICS

48-HOUR OBSERVATIONS

Loeffler medium—

Variant I—Pleomorphic, swollen acidfast bacilli and oval bodies, only a few long acidfast rods; a number of long, slender, non-acidfast rods (figure 1, 10).

Variant II—Mainly long filamentous non-acidfast organisms with numbers of swollen acidfast and non-acidfast granules, and a suggestion of branching forms (figure 1, 13).

Egg medium, and glycerol agar—

Variant I—Swollen, long, acidfast rods; numbers of non-acidfast slender rods of various sizes (figure 1, 3).

Variant II—Very similar to variant I.

Plain agar medium—

Variant I—Mostly non-acidfast rods; occasional acidfast oval bodies and swollen bacilli (figure 1, 6).

Variant II—Mostly coccoid, acidfast bodies with occasional slender non-acidfast rods.

Litmus milk medium—

Variant I—Swollen short, strongly acidfast rods; only a few non-acidfast granules (figure 1, 7).

Variant II—Pleomorphic rods, some short and swollen, others long and beaded, only a few filamentous, long, non-acidfast rods (figure 1, 11).

Pleural fluid broth—

Variant I—Pleomorphic acidfast and non-acidfast rods.

Variant II—Uniform medium sized acidfast rods.

Glycerol potato medium—

Variant I—Acidfast and non-acidfast rods.

Variant II—Acidfast rods of approximately uniform size; some of the bacilli beaded.

Ten days after seeding, the tinctorial characteristics were somewhat modified, and all cultures revealed moderately to strongly acidfast rods of various sizes. Filamentous bacilli were no longer present. The only difference noted was on plain beef agar cultures where the individual organism was of cocco-bacillus form (figure 1, 4).

Eighteen day cultures showed modifications only on Loeffler's medium where the organism had again lost its acid fast properties, giving a similar picture to the 48-hour observation, variant II developing in filamentous form (figure 1, 14). The remaining cultures were composed as acidfast bacilli, cocci and granules of various sizes and forms.

HYDROGEN ION DETERMINATION

Hydrogen ion concentration studies were made on glycerol beef broth of approximately p_H 7.3. At the end of 15 days both variants developed alkaline reactions—variant I from p_H 7.3 to p_H 7.8, and variant II from p_H 7.4 to p_H 8.00. This is rather a typical reaction observed with all acidfast saprophytes.

ANIMAL INOCULATION

Guinea pigs were inoculated intratesticularly with graded doses of the two variants. Such animals became sensitized to a small degree to old tuberculin and reacted moderately in 3 weeks to a tuberculin prepared from the organism used for inoculation and sensitization. No difference in the two variants was noted. Guinea pigs inoculated with variant I reacted with the same intensity to tuberculin prepared from variants I and II and vice versa. The animals were killed after 3 months and no pathological lesions were found.

Rabbits, chickens and white mice were also inoculated by the usual routes with graded doses of the variants without producing disease, and on microscopic examination of the organs no acidfast organisms could be demonstrated.

SEROLOGICAL STUDIES

Rabbits were sensitized intravenously on three occasions 3 days apart with 0.5 cc. of a milky suspension of the two variants. After 3 weeks they were bled, and the serum tested for agglutinins, precipitins and complement-fixing antibodies. At 3 weeks' time no agglutinins or precipitins were demonstrated in these rabbits, but complement-fixing antibodies were present in all in fair concentrations. Only slight specificities were noted. Rabbits sensitized with variant I reacted more strongly to its homologous and less to the heterologous antigen. The same was true with variant II.

It is not surprising that there were no agglutinins or precipitins in these rabbits' serums as it is known that such antibodies develop later in due time after the complement-fixing antibodies have appeared.

MYCOBACTERIUM "M"

This organism was isolated by Prof. Lyle Cummins from a case that presented a similar clinical picture to that from which the "I.P." strain was isolated. Extensive studies have been reported by Cummins and Griffith[6] on the undissociated strain. The similarity of this organism to strain "I.P." suggested a further study based on dissociation phenomena.

DISSOCIATION OF "M" STRAIN

The culture was received on a glycerol agar slant. A suspension for single colony isolation[7] was made and inoculated on the surface of gentian violet egg medium. Colonies appeared within 5 days, but no differentiation could be made until the end of the second week, when two distinct variants were noted. These were fished out, suspensions prepared, and subinoculated on fresh flasks. After 2 weeks these subcultures revealed colonies similar to the original from which the subinoculations were made. a. Variant I (figure 2, 2) was raised, wrinkled, dry, with clear-cut periphery and cream-colored. b. Variant II (figure 2, 8) was spreading, smooth, moist, with extending periphery, and also cream-colored. Both variants had a tendency to become slightly darker after several days at room temperature.

Variant I (figure 2, 1) on glycerol tomato broth at 17 days was very dense and wrinkled, white, with no thin filaments appearing on the surface, while variant II showed no surface growth, but grew well at the bottom of the medium and was very tenacious. On synthetic medium at the same period of incubation the growth of variant I (figure 2, 5) appeared as a dense white mass, with a few small veil-like filaments between the islands, while variant II (figure 2, 9) was white, veil-like and wrinkled, the growth creeping up the sides of the flasks.

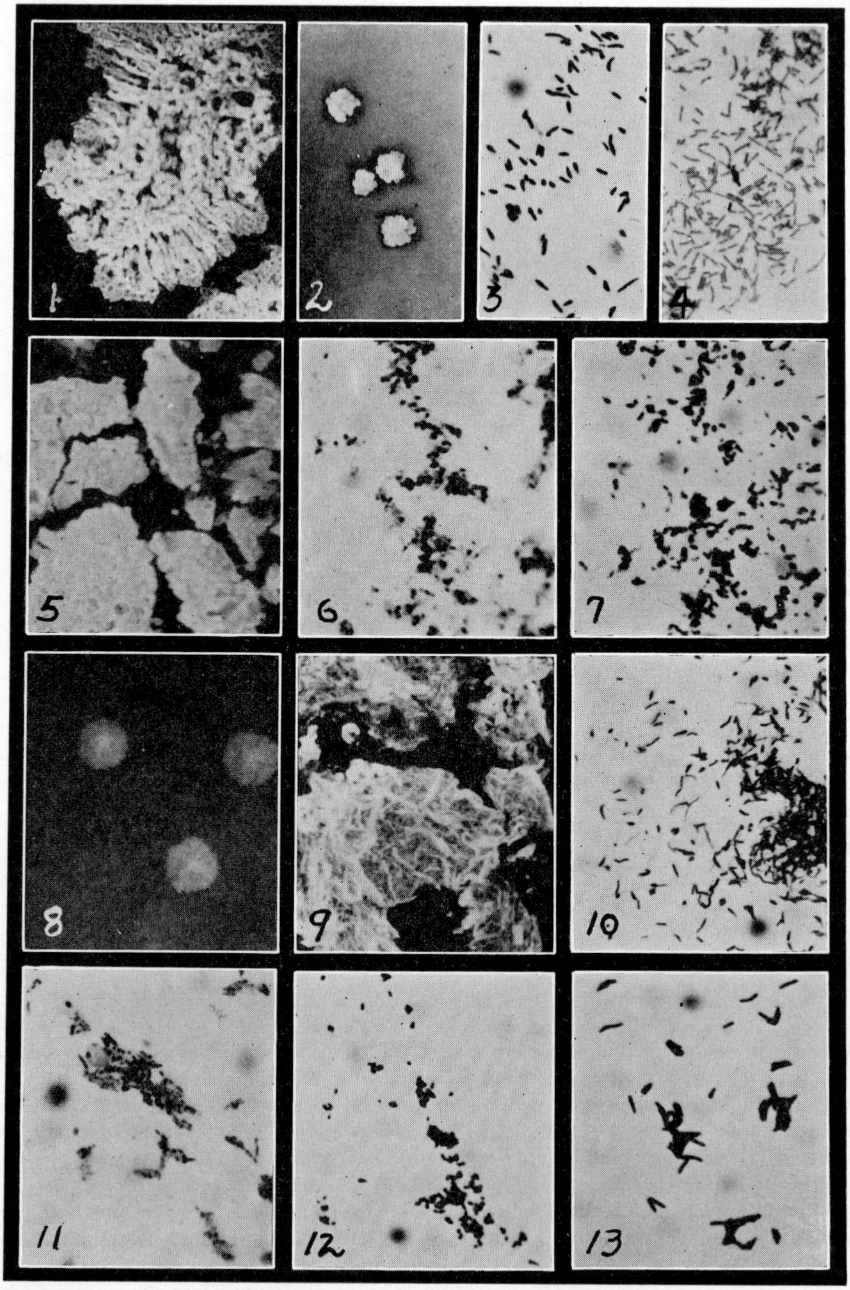

Figure 2. "M"

In each case growth appeared more rapidly and more profusely at 37.5 C. than at 20 C. and no growth occurred at 55 C. cultures that had been kept at 55 C. for 10 days and then transferred to 37.5 C. still failed to exhibit growth.

Glycerol beef broth—Moderate white flocculent growth developed under the surface in both variants after 3 to 4 days. The surface growth was white, delicate and veil-like. After 35 days, growth was very profuse in both, but somewhat darker for variant I.

Non-glycerol beef broth—Growth characteristics were identical with those on glycerol beef broth, except that it was slightly more tardy and not so profuse.

Glycerol synthetic broth—Moderate moist growth appeared with the same features as on beef broth. No chromogenicity.

Non-glycerol synthetic broth—No growth was obtained at any time with either of the variants at any of the temperatures studied.

Pleural fluid broth—Growth was slight and tardy, and occurred mostly in the depths of the medium.

Litmus milk—Only slight growth appeared at the bottom of the tubes, with the development of slight alkalinity.

Glycerol potato slants—Growth was somewhat tardy at first, but after 8–12 days grew rapidly, and in both variants was dry, heaped and closely corrugated with sharp periphery.

Plain agar slants—Moderate growth appeared, white, spreading, dry and gently wrinkled.

Glycerol beef agar slants—Similar to plain agar slants.

Glycerol egg slants—Growth was profuse, appeared early and was very stable—dry, rough and wrinkled, with sharp periphery and white to cream in color.

With both variants on exposure at room temperature the development of chromogenicity was very slight, except a few cultures of variant I which became brownish after several days' exposure to light.

MORPHOLOGY AND TINCTORIAL CHARACTERISTICS

5-DAY OBSERVATIONS

When grown on gentian violet medium for 11 days, variant I (figure 2, 3) displayed acidfast rods, a few ovoid bodies and non-acidfast forms, whereas variant I (figure 2, 10) was composed of short and long, more slender, acidfast rods.

Glycerol beef broth—

Variant I—Pleomorphic, short and stumpy acidfast rods and cocco-bacillary forms.

Variant II—Short, slender straight acidfast rods.

Non-glycerol beef broth—

Variant I—Acidfast coccobacilli.

Variant II—Short and long slender acidfast rods and coccobacilli.

Glycerol synthetic broth—

Variant I—Short, stumpy acidfast rods.

Variant II—Acidfast and non-acidfast coccobacilli.

Figure 2. "M"

1. Variant I—17 days on glycerol tomato broth. ×2.
2. Variant I—21 days on gentian violet medium. ×2.
3. Variant I—11 days on gentian violet medium, Ziehl Neelsen. ×865.
4. Variant I—5 days on glycerol beef slants, Ziehl Neelsen. ×865.
5. Variant I—17 days on synthetic medium. ×2.
6. Variant I—12 days on glycerol beef slants, Ziehl Neelsen. ×865.
7. Variant I—36 days on glycerol egg slants, Ziehl Neelsen. ×865.
8. Variant II—21 days on gentian violet medium. ×2.
9. Variant II—17 days on synthetic medium. ×2.
10. Variant II—11 days on gentian violet medium, Ziehl Neelsen. ×865.
11. Variant II—8 days on glycerol potato slants, Ziehl Neelsen. ×865.
12. Variant II—12 days on glycerol egg slants, Ziehl Neelsen. ×865.
13. Variant II—36 days on non-glycerol beef slants, Ziehl Neelsen. ×865.

Pleural fluid broth—
Variant I—Short, stumpy acid-fast rods.
Variant II—Long and short, straight and slender acidfast rods.
Glycerol potato medium—
Variant I—Short, acidfast and non-acidfast rods.
Variant II—Long and short, straight slender acidfast and non-acidfast rods.
Plain agar medium—
Variant I—Acidfast and non-acidfast coccobacilli.
Variant II—Slender and swollen acidfast and non-acidfast coccobacilli.
Glycerol beef slants—
Variant I—Short, slender acidfast and non-acidfast rods and beaded forms (figure 2, 4).
Variant II—Short, slender acidfast and non-acidfast rods with slight beading and coccobacilli.
Glycerol egg slants—
Variant I—Short, slender acidfast rods and coccobacilli.
Variant II—Short, slender, acidfast and non-acidfast rods and coccobacilli.

With increase of the time after seeding, the tinctorial characteristics were modified. As the cultures became older there were more non-acidfast forms in both variants up to 12 days, and thereafter only in variant I. There was a tendency for more coccobacillary forms to develop at 20 C. than at 37.5 C. Clubbed forms also developed with age of the organisms, as also the presence of more curved and beaded forms of the acidfast rods. Pleomorphism was a greater feature in cultures grown at 20 C. (figure 2, 6, 7, 11, 12, 13).

HYDROGEN ION DETERMINATION

p_H curves for both variants were identical, using glycerol beef broth at p_H 7.3 as the starting point. At the end of 15 days' growth the broth reached a p_H of 8.00, without any change for 5 days thereafter.

ANIMAL INOCULATION

a. *Guinea pigs* were inoculated intratesticularly with 0.5 cc. suspension containing 0.2 mgm. of the variant in each case. These animals developed no sensitivity to old tuberculin at any time up to 113 days, when the animals were killed. However, they developed slight hypersensitiveness to a tuberculin prepared from the variants, but there was no specificity between the two types. At necropsy in no case was there any gross or microscopic evidence of disease.

b. *White mice* were inoculated intravenously and intraperitoneally with 0.5 cc. suspension containing 0.2 mgm. Half of the mice were killed after 6 days, and in those inoculated with variant I at necropsy there were no macroscopic lesions. Smears from the spleen, bone marrow and kidneys revealed the presence of short and plump acidfast rods with a few non-acidfast forms. Those inoculated with variant II presented a few minute greyish nodules in spleen, kidneys and lungs. Smears from these lesions revealed slender, slightly curved, long and beaded acidfast rods, a few short and plump, and others with clubbed ends. A number of the rods were non-acidfast. Fourteen days after inoculation, at necropsy small white tubercles were found in the spleens of mice inoculated with both variants. Smears from these lesions revealed acidfast organisms of the same morphology as on the 6th day.

c. *Chickens* were inoculated intravenously with 0.5 cc. suspension containing 0.2 mgm. of the variants. The chickens were killed after 111 days and in no case was there any macroscopic or microscopic evidence of disease. Smears from the organs were negative for acidfast bacilli. At no time was any hypersensitiveness produced to avian tuberculin or tuberculin prepared from the variants.

d. *Rabbits* were inoculated intravenously with 0.5 cc. suspension containing 0.2 mgm. of the variant in each case. These animals were killed after 114 days. Those inoculated with variant I showed small white tubercles in the lungs of one animal, some had a white, diffuse fibrous lower border to the liver, and there were no macroscopic lesions in the spleen, kidneys, or joint spaces. Smears from these lung lesions revealed the presence of long and short, straight and curved, beaded acidfast rods and coccobacilli.

In those animals inoculated with variant II, one animal had a solitary abscess in the lung about the size of a pea, filled with cheesy pus, and containing acidfast coccobacilli. Another animal had a large subcutaneous abscess the size of a hen's egg over the abdominal wall involving the fascial plane and containing thick yellow pus with numerous acidfast, short and long rods, beaded forms, some slender, and coccobacilli. Acidfast coccobacilli were also found in a diffuse fibrous lesion along the lower border of the liver. There were no lesions in the spleen, kidneys or joint spaces.

SEROLOGICAL STUDIES

Rabbits were sensitized intravenously on three occasions 3 days apart with 0.5 cc. of a milky suspension of heat-killed variant. After 3 weeks they were bled and the serum tested for agglutinins, precipitins and complement-fixing antibodies. No agglutinins or precipitins could be demonstrated, but complement-fixing antibodies were present in all in fair concentrations. Only slight specificities were noted. Rabbits sensitized with variant I reacted more strongly to its homologous and less to the heterologous antigen. The same was true for variant II.

The preceding two organisms as previously stated were isolated from human sources. Although the third organism, about to be described, was not isolated from a human source, it seemed appropriate to report it, as it had some unusual characteristics not encountered in ordinary saprophytic acidfast organisms, viz. its longer lag period of growth and its peculiar stages of chromogenicity.

MYCOBACTERIUM "BG"

This strain of acidfast bacillus was isolated by one of us (W.S.) from a BCG culture which was treated by the usual dissociation method, the suspension being inoculated on the surface of several gentian violet egg flasks. After one month of incubation at 37.5 C., in one of the flasks, which had never been opened since seeding, a small chromogenic colony developed on the surface of one BCG colony. This colony was fished out and streaked on the surface of a plain egg medium slant. The organism did not grow as rapidly as ordinary saprophytes, a characteristic which stimulated our interest for a more complete study.

DISSOCIATION OF "BG"

Further plating was done with the object of dissociation. Single colonies which were uniform in size and character, developed at 37.5 C. at the 10th day. Two distinct types of colonies which were best separable at the 25th day (figure 3, 3) were present—chromogenic and white, respectively. These were subcultured on plain gentian violet. Variant I (figure 3, 1) was dry, spreading, with nippled center, orange in color. Variant II (figure 3, 8) was dry, wrinkled, spreading with nippled center, white at first, but becoming salmon-pink after 5 to 7 days at room temperature. An original white colony culture aged for 120 days at incubator temperature developed a secondary growth (figure 3, 7) which was chromogenic and remains chromogenic, and on subculture had the same topography as variant I.

CULTURAL CHARACTERISTICS

Both variants were seeded on various culture mediums, and growth characteristics observed at 20 C., 37.5 C., and 55 C. Growth generally appeared first after 6 days with both variants, was more profuse with variant I (chromogenic), and occurred more profusely at 20 C. than at 37.5 C. for variant II (white), while there was little or no difference with variant I (chromogenic) at 20 C. and 37.5 C. No growth occurred with either at 55 C.

A 17-day growth on glycerol tomato broth of variant I (figure 3, 2) was dense brittle, chromogenic, whereas variant II (figure 3, 9) was wrinkled and tenacious, white at first but became pinkish after several days at room temperature.

Glycerol beef broth—Moderate growth appeared. With variant II the surface growth was white, veil-like and wrinkled, with white flocculation in the depths, whereas variant I surface growth was orange-colored and wrinkled, and had flocculation in the depths. These characteristics were brought out more with the age of the cultures.

Non-glycerol beef broth—Moderate growth appeared with the same characteristics as on glycerol beef broth.

Glycerol synthetic broth—Variant I, slight growth after 9–14 days, orange-colored, veil-like surface, with flocculation in the depths. Variant II, no growth at 20 or at 37.5 C.

Non-glycerol synthetic broth—No growth for either variant at 20 C. or at 37.5 C.

Pleural fluid broth—Variant I, moderate chromogenic growth after 6–9 days. Variant II, moderate white growth after 9–12 days.

Litmus milk medium—Variant I, chromogenic growth at the bottom of the tubes after 9–14 days, with the development of slight alkalinity. Variant II, no growth at 20 or at 37.5 C.

Glycerol potato slant—Variant I (chromogenic), no growth. Variant II (white), growth only appeared after 23 days at 20 C., dry, rough, corrugated pinkish-white.

Plain beef agar slant—Variant I, slight growth after 14 days at 20 C. while no growth at 37.5 C. Variant II, slight growth after 14 days at 20 C., chromogenic—no growth at 37.5 C.

Glycerol beef agar—Variant I, no growth. Variant II, no growth at 20 C., slight growth after 6–9 days at 37.5 C., salmon-pink in color and dry.

Glycerol egg slant—Variant I, moderate growth after 3–6 days, becoming very profuse with age and orange-colored. Variant II, moderate growth after 3–6 days at 37.5 C. and after 9–14 days at 20 C. becoming more profuse with age, salmon-pink rough and dry.

MORPHOLOGY AND TINCTORIAL CHARACTERISTICS

After 11 days on gentian violet egg medium variant I ((chromogenic) figure 3, 6) revealed uniformly moderate sized acidfast rods, no non-acidfast forms present. Variant II ((white) figure 3, 11) appeared as long, filamentous, very pleomorphic acidfast organisms, a few short ovoid acidfast forms and a few non-acidfast forms. With increase of time, pleomorphism increased at first but there were no filamentous forms, and many non-acidfast forms appeared.

At 21 days, variant I (figure 3, 5) was very pleomorphic. There were long and short, club-shaped, ovoid acidfast forms, and some non-acidfast forms.

At 35 days, with variant I (figure 3, 4) there were long and short acid-fast bacilli, round and ovoid bodies, and at least 50 per cent non-acidfast forms. Colonies from variant II (figure 3, 10) showed a few short bacilli with a predominance of round acid-fast bodies, and also many non-acidfast bacillary and coccoid forms.

HYDROGEN ION DETERMINATION

p_H determinations were the same as those for strains "M" and "I.P.," alkaline reaction having developed.

ANIMAL INOCULATION

Guinea pigs were inoculated intratesticularly with 0.5 cc. suspension containing 0.22 mgm of the variants. These animals developed no hypersensitiveness to 5 per cent old tuberculin, and only slight reactions were produced on testing them with tuberculins prepared from the respective variants, but there was no specific difference between the two types. The animals were killed after 80 days, and in no case was there any gross or microscopic evidence of disease.

Figure 3. "Bg"

1. Variant I—25 days on gentian violet medium. ×2.
2. Variant I—17 days on glycerol tomato broth. ×2.
3. Undissociated Bg—25 days on gentian violet medium. ×2.
4. Variant I—35 days on gentian violet medium, Ziehl Neelsen. ×865.
5. Variant I—21 days on gentian violet medium, Ziehl Neelsen. ×865.
6. Variant I—11 days on gentian violet medium, Ziehl Neelsen. ×865.
7. Variant II with secondary chromogenic (variant I) growth—120 days on gentian violet medium. ×2.
8. Variant II—25 days on gentian violet medium. ×2.
9. Variant II—17 days on glycerol tomato broth. ×2.
10. Variant II—35 days on gentian violet medium, Ziehl Neelsen. ×865.
11. Variant II—11 days on gentian violet medium, Ziehl Neelsen. ×865.

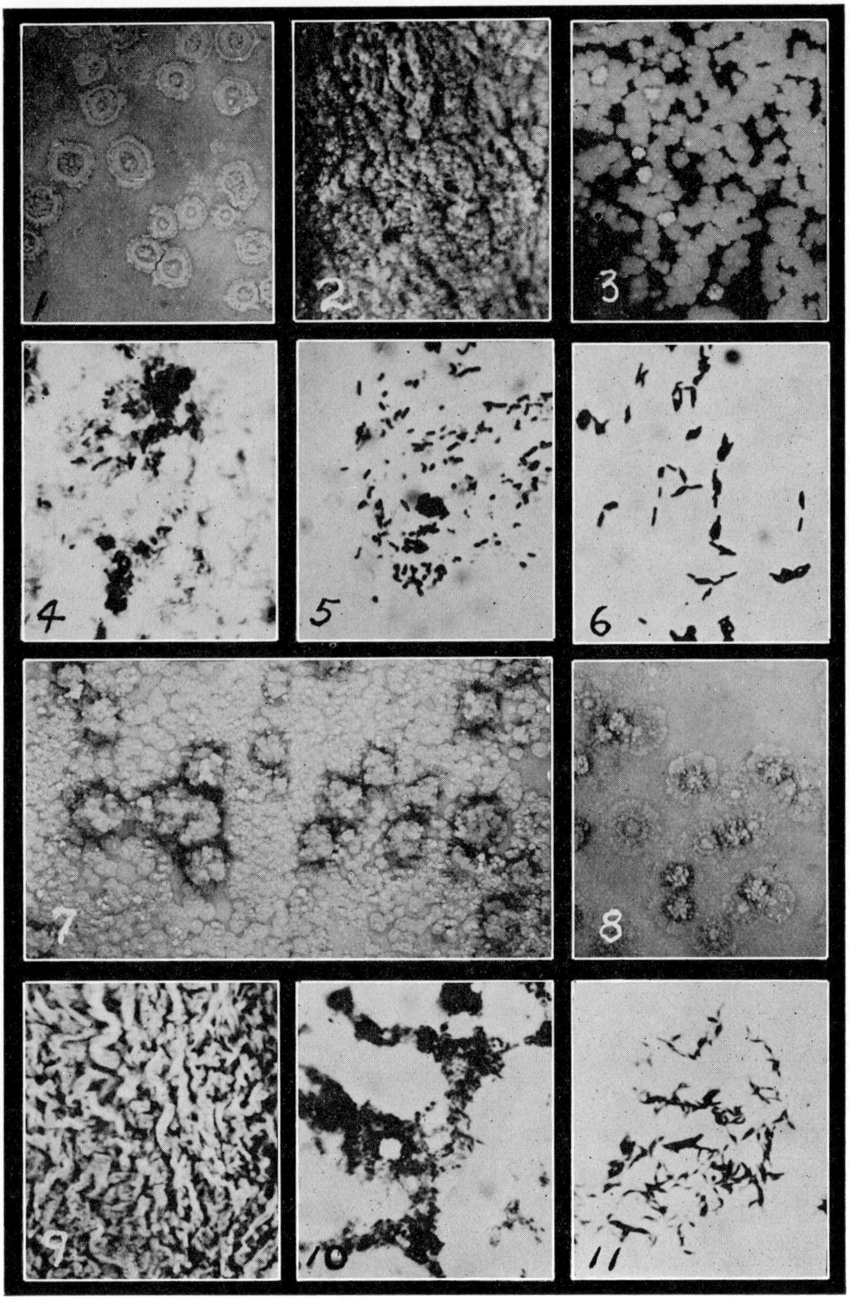

Figure 3. "Bg"

White mice inoculated intraperitoneally with 0.5 cc. suspension containing 0.22 mgm. of the variants also showed no evidence of disease, after 3 weeks, nor could acidfast organisms be demonstrated in smears prepared from the organs.

Chickens were inoculated intravenously with 0.5 cc. suspension containing 0.22 mgm. of the variants. No hypersensitiveness developed to 50 per cent avian tuberculin nor to tuberculin prepared from both variants. Further there was no evidence of disease on gross or microscopic examination of the organs when the animals were killed after 80 days.

Rabbits inoculated intravenously with the same dose, and killed after 81 days, showed no evidence of disease macroscopically or microscopically, nor the presence of acidfast organisms on direct smears from the organs.

SEROLOGICAL STUDIES

Again, as with the other two strains of organisms studied, in rabbits sensitized intravenously with heat-killed organisms, complement fixing antibodies could be demonstrated in fair concentration in the serum after an interval of 3 weeks, with a certain degree of specificity, but no agglutinins or precipitins were demonstrable at this time.

SUMMARY AND CONCLUSIONS

In the preceding pages we have described three strains of acidfast organisms, two isolated from human sources and one probably a contaminant. Each strain was dissociated into at least two variants possessing distinct topographical and other biological characteristics. Some of the variants in the early stages of colony development appeared to be white, but as they aged, when left at room temperature and exposed to light, invariably developed chromogenicity. All the variants propagated at 37.5 C. as well as at 20 C.; however, at the former temperature their growth was more profuse. Their morphological and tinctorial characteristics could not be used as a means of differentiation. Non-acidfast forms could be demonstrated in very young and again in older cultures. They were all very pleomorphic. These studies definitely show that environmental conditions play no small part in morphological variation. They were non-pathogenic for laboratory animals except in the case of "M" which displayed some pathogenicity for mice and rabbits. It may be that larger doses are required, or it is possible that their virulence will be enhanced after several animal passages. They were weak antigens producing complement-fixing antibodies with some degree of specificity. Specific tuberculins could be prepared from each strain, and animals inoculated with the strain reacted more strongly to the homologous than to the heterologous tuberculin.

The interpretation of the significance of the various so-called non-pathogenic acidfast organisms isolated from human sources is at present still a speculative one. It seems, however, that we cannot regard them merely as saprophytes, although there are certain similarities, viz., their behavior on artificial mediums, the production of chromogenicity, the p_H curves, and their pleomorphic morphology in different environments. It seems highly probable, however, that these organisms may, under certain circumstances, be responsible for the production of disease in man.

OXIDATION-REDUCTION POTENTIALS IN SALMONELLA CULTURES

II. CHARACTERISTIC POTENTIALS PRODUCED BY MEMBERS OF THE SUIPESTIFER AND ENTERITIDIS GROUPS

WILLIAM BURROWS

AND

EDWIN O. JORDAN

CHICAGO

In a previous paper[1] we have shown that the oxidation-reduction potentials developed in cultures of certain bacteria of the Salmonella group differed within the group but were correlated with bacterial type. The potential levels attained after the first few hours of incubation and maintained for several days thereafter were constant among strains of a single type but the main Salmonella types differed from one another in the degree of reducing intensity produced in their cultures. It was possible, by means of a considerable number of experiments, to accumulate sufficient data for mathematical analysis and to show that the types of bacteria examined, although in some cases quite near one another in oxidation-reduction potential, were nevertheless significantly different[2] in this respect. The present paper deals with the determination of characteristic potentials of additional Salmonella types.

The characteristic oxidation-reduction potentials reported here are those of S. paratyphi C, S. cholerae-suis var. kunzendorf, and S. sendai. These bacteria, together with those previously studied, represent four of the five serological groups recognized in the Kauffmann-White schema:[3] Group A (S. paratyphi A); group B, containing S. paratyphi B (S. schottmülleri); group C or the Suipestifer group containing S. cholerae-suis (American suipestifer), S. cholerae-suis var. kunzendorf (European suipestifer) and S. paratyphi C (Eastern or Hirschfeld type); and group D, the Enteritidis group in which the schema places S. enteritidis, S. sendai, and S. typhi. Other Salmonella types attached to these main groups will be discussed in a later paper.

The technic used in these experiments has previously been described in detail.[1] The organisms were grown in nutrient broth buffered with M/30 phosphate at p_H 7.10 to 7.12 at $37 \pm .02$ C. The strains used in the present experiments form a part of the Jordan Collection and have been thoroughly

---

Submitted for publication, August 15, 1935.

From the Department of Hygiene and Bacteriology of the University of Chicago.

This work was aided by a grant to the University of Chicago from the Rockefeller Foundation.

1. J. Infect. Dis. **56:** 255, 1935.
2. In the statistical sense of "significant difference."
3. J. Hyg. **34:** 333, 1934.

studied and carefully identified by detailed biochemical and serological methods. Their histories are as follows:

Kunzendorf—Three strains were isolated from the blood in human infections, one from food epidemiologically implicated in a food poisoning outbreak, one from hog cholera "virus blood"; two strains were obtained from the National Collection of Type Cultures and three from the Pribram-Kral Collection. The first five were isolated in the United States, the other five are of European origin.

Paratyphi C—Two strains ("Witte" and "Bagdad 41") were received from Dr. F. W. Andrewes, four ("Hirschfeld", "Bagdad, 31, 782, 1251") from the National Collection.

Sendai—Eight strains were received from Dr. Aoki.

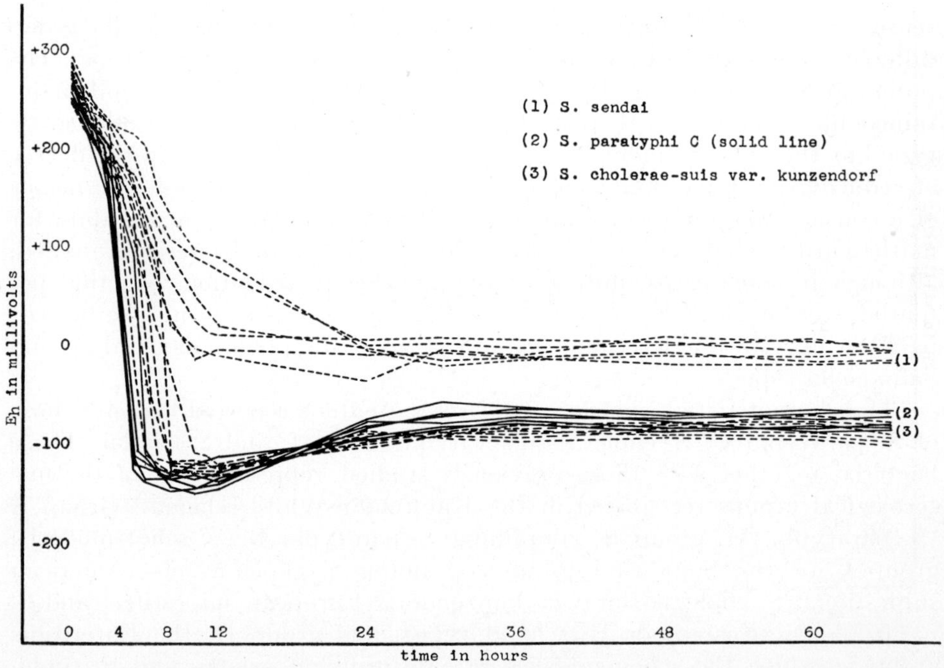

Fig. 1.—Time-potential curves produced by S. sendai, S. paratyphi C and S. cholerae-suis var. kunzendorf.

The results of these experiments are summarized in figures 1 and 2. Figure 1 shows the rapid negative drift at the beginning of the experiments and the final flattening out of the time-potential curves to a characteristic level. The tendency for strains of a single type to attain a characteristic potential is apparent again as in experiments previously reported. While S. sendai is considerably different from the other types studied, S. cholerae-suis var. kunzendorf and S. paratyphi C are indistinguishable from one another in characteristic potential. Figure 2 shows the relation of the characteristic potentials of the types here reported to those which have been previously discussed. The data at 36, 48, 60, and 72 hours were considered as making up the significant portion of the time-potential curve. These data were treated statistically, and regression lines fitted to the means by the usual method of a regression of Y on X. The method of treatment has been previously described.[1]

The difference in characteristic potential between S. paratyphi A and S. sendai is of particular interest since these two types have the specific H-antigen *a* in common but differ in the O-antigen and in the fact that non-specific H-antigens are absent in S. paratyphi A. On the other hand the Sendai strains, which in the Kauffmann-White schema are placed in the Enteritidis group (group D), because of their common possession of the O-

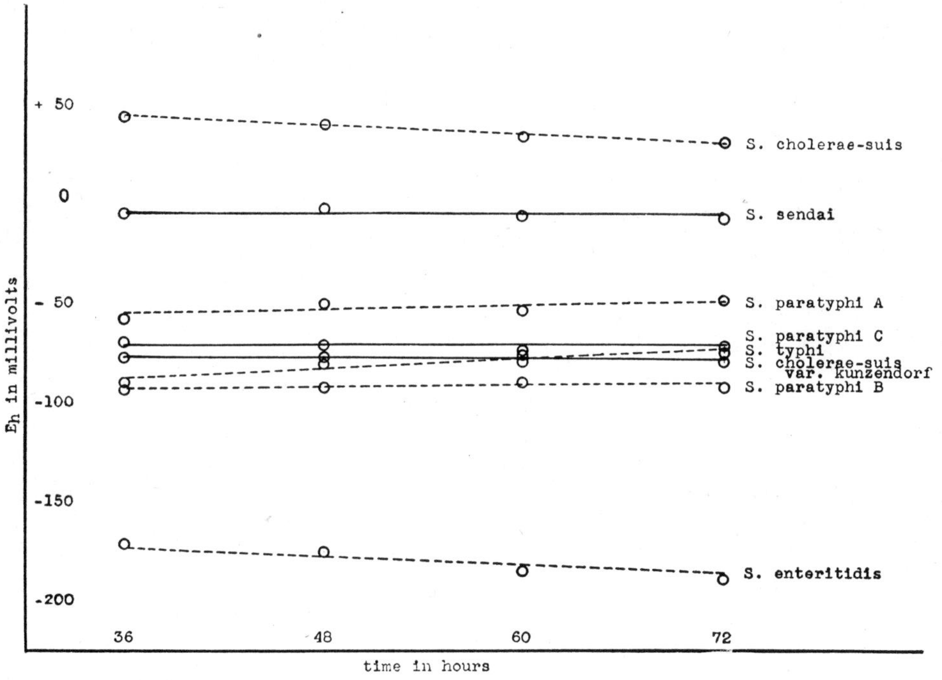

Fig. 2.—Oxidation-reduction potentials produced by various Salmonella types as shown by fitted regression lines.

The types reported in the present paper are shown by solid lines; those previously discussed by dotted lines.

antigen IX, are farther removed from this group in their characteristic potential levels than they are from the Paratyphi A strains.

The characteristic potentials of S. cholerae-suis var. kunzendorf and S. paratyphi C are very close to one another, so close as not to be significantly different. This observation is in keeping with the close biochemical and serological similarities of these two types. There is, however, a marked discrepancy in the potential level maintained by these two types as compared with that of S. cholerae-suis (figure 2). This cannot be explained in the light of our present knowledge.

It is worth noting, however, that the "American" Cholerae suis strains do not produce hydrogen sulfide demonstrable in lead acetate medium, while the Kunzendorf and Paratyphi C strains do blacken lead acetate agar. The latter types are in fact farther removed in their potential levels from the Cholerae Suis types than are the Sendai and Paratyphi A strains (figure 2). Since both the Sendai and Paratyphi A types are non-producers of hydrogen sulfide in cultural tests it is tempting to conclude that the potential levels of these organisms are correlated with important differences in their metabolic activities. Preliminary tests of Pullorum strains, however, not included in this paper, have given a lower potential than the Kunzendorf strains, although this type of Salmonella, if it is properly a Salmonella, does not produce hydrogen sulfide. It would appear that no single metabolic or antigenic factor determines the potential level.

EXPERIMENTAL MENINGOCOCCAL INFECTION IN THE MOUSE

C. PHILLIP MILLER

AND

RUTH CASTLES

CHICAGO

METHOD OF PRODUCTION

The method described below developed out of a long series of attempts to infect some easily available laboratory animal with gonococcus. To the reader interested in the evolution of technical procedures, it may not seem superfluous to recount briefly the preliminary steps leading to its adoption as a means of studying experimental meningococcal infection.

After a fruitless effort to establish gonococcal infection in rabbits and guinea pigs, an attempt was made to "adapt" a freshly isolated strain of gonococcus to the mouse by rapid animal-to-animal passage without intermediate growth on artificial mediums. To avoid contamination, the peritoneal cavity was chosen as the site of inoculation and exudate was transferred from recently succumbed or moribund mice directly to normal animals within the briefest possible time. It was hoped that in the course of many transfers the strain might acquire virulence for the mouse. During the experiments it was found that multiplication of the organisms failed unless a sufficient quantity of fluid was maintained within the animal's peritoneal cavity. The liquids ordinarily used for suspending inocula—buffered saline, Ringer's and broth—were rapidly absorbed. These facts clearly indicated protein solutions as more suitable vehicles, and various serums, egg albumin, etc. were employed.

The gonococcus ordinarily begins its invasion of a new host by multiplying on the surface of a mucous membrane, i.e., an epithelial structure coated by a film of mucus. It seemed possible, therefore, that mucus, preferably human mucus, might furnish a suitable environment for the initiation of growth within the peritoneal cavity of the mouse. The impracticability of obtaining sterile human mucus* forced us to attempt the isolation of mucin from saliva and from the gastro-intestinal mucosa from fresh autopsy material, but the yields proving insufficient for the needs of the investigation, a commercial preparation of hog's gastric mucin, was tried out. While this did not serve the purpose for which it was intended, it did prove to be highly satisfactory as a menstruum in which to inoculate mice with meningococcus, with which trial inoculations had been carried in parallel. This had been done

Received for publication, August 29, 1935.

From the Department of Medicine and the A. B. Kuppenheimer Research Foundation, University of Chicago.

* It should be mentioned in passing that synovial fluids from two cases of acute gonococcal arthritis failed to stimulate growth of gonococci in vivo and in vitro.

because it seemed prudent to control the method with a closely related but somewhat more virulent organism.

The commercial preparation of hog mucin made it possible to initiate a lethal infection in mice with less than 100 meningococci.[1] Difficulties were encountered[2] which for several months prevented repetition of the published results. It was eventually determined that the fault lay in the newer lots of mucin, and after the manufacturers (The Wilson Laboratories, Chicago) very kindly made up a special preparation for our purpose the method was found to be as effective as before. This material is now available under the label "Granular Mucin."

While the earlier of these studies was in progress, Nungester, Wolf, and Jourdonais[3] were independently at work on the effect of gastric mucin on phagocytosis. Their observations led to the finding that the lethal action of pneumococci, streptococci and staphylococci for mice is enhanced by mucin. Nungester has also used the method for the inoculation of mice with the virus of poliomyelitis.[4]

METHODS

The suspension of mucin.—Of the mucin now employed a 5% suspension has been found most satisfactory. It is prepared by pouring enough of the measured volume of distilled water onto the weighed quantity of mucin to moisten it thoroughly. After having stood about half an hour the sticky mass is rubbed free of lumps and the rest of the water is added slowly while rubbing and then stirring continues, until the suspension is uniformly distributed. It is quite acid, p_H about 5.0, at which reaction it has been found to be least harmed by the heat of sterilization. It is now distributed into suitable containers and autoclaved at 15 pounds pressure for 15 minutes. After cooling, its reaction is adjusted with sodium hydroxide to p_H 7.3.

As the product now being used contains insoluble particles of sufficient size to occlude fine hypodermic needles, it has been found convenient to withdraw the supernatant from this coarse sediment which falls to the bottom of the container within a short time and is easily visible to the naked eye. The supernatant, hereafter designated the "mucin suspension," is incubated for one day to insure sterility and is then ready for use. It should be noted that this suspension tends to settle on long standing, particularly in the cold, and should always be thoroughly mixed by gentle agitation before use to insure its uniform composition in all experiments.

Inoculation.—Stock cultures of meningococci are maintained on solid medium consisting of equal parts of meat infusion broth and buffer solution (containing 6.6 gm. of $Na_2HPO_4 \cdot 12H_2O$ and 0.83 gm. of $NaH_2PO_4 \cdot H_2O$ and 8.8 gm. NaCl per liter), 1% dextrose, 1% peptone, 1% corn starch and 2% agar. Its reaction is adjusted to p_H 7.3 to 7.4. Inoculated agar slants are kept stoppered with corks. Although stock cultures are transplanted only twice a

1. Miller, C. P.: Science **78:** 340, 1933.
2. Miller, C. P.: Proc. Soc. Exper. Biol. & Med. **32:** 1136, 1935.
3. Proc. Soc. Exper. Biol. & Med. **30:** 120, 1932.
4. Proc. Soc. Exper. Biol. & Med. **30:** 1128, 1933.

week, a strain which is to be used for mouse inoculation is subcultured at least twice at daily intervals before the final culture is inoculated. This seems necessary to insure satisfactory growth. The final transplant is allowed to grow no longer than 5 hours, for it has been found repeatedly that the number of meningococci required to initiate a lethal infection rises steadily after the 5th hour of growth on the medium described, an indication that the bacterial population contains the maximum number of vigorous individuals at that time.

The bacterial growth is recovered from the slant by washing with a few cc. of saline and is mixed in a test tube to insure uniform suspension. It is then diluted with saline to a density which experience has shown to indicate a concentration of approximately a billion organisms per cc. When checks are desired, as they were in most of the earlier experiments, samples are taken at this point for enumeration. The actual counting, which is done both by the Wright method and by means of a bacterial counting chamber, is postposed until after the inoculations. Titrations are then made by progressive 10-fold dilution in mucin suspension and mice are inoculated intraperitoneally as rapidly as possible with amounts of 1 cc.

RESULTS

By this method it was regularly possible to initiate lethal infections in mice with very few meningococci. Five of 13 strains studied required approximately 10 organisms. All of these highly virulent strains belonged to type I–III. The minimum fatal doses of the other strains ranged from approximately 100 to several thousand organisms. No instance has thus far been encountered of loss of virulence by cultivation on artificial medium. One strain whose M F D has repeatedly been below 10 organisms has been under cultivation for over three years.

With saline suspensions of our most virulent strains of meningococci the numbers of organisms required to insure a fatal outcome ranged from 100 millions upwards.

PRACTICAL APPLICATION OF THE METHOD TO THE BACTERIOLOGICAL DIAGNOSIS OF EPIDEMIC MENINGITIS

On two occasions within a short time the method has facilitated identification of the infecting organism in the spinal fluids of patients suffering from meningococcus meningitis. In both instances mice were inoculated intraperitoneally with the centrifuged sediment of spinal fluid (plus mucin) at the same time that smears and cultures were made. In one case meningococci were identified in the peritoneal exudate of the mouse before the cultures had grown out. In the other instance the organisms were so scarce in the sediment of the spinal fluid that none could be found in smears, and cultures remained sterile; but the peritoneal exudate of the mouse contained an abundance of typical meningococci.

DISCUSSION OF METHOD

Heretofore it has been impossible to study meningococcal infection (strictly speaking) in a small laboratory animal because means were lacking to induce a few organisms introduced into such a host to multiply and invade its tissues. Unusual credit is therefore due the investigators who have, notwithstanding, been able to advance so far our knowledge of the bacteriology and epidemiology of cerebro-spinal fever and to provide us with a specific therapy.

Except for Branham's recent work[5] previous attempts to infect small laboratory animals intraperitoneally with meningococci have succeeded only when large numbers of organisms were used.[6] In our own experience several hundred millions are required to kill a mouse by intraperitoneal inoculation without mucin. Such numbers are not far below the lethal dose of killed organisms and suggest that "infection" here is incidental to a primary intoxication.

Quite recently Branham[5] has reported the production of experimental infection in mice by the intraperitoneal injection of meningococci of unusually high virulence. While she does not give the numbers of organisms constituting the minimum lethal doses of her various strains, she does state that those which required more than 10,000 organisms were regarded as unsatisfactory for her purpose. This seems to be the most successful attempt thus far reported to infect mice with meningococci alone; but Branham encountered the same difficulty which others have noted—that the virulence of most strains could not be long maintained.

The experimental disease produced in mice by the method we describe simulates only the initial stages of invasion and generalized bacteremia with which cerebrospinal fever in man begins, for no evidence has been observed of localization of the infection to the meninges of the mouse. Occasionally an animal has exhibited peculiarities of behavior after recovery, but these occurrences have seemed not more numerous than after recovery from in fection with other microörganisms.

The effectiveness of the method for the production of experimental meningococcal infection has been confirmed by the publications of Rake[7] and Cohen.[8] Rake[9] has also applied the method with success to the typhoid bacillus.

It was surprising to find that cultivation on artificial medium failed to lower the virulence of the strains which have been studied; for at the time of his preliminary report[1] the author was under the impression that recently isolated strains were especially virulent, and he so expressed himself, by inference. But one of the strains (the other has been lost) which gave rise to this idea is still, three years later, one of our most effective. Cohen[8] mentions one stock strain 15 years old which proved virulent for mice by this method.

5. Pub. Health Rep. **50:** 768, 1935.

6. For a review of the literature consult the excellent monograph by E. G. D. Murray: The Meningococcus, Medical Research Council Special Series, No. 124, London, His Majesty's Stationery Office, 1929.

7. J. Exper. Med. **59:** 553, 1934: Proc. Soc. Exper. Biol. & Med. **32:** 1175, 1935.

8. J. Immunol. **29:** 61, 1935.

9. Proc. Soc. Exper. Biol. & Med. **32:** 1523, 1935.

THE COURSE OF EXPERIMENTAL MENINGOCOCCAL INFECTION IN THE MOUSE AND THE ROLE OF MUCIN IN ITS PRODUCTION

Mice inoculated with lethal doses of meningococci by the method described in the preceding paper sicken rapidly and succumb within 48 hours, usually in 16–24 hours. They sit quietly in their cages, their fur ruffled, show increasing indisposition to move about take no interest in food; their eyes are kept closed and the lids finally become glued together by the mucous secretion which accumulates. In short, they look like mice suffering from a generalized infection with some other organisms, e.g., pneumococcus or hemolytic streptococcus, highly virulent for this species. We observed none of the symptoms which Branham[5] noted and interpreted as indicative of meningeal involvement. The only evidence we obtained on this point was the appearance once in a great while of an individual among the recovered mice which exhibited peculiarities of behavior. Experiments are now in progress to determine whether localization of the infection in the meninges can be encouraged by lengthening the period of infection by the administration of small doses of antiserum. Thus far these experiments have been unsuccessful.

METHODS

The progress of the infection was followed by examining the blood and peritoneal exudate at intervals during its course. Blood for cultures was obtained from the end of the tail, after cleansing it with alcohol, by snipping it across with a pair of sharp sterile scissors and allowing a drop of blood to accumulate in the end of a finely drawn capillary pipette placed in the center of the wound; with a little practice it was possible to obtain blood without its coming into contact with the skin of the tail. It was found necessary to use pipettes made from glass tubing which had been carefully cleaned and to rinse them with sterile saline just before drawing the blood. The drop of blood was expressed from the pipette onto the surface of a freshly poured blood agar plate and distributed by means of a sterile loop. After incubation the number of colonies was counted and recorded in terms of plus marks. This means of estimating the microbic content of samples of blood, admittedly inexact, was adequate for the purposes at hand and actually more dependable than the ordinary method of poured plates. On a number of occasions animals whose blood had just been cultured from the tail were sacrificed in order to culture their heart's blood as a check on the reliability of the method.

Peritoneal exudate was obtained by aspirating a drop with a fine hypodermic needle attached to a syringe. It was either cultured on the surface of freshly poured blood agar plates or spread into films and stained for microscopic examination. This method was checked from time to time by withdrawing the entire fluid content of the peritoneal cavity of a sacrificed mouse, mixing it thoroughly and examining it by means of cultures and smears.

BACTERIOLOGICAL EXAMINATION OF PERITONEAL EXUDATE AND BLOOD

The following type experiment illustrates the findings obtained by the methods just described:

Experiment 1.—Four mice were injected intraperitoneally with 1 cc. each of mucin suspension containing different numbers of meningococci, as indicated in table 1. During the course of the next 13 hours four samples of peritoneal exudate from each animal and as many of peripheral blood were cultured. The results of these cultures are shown in the tabulated protocol. It will be seen that on each occasion cultures of the peritoneal exudate of

TABLE 1.—*Cultures of Peritoneal Exudate and Blood during the Course of Infection*

Inocula		Cultures of peritoneal exudates at:				Culture of (heart's) blood at:				Time of death
Dilution	Number of Organisms	1 hr.	3 hr.	5 hr.	13 hr.	45 min.	$2\frac{1}{4}$ hr.	$4\frac{1}{2}$ hr.	13 hr.	
10^{-3}	2,410,000	+++	++++	++++	++++	+	++	++++	++++	20 hr.
10^{-4}	241,000	+++	+++	+++	++++	+	++	+++	+++	24 hr.
10^{-6}	2,410	+	++	+	++++	+	++	+	0	48 hr.
10^{-8}	24	0	0	0	dry tap	0	+	+	+	20 hr.

0 no growth
\+ few colonies
++ many colonies
+++ innumerable colonies
++++ confluent growth

the two mice receiving the largest inocula showed either innumerable colonies or confluent growth. The growth from the exudate of the mouse infected with 2,400 organisms was scant until the thirteenth hour and the cultures from the mouse receiving only 24 organisms failed to grow. The aspiration attempted at 13 hours yielded no fluid.

The initial (45 minute) blood cultures of the first three mice were positive while that of the mouse receiving only 24 organisms was negative. It is of interest to note that the 13-hour blood culture of the third mouse was sterile and that this mouse died many hours later than the others. This would have been attributed to faulty technic but for a somewhat similar occurrence of another experiment (vide infra).

From this and other experiments it is clear that the number of meningococci within the peritoneal cavity does not begin to increase until four or five hours have elapsed. Nevertheless the blood stream is rapidly invaded, for it was found that when very large numbers of organisms (a million or more) were injected into the peritoneal cavity, positive blood cultures were usually obtained within a few minutes. When the inocula exceeded a thousand the cultures were often positive within an hour. The inoculation of smaller numbers was often followed by negative blood cultures for several hours; but once they had become positive they usually continued to be so throughout the remaining period of life. Two exceptions to this generalization were encountered: one has already been noted in the foregoing experiment; the other, which deserves mention in passing, was an animal which survived infection with 1,000 minimum fatal doses of a highly virulent strain. Its blood cultures were positive until the 24th hour when they became negative and remained so although the animal appeared to be moribund from the 24th to the 30th hour.

MICROSCOPIC EXAMINATION OF PERITONEAL EXUDATES DURING THE COURSE OF INFECTION

Experiment 2.—Six mice were injected intraperitoneally with 1.0 cc. each of a 10^{-6} dilution of a virulent strain of meningococcus suspended in mucin.

Six control mice were also injected with an equal quantity of uninoculated mucin. At intervals of 3, 6, 9, 11, and 24 hours thereafter one mouse in each series was sacrificed, its peritoneal exudate removed, mixed and spread in thin films on a number of slides. Of the several stains employed, Gram's and Wright's proved the most satisfactory. It was found necessary to exercise more than ordinary care to prevent overstaining, as the structural details of certain highly chromophilic cells were visible only in faintly stained preparations.

In the following descriptions of the films the term "granular material" has been applied to the particles of various sizes and shapes contained in the mucin suspension. Many of these resembled cocci so closely that it was difficult not to mistake them for meningococci and careful comparison of the smears of infected and uninoculated exudates was necessary to avoid this error. Their real nature has not been determined, but considering the origin of mucin, it seems quite probable that some of them are in fact the bodies of dead bacteria.

INFECTED EXUDATES

Three hours: Very much "granular material," few cells (about 2 per high power field), mostly small round cells with deeply stained nuclei and little or no cytoplasm. A few larger cells with round pale, nuclei and abundant cytoplasm. Only an occasional polymorphonuclear and an occasional cell with elongated, pale, vesicular nucleus and abundant cytoplasm.

Six hours: Slightly less "granular material." Cells more numerous, about $\frac{2}{3}$–$\frac{3}{4}$ of them polymorphonuclear leukocytes, most of which are normal in appearance. No phagocytosis of meningococci but some of the "granular material." Mononuclear cells are mostly large with moderate amounts of cytoplasm. Small round cells are rare. Few organisms visible.

Nine hours: Much less "granular material." Numerous organisms. Many cells, at least $\frac{3}{4}$ of them polymorphonuclear leukocytes, more than in the uninoculated mucin. A larger proportion of them appear normal than in the uninoculated mucin.

Eleven hours: Polymorphonuclears more abundant than in uninoculated mucin. A considerable portion of them are swollen, vacuolated and are poorly stained. Many organisms. Very few within polymorphonuclears.

Twenty-four hours: Every field crowded with organisms and cells, mostly polymorphonuclears, about $\frac{1}{3}$ of these are swollen and vacuolated. Very few contain organisms. No granular material.

UNINOCULATED MUCIN

Three hours: Very much "granular material." Fewer cells than in infected mucin. Almost all of them are small round cells.

Six hours: Similar to 6 hours smears of infected mucin, except that a larger portion of the polymorphonuclears are shrunken and deeply stained.

Nine hours: Cells very numerous, about $\frac{3}{4}$ of them polymorphonuclears; of these many are poor in cytoplasm with their nuclear lobes tightly tacked together so that they are difficult (some impossible?) to distinguish from medium sized round cells.

Eleven hours: Very little "granular material." Increased number of cells.

Twenty-four hours: No "granular material." Very many cells, about $\frac{2}{3}$ polymorphonuclear, ranging in size from the shrunken deeply stained ones described above, to swollen, poorly stained, vacuolated cells. A much larger proportion of healthy polymorphonuclears than before. Much phagocytosis of "granular material." The mononuclears vary in size from small round cells without visible cytoplasm to large cells with abundant cytoplasm.

To summarize: cellular elements did not begin to accumulate in the peritoneal cavity until after 3 hours after inoculation and were not abundant until the 9th hour. At first they consisted chiefly of small round cells, the proportion of polymorphonuclears rising during the second 3-hour period to $\frac{2}{3}$ to $\frac{3}{4}$ of the total. Meningococci became numerous at 9 hours. Very little phagocytosis was apparent at any time.

Comparison of the infected and uninfected exudates brought out, in addition to the presence of meningococci in the former, only two striking differences: (a) the greater number of healthy-looking polymorphonuclear leukocytes in the infected; and (b) the difference in appearance of the degenerated polymorphonuclears, which in the infected exudates were mostly swollen as if falling apart, and in the uninoculated exudates compressed and shrunken.

It should be mentioned at this point that in similar experiments with meningococci belonging to less virulent strains phagocytosis of large numbers of organisms by polymorphonuclears was observed.

Comparison of the infected and uninfected exudates and comment on their cytology is reserved for a subsequent section dealing with the role played by mucin in facilitating the infection.

DURATION OF THE EFFECTIVENESS OF MUCIN IN FACILITATING INTRAPERITONEAL INFECTION

In view of the foregoing observations it was not surprising to find that sterile mucin introduced into the peritoneal cavity was able to promote infection with meningococci (suspended in saline) introduced several hours later. This capacity was not maintained undiminished for long, however, as shown by the following experiment.

Experiment 3.—Each of six mice was injected intraperitoneally with one cubic centimeter of mucin suspension. At intervals of two, and then one hour thereafter, other groups of mice were similarly treated. Immediately after the fourth group had received its injection of mucin all of the mice were inoculated intraperitoneally with graded doses of meningococci suspended in saline. Each mouse received the dose indicated by the dilution factor at the top of its column (see table 2). In this as in all experiments in which saline suspensions of meningococci were employed, inoculation was carried out as quickly as possible after the suspension had been made to minimize the toxic effect of this menstruum on the organisms.

The results shown in table 2 indicate that the effectiveness of mucin began to diminish three hours after its introduction into the peritoneal cavity.

Since these results might be explained by the absorption of mucin from the peritoneal cavity or its destruction or denaturation in situ, the question naturally arose of whether mice which had been injected with sterile mucin

TABLE 2.—*Duration of Infection-promoting Action of Mucin*

Interval between mucin and organisms*	Dilutions of suspension of meningococci						
Hours	10^{-4}	10^{-5}	10^{-6}	10^{-7}	10^{-8}	10^{-9}	10^{-10}
5	18	18	19	24	S	S	
3		18	18	24	24	S	S
1		18	18	20	36	24	S
0		18	24	24	24	24	S

* Meningococci suspended in saline injected intraperitoneally.
In this and subsequent tables figures indicate time of death in hours after inoculation.
S=Survived.

regained their normal susceptibility after its infection-promoting action had worn off. The following experiment demonstrated that this was not the case:

ACTION OF MUCIN IN DEVELOPING LOCAL RESISTANCE TO INFECTION

Experiment 4.—Three series of mice which had been prepared by intraperitoneal injection of sterile mucin 29, 24, and 2 hours before, were inoculated, along with a control series, with varying dilutions of meningococci suspended in mucin. As the culture employed had been grown longer than the customary five hours, its M F D was one dilution lower than usual for this strain. The results (shown in table 3) indicate that the mice which had received sterile mucin only two hours before were as susceptible to infection as were the controls, but that those which had received this preliminary treatment 24 and 29 hours before inoculation resisted 1,000 minimum fatal doses.

TABLE 3.—*Effect of Preliminary Injections of Mucin*

Interval between preliminary injection and inoculation*	Dilution of original suspension of meningococci						
Hours	10^{-4}	10^{-5}	10^{-6}	10^{-7}	10^{-8}	10^{-9}	10^{-10}
29	18	S	S	S	S	S	
24	18	S	S	S	S	S	
2		18	22	24	36	S	S
0		18	18	22	18	S	S

* Inoculation carried out with meningococci suspended in mucin.

From this and the preceding experiment, it seems clear that although the ability of intraperitoneal mucin to facilitate infection with meningococci is maintained for several hours, the subsequent loss of this ability is followed by a refractory state. This increased resistance to infection, which could be augmented by multiplying at daily intervals the number of intraperitoneal injections of sterile mucin, was regarded as a local stimulation of the defense mechanism, for no evidence was obtained suggesting the development of humoral immunity. Repeated subcutaneous injections of mucin failed to alter the susceptibility to infection and the serum of rabbits which had been injected intravenously with mucin until their precipitin titers reached 1:10,000 afforded no passive protection whatever.

EFFECT OF INTRAPERITONEAL MUCIN ON MICE INOCULATED BY OTHER ROUTES

In all of the foregoing experiments meningococci were introduced directly into the peritoneal cavity already containing or about to contain mucin suspension. A number of experiments were made, however, in which mice were injected intravenously and subcutaneously. The results may be summarized as follows:

Intravenous inoculations.

A. With mucin suspensions of organisms.

It usually required somewhat larger numbers of meningococci to initiate a lethal infection by intravenous inoculation (organisms suspended in mucin) than by the intraperitoneal route. The difference varied from ten to 1,000 M F D. However, mice containing recently injected mucin in their peritoneal cavities succumbed to intravenous inoculation of doses more nearly approaching the M F D determined by the intraperitoneal method.

B. With saline suspension of organisms.

To infect mice intravenously with meningococci suspended in saline required relatively enormous numbers (a million or more M F D). Much smaller doses sufficed, however, if the animals contained sterile mucin within their peritoneal cavities. In other words, the presence of mucin in the peritoneal cavity facilitated infection by organisms introduced directly into the blood stream.

Examination of the intraperitoneal mucin showed that it becomes infected with meningococci very soon after their introduction into the circulation. This fact, together with the observation that organisms injected into the peritoneal cavity quickly invade the blood stream, suggests that mucin renders permeable to these bacteria the barrier between the peritoneal cavity and the vascular system.

Subcutaneous inoculations.

Organisms suspended in mucin and injected subcutaneously produced fatal infections only when quite heavy inocula were employed. We were uniformly unsuccessful in infecting mice by this method with organisms suspended in saline.

DISCUSSION

It was originally supposed by the authors that the mucin acted as a satisfactory culture medium which remained in the peritoneal cavity long enough to permit the multiplication of meningococci to numbers sufficient to overwhelm the mouse's resistance to invasion; or more briefly, that the mucin served merely as culture medium and the mouse as incubator. This simple and obvious explanation seemed reasonable at the time, because meningococci would grow in vitro in the particular lot of mucin then employed. It was subsequently found, however, that other preparations of mucin behaved differently in this respect; in fact the one which has been found most effective in promoting infection in the mouse, fails altogether to support growth in the test tube.

The assumption that mucin might function as a kind of aggressin was rendered untenable by the observation that anti-mucin serum failed to protect mice against infection and by the fact that mucin injected subcutaneously failed to immunize against infection.

No relationship, detectable by immunological methods, was found between mucin and meningococcus analogous, for instance, to the relationship discovered by Heidelberger, Avery and Goebel[10] between gum arabic and pneumococcus type II. Antimeningococcus serum always failed to give precipitin reactions with mucin, and conversely, anti-mucin serum with titers of 1:10,000 precipitated no antigens prepared from meningococci. Nor were the titers of antimeningococcus serums reduced after absorption with mucin in any concentration.

Our experimental data have thus far failed to support the notion that mucin enhances the virulence of meningococci, unless one takes liberties with the conventional concept of virulence. For organisms recovered from exudates or blood of moribund mice proved no more virulent when titrated with saline than cultures grown on artificial mediums. Nor have consistent differences been observed in the colonial structure of organisms used for inoculation and those recovered from the peritoneal cavity or blood stream of infected animals.

The material presented in this paper seems rather to indicate that mucin interferes in some way with the host's defense mechanism. This interference is a local one, for subcutaneous injections of mucin were ineffective in promoting infection with organisms introduced intravenously or intraperitoneally. The microscopical examination of peritoneal exudates described in experiment 2 revealed degenerative changes in many of the cells, and ingestion by some, especially polymorphonuclears, of the insoluble particles contained in the mucin. It is obvious, therefore, that a certain number of the phagocytic cells were put out of commission by the mucin; but not all, for the infected exudate contained numerous healthy looking polymorphonuclears. It might be supposed that these had been somehow restrained by the mucin from engulfing meningococci, were it not for the fact that organisms belonging to certain other strains were readily taken up by them. Furthermore, the appearance of the polymorphonuclears in the peritoneal exudates of mice protected by immune serum present a very similar appearance to those already described, except that more of them contained meningococci. Its effect on the mobile phagocytes (polymorphonuclears) must, therefore, represent only a part of the action of mucin. There remain the fixed tissue phagocytes of the peritoneal cavity. As they constitute in part the barrier between it and the vascular system, a barrier which is rendered easily permeable to organisms by the presence of mucin, it seems likely that injury to them is also an important feature of its action in promoting invasion of the host.

It seems probable that in the struggle between the infecting organism and its host the presence of mucin may interfere just enough with the latter's defense mechanism to tip the scales in favor of the microbic invader.

---

10. J. Exper. Med. **49:** 847, 1929.

The action of immune serum in experimental meningococcal infection in the mouse—One of the uses to which experimental meningococcal infection in mice[1] has been put is a study of the effectiveness of immune serums. Our observations on this point will be considered under three headings:

(a) The protective action of monovalent rabbit immune serums.

(b) The effect of immune serums on the course of the experimental disease.

(c) The protective action of commercial polyvalent serums marketed for therapeutic use.

METHODS

Preparation of rabbit serum.—Monovalent serums were prepared from 17 strains of meningococci, of which 2 had been recently isolated, 8 had been carried in the laboratory on artificial medium from 1 to 14 months, and 7 were strains generously supplied by Dr. Sara E. Branham of the National Institute of Health.

Rabbits were immunized by the intravenous injection of saline suspensions of organisms grown on the solid medium described in the first paper in this series. A few rabbits received only living organisms from freshly grown young cultures; for the rest stock suspensions were made up and kept in the ice box. No great difference was observed in the rapidity with which agglutinative or mouse-protective substances were engendered by these two kinds of antigens and the latter method afforded a considerable economy of time. Rabbits were usually injected on three successive days each week, for three or four weeks, beginning with one half cc. and increasing rapidly to 1 cc. of a suspension containing $\frac{1}{5}$ of a slant to the cubic centimeter. No attempt was made to produce serums of particularly high titer.

Method of administration.—Preliminary experiments showed that intravenous and intraperitoneal injections of serum were equally effective, but that the subcutaneous route was appreciably less so. In most experiments the intraperitoneal route was therefore used because it was the easier.

It was found convenient to keep the volume of serum constant at 0.5 cc. and to vary the dosage by diluting the serum appropriately with normal salt solution. Unless otherwise stated, the serum was injected intraperitoneally about half an hour before the mice were inoculated.

TITRATION OF RABBIT IMMUNE SERUM

The results of an experiment (experiment 5) demonstrating the protective action of rabbit immune serum is presented in table 4. The meningococcus used for inoculation was a highly virulent strain; the immune serum was homologous. It will be seen that the number of lethal inocula from which mice recovered was (roughly) proportional to the quantity of serum used and that even 0.000,125 cc. and 0.000,06 cc. (the 1:4,000 and 1:8,000 dilutions of serum, respectively) afforded some degree of protection. Certain of our heterologous serums belonging to the same type (I–III) protected quite as well in the higher concentrations but usually failed to protect in doses smaller than 0.000,25 (1:2,000 dilution). Not all serums were equally effective but as only one rabbit (sometimes a pair) was immunized against each strain, differences in potency were attributed, at least among the type I–III serums, to individual variation in the ability of the animals to produce antibodies. Judgment is reserved in the case of type II for none of our three strains belonging to this type engendered mouse-protective antibodies as readily as most of our type I–III strains—a coincidence which may or may not have been fortuitous.

TABLE 4.—*Titration of Protective Action of Monovalent Serum*

Dilutions of serum	Dilution of original suspension of meningococci									
	10^{-2}	10^{-3}	10^{-4}	10^{-5}	10^{-6}	10^{-7}	10^{-8}	10^{-9}	10^{-10}	10^{-11}
1:4	S	S	S							
1:64	S	S	S	S						
1:250		S	S	S	S					
1:500		22*	S	S	S	S				
1:1000		<18	S	S	S	S				
1:2000			<18	S		S	S	S		
1:4000			22	22	S	S	S	S		
1:8000				22	36	S	S	S		
Controls						<18	23	22	S	S

* Figures indicate time of death in hours after inoculation.
S = Survived.

THE ACTION OF IMMUNE SERUM

Inquiry into the means by which immune serum protected was made by studying the blood and peritoneal exudates of serum-treated and control mice during the course of their infection by the methods used in experiment 1.

Two series of 5 mice each were inoculated intraperitoneally with 100 minimum fatal doses of meningococci suspended in mucin. One series had just received a large dose, 0.5 cc. of a 1:64 dilution (=0.0078 cc.) of potent immune serum. At intervals of approximately 2 hours thereafter one mouse in each series was sacrificed, its heart's blood and peritoneal exudate cultured and the latter also examined microscopically in stained smears.

TABLE 5.—*Cultures of Heart's Blood and Peritoneal Exudate of Mice Infected with 100 M F D*

Interval after inoculation	Serum treated		Controls	
Hours	Blood	Exudate	Blood	Exudate
2	0	++	++++	++++
4	0	++	++++	++++
6	0	0	++++	++++
$8\frac{1}{2}$	0	0	+++	++++
10	0	0	++++	++++

0 no growth.
\+ few colonies.
++ many colonies
+++ innumerable colonies.
++++ confluent growth.

The results presented in table 5 show that the immune serum prevented invasion of the blood stream, which in the controls occurred promptly, and enabled the local defenses of the host to sterilize the peritoneal cavity within 6 hours.

DURATION OF PASSIVE PROTECTION

Experiment 6.—Each of six mice was injected intraperitoneally with 0.125 cc. of rabbit immune serum diluted to 0.5 cc. Two days later a second series was similarly injected, 4 days after that a third, and so on until six series had been thus treated over a period of three weeks. One day after the last injection they were infected by intraperitoneal inoculation, each mouse receiving the dose of organisms represented by the dilution factor at the head of its column (see table 6). The results indicate that mice which had received immune serum seven and ten days before inoculation survived a million minimum fatal doses and those which had received it two weeks before survived 10,000 M F D. In other words, protection persisted in high degree for about two weeks and then fell off.

TABLE 6.—*Duration of Passive Protection*

Days between serum administration and inoculation	Dilution of original suspension of meningococci							
	10^{-2}	10^{-3}	10^{-4}	10^{-5}	10^{-6}	10^{-7}	10^{-8}	10^{-9}
1	S	S	S	S	S			
3	<18	S	S	S	S	S		
10	<18	S	S	S	S	S		
14	<18	<18	<18	S	S	S	S	S
18	<18	<18	23	S	S	S	26	S
20	<18	26	23	36	36	S	23	26

SPECIFICITY OF THE MOUSE PROTECTIVE ACTION OF SERUM

Cross-protection tests have been carried out with a considerable number of serums and strains. In no instance has a type I–III serum failed to protect against many more M F D of meningococci belonging to this type than to type II organisms and vice versa. In other words, we have found, among the strains examined, quite a high degree of type specificity. Our single type IV strain is of such low virulence that protection experiments in which it served as the infecting organism have been inconclusive. The serum prepared from it had a fairly high agglutination titer but failed altogether to protect against infection with organisms belonging to the other types.

A sample protocol is given in table 7.

TABLE 7.—*Protection of Mice by Serums of Various Types Against Infection with Meningococci type I–III and type II*

Infecting Strain	Type of Immune Serum*	Dilution of original suspension of meningococci						
		10^{-2}	10^{-3}	10^{-4}	10^{-5}	10^{-6}	10^{-7}	10^{-8}
Type I–III	I**	S	S	S				
	II	<18	<18	24	<18	22	28	28
	III**	S	S	S				
	IV	<18	<18	<18	<18	<18		
Type II	I**			<18	22	20	28	
	II	S	S	S	S	S	S	
	III**			<18	<18	19	S	
	IV			<19	19	20	24	

* One half cc. of 1:10 dilution injected intraperitoneally into each mouse shortly before inoculation.

** Serums prepared from strains very kindly supplied by Dr. Sara E. Branham of the National Institute of Health. The type I strain was number 331; the type III, number 146. They represent extremes of the group I–III. Considerable information regarding their serological properties is contained in the report of her exhaustive study of agglutination of meningococci.[11]

No protection whatever against meningococcal infection was afforded by anti-gonococcus serum which precipitated meningococcus protein and carbo-

11. J. Immunol. **23:** 49, 1932.

hydrate in very high dilution. Nor was any evidence of cross-protection found between meningococcus and anti-pneumococcus serum type III or vice versa, although an immunological relationship between these organisms has been described.[12]

EFFECT OF SERUM ADMINISTERED DURING THE COURSE OF THE INFECTION

Experiment 7.—Seven groups of mice were injected by intraperitoneal inoculation with mucin suspensions of meningococci so that each series constituted a titration, the dose of organisms received by each mouse being indicated in table 8 by the dilution factor at the top of its column. Immediately after inoculation one group of animals was given 0.5 cc. of a 1:200 dilution (=0.0025 cc.) of rabbit immune serum intraperitoneally. Two hours later

TABLE 8.—*Protective Action of Rabbit Immune Serum Administered after Inoculation*

Interval between culture and anti-serum	Dilution of original suspension of meningococci									
	10^{-1}	10^{-2}	10^{-3}	10^{-4}	10^{-5}	10^{-6}	10^{-7}	10^{-8}	10^{-9}	10^{-10}
0	10	21	S	S	S	S				
2 hr.	10	9	S	S	S					
4 hr.		21	10	S	S	S				
7 hr.			21	21	21	S	S			
9 hr.			21	21	21	S	S	S		
$10\frac{1}{2}$ hr.			10	10	21	S	S	S		
Controls					21	21	21	21	21	S

another group was similarly treated and this process was repeated at intervals up to $10\frac{1}{2}$ hours. As shown in table 8, serum administered two hours after inoculation protected against as many organisms as did serum administered immediately after inoculation, viz., against a million M F D. Serum injected four hours after inoculation protected against 100,000 M F D and mice receiving serum as late as $10\frac{1}{2}$ hours after inoculation survived 1,000 M F D. That the infection was by that time well developed is demonstrated by the fact that all of the controls had succumbed 10 hours later.

TITRATION OF THE PROTECTIVE ACTION OF POLYVALENT THERAPEUTIC SERUMS

Packages of anti-meningococcus serums prepared by 6 commercial firms and distributed for clinical therapeutic use were purchased in the open market. They were all polyvalent and some "concentrated." Titrations of their mouse-protective action showed 4 of them to be quite as effective as our most potent monovalent rabbit serums; another nearly so. Text figure 1 summarizes graphically the results of 8 typical protection experiments in which 4 rabbit serums and the 4 most effective commercial serums were employed. The curves also show that although protective action is roughly proportional to the dose of serum, a point is reached beyond which increments of serum fail to protect against further increase in the number of infecting organisms.

12. Boor, A. K., and Miller, C. P.: Proc. Soc. Exper. Biol. & Med. **28:** 1050, 1931; J. Exper. Med. **59:** 63, 1934.

EFFECT OF NORMAL SERUM

We have been unable to confirm Branham's observation[5] that some normal horse serums protect against meningococcal infection. Of 8 serums each from a different horse which had not been subjected to any immunization none was found to afford any protection in doses of 0.1 cc. and 0.5 cc. Tests with several normal rabbit serums were also negative.

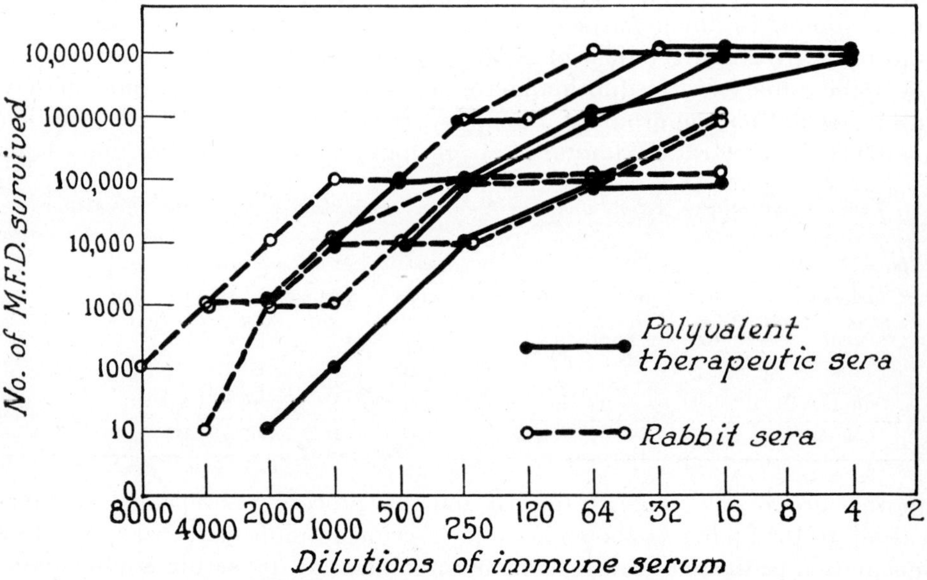

Fig. 1.—Titrations of Mouse-Protective Action of Four Monovalent Rabbit Serums (Type I–III) and Four Polyvalent Therapeutic Serums.

SUMMARY

It was possible to initiate fatal infections regularly in mice by the intraperitoneal inoculation of very few meningococci suspended in mucin prepared from hog's gastric mucosa. With our most virulent strains approximately ten organisms sufficed.

Multiplication of meningococci inoculated into the peritoneal cavity in mucin suspension did not occur during the first few hours, after which it proceeded rapidly. The blood stream was always invaded at some time during the course of the infection, within the first hour if the infecting dose were large. Very little phagocytosis was observed in the peritoneal exudates of animals infected with virulent strains; but considerable in those inoculated with less virulent organisms. The ability of mucin to facilitate intraperitoneal infection with meningococci persisted for several hours and was followed by a state of increased resistance. The presence of sterile mucin in the peritoneal cavity also promoted infection by the intravenous route. Mucin in the subcutaneous tissues failed to do so. No evidence was found that mucin raises the virulence of meningococci. The apparent enhancement of their invasiveness seems to be due to local interference with the defense mechanism of the host.

Monovalent rabbit anti-meningococcus serums were found to protect mice effectively against inoculation with numbers of meningococci many times the minimum fatal dose. Below a maximum of 10 million M F D these multiples were roughly proportional to the quantity of serum administered. Among the serums tested, those belonging to type I–III protected (within the limits of their potency) against all the strains of this type. Similarly the three type II serums examined were effective against the three strains of this type. Serums of either type protected poorly or not at all against strains belonging to the other. In short, the monovalent serums examined were type-specific in their protective action. The protection afforded by a large dose of serum persisted in quite high degree for about two weeks. Immune serum averted a fatal outcome even when administered after the infection was quite well developed. Four of six polyvalent therapeutic serums tested were as effective as our most potent rabbit serum, and another nearly so. The mouse-protected test is suggested as a means of standardizing therapeutic serums.

THE SEROLOGIC CLASSIFICATION OF THE BRUCELLA GROUP

LYLE VEAZIE

AND

K. F. MEYER

SAN FRANCISCO

Contemporaneous publications and reviews on the Brucella group (Hofmann and Bartsch[1]) continue to convey the impression that a serological classification by means of the agglutination and agglutinin absorption tests is impractical and impossible. On the other hand, some noteworthy progress has been made since Wilson and Miles[2] pointed out some of the technical difficulties inherent in the Brucella absorption tests. Furthermore, in view of the reported serologic classifications, workers have now become more and more confused on account of the fact that the types established by the dye and H_2S tests quite frequently belong to different serologic races. Certain reasons for these discrepancies have been discussed by Meyer.[3] In fact, the historical data and recent papers have been reviewed in the critical summary and require little amplification. Independent studies by Wilson and Miles,[2] by Francis,[4] by Olin[5] by Habs[6] and by the authors have shown that 2 properly absorbed antiserums prepared with smooth Brucella strains may quickly place a culture into the abortus (bovine and porcine types) or the melitensis group.

In conjunction with the studies of Meyer and ZoBell on the behavior of an international collection of Brucella strains toward dyes, H_2S production and nitrate reduction, a total of 447 cultures has been serologically classified. The studies were made in 1931 and 1932, and have since been enhanced by continuous retesting of old and the examination of new strains. It is the purpose of the paper to detail briefly the findings and offer evidence that a serologic classification is most valuable as an aid in recognizing epidemiologically interesting strains.

TECHNICAL PROCEDURES

The technic used for all the experiments was essentially the same. The antigens for absorption were grown on liver hormone agar slants for 48 hours, and the growth from these was used to inoculate Blake bottles containing

---

Received for publication, October 9, 1935.

From the George Williams Hooper Foundation and the Department of Bacteriology, University of California Medical School.

1. Zentralbl. f. Bakteriol., I. Abt., Orig. **129:** 449, 1933.
2. Brit. J. Exper. Path. **13:** 1, 1932.
3. Fifth Pacific Science Congress, B3, **15:** 3023, 1934.
4. Pub. Health Rep. **46:** 2416, 1931.
5. Acta Soc. Med. Suecanae **61:** 7, 1935.
6. Zentralbl. f. d. ges. Hyg. **28:** 481, 1933.

the same medium. These were incubated 48 hours, washed off in saline containing 0.1 per cent formaldehyde, and the heavy suspensions put back in the incubator until sterile. They were stored in the ice box. Antigens for the agglutination tests were made by washing off the growth of 48 hour liver agar slants in 0.25 per cent formaldehyde-saline, and when sterile, diluting to the desired opacity with saline. The standardization was done in a nephelometer, a 0.06 per cent suspension of Brucella prepared in a Hopkins tube being used as a standard of opacity. This proved a rapid and accurate method of standardizing large quantities of antigen.

Serums were obtained by injecting rabbits with formalinized suspensions. One injection of 1 cc. of a 0.5 per cent suspension was usually sufficient to produce a satisfactory titer in 6 or 7 days. The rabbits were bled when a titer of 1–1,280 was reached. The serums were preserved with an equal quantity of glycerine, and thus the titer was reduced to 1–640. This is considered the most satisfactory for absorption (Evans, Francis), and was consequently chosen for the experiments.

Absorptions were carried out in the following manner: The heavy suspensions prepared from Blake bottles were washed once in saline, and packed in the centrifuge. The supernatant fluid was discarded and serum, equal in volume to the mass of packed cells, was added with four times the quantity of saline. The cells were thoroughly suspended in the fluid, and the mixture placed in the incubator for 18 hours. It was centrifuged again, and the supernatant fluid used for the agglutinations. This procedure always proved sufficient to exhaust the serum of agglutinins for the absorbing strain. Parallel absorptions were made for the first series of experiments with fresh, live organisms. The results were identical with those obtained with formalin-killed antigens, so the latter were employed for the remainder of the tests.

The serum dilutions were made directly in the antigen, 0.5 cc. of serum being added to a tube containing 1.5 cc. of antigen and 1 cc. of this, after thorough mixing, being transferred to a second tube containing 1 cc. of antigen, and so on. Five tubes and a control were used with final serum dilutions of 1–20, 1–40, 1–80, 1–160 and 1–320. Duplicate sets of antigen were made for agglutination with the various test serums. The tubes were placed in a water-bath at 37 C. for 18 hours and were then read. Second readings after 24 hours at room temperature may be made if desirable.

At the beginning of the studies, 24 strains of various origins were selected at random for reciprocal absorption tests. Serums were prepared from 12 of them, and these were absorbed by all the strains, each antigen being tested with all the absorbed serums. It was found that all the strains fell into 2 main groups, with 1 small subgroup which is designated as the "intermediate." The characteristics of this group will be discussed later. The 2 main types corresponded to the melitensis and the abortus-suis types found by other investigators. For the remainder of the investigation, monospecific serums were prepared from typical strains of each of the 2 main types, and the entire collection of 447 strains was agglutinated with the 2 serums.

The strains used for preparation of the monospecific serums were No.

80, a suis type, No. 428 (Evans),[7] a melitensis type and "Tunis Green," a human strain as the "intermediate" (probably the "transitional" of Wilson and Miles)[2] type. In order to assure the purity and smoothness of these strains, plates were streaked from each culture, the colonies examined under the microscope and a single, perfectly smooth colony picked to streak another plate. This was repeated 6 times for each culture until the final plates showed no dissociating colonies. Antigens were then made from the resulting pure cultures and serums prepared. These were absorbed by a heterologous antigen in order to secure a monospecific test serum. The "Tunis Green" strain was not used in the preparation of monospecific serums, but was employed as a control antigen with each set of agglutination reactions which was made.

RESULTS

In the manner outlined, 447 strains were tested; of these, 427 were sufficiently smooth to be classified. Seventy-eight or 18.2 per cent were agglutinated only by the monospecific melitensis serum, 323 or 75.6 per cent only by the monospecific abortus and 26 or 6 per cent by both, thus reacting as "intermediates." The table shows the distribution of the strains by host and country.

TABLE 1.—*Serological Classification of Brucella Types by Host and Geographic Origin*

Serological Group Origin	Number	Abortus						Melitensis				Intermediate			Rough				
		Bovine	Porcine	Caprine	Human	Ovine	Equine	Bovine	Caprine	Human	Equine	Bovine	Caprine	Human	Bovine	Porcine	Caprine	Human	Ovine
Africa	7	1			5					1									
Algeria	3				1					2									
Argentina	22	7	1					5	4						4	1			
Austria	1				1														
Canada	1				1														
Denmark	43	22	6		15														
England	9	6			2					1									
Esthonia	6	4						2											
France	16	8				1	2								3		1		1
Germany	25	14			10					1									
Hungary	4	4																	
Italy	47	18			5			1		12		1		8				2	
Malta	6			4					1	1									
Palestine	2	1													1				
Russia	10													8				2	
Sardinia	6								1			3	1				1		
Sweden	6				6														
Switzerland	16		5		8									1				2	
Tunis	6			1					2				3						
U.S.A.	211	51	38		68		7	13	17	12	1			[1]	1			2	
Total	477	136	50	5	122	1	9	21	25	30	1	4	4	18	9	1	2	8	1

The strains used for serological tests had previously been classified as bovis, suis or melitensis types by means of H_2S production, nitrate reduction and the modified dye test originated by Meyer and ZoBell in this laboratory. A table is given showing the correlation between the methods.

Of the 407 strains which could be classified by both reactions, 357 or 87.4 per cent fall into the same groups by both methods and 24 or 5.8 per cent disagree. The 26 "intermediate" strains, which form 6.3 per cent of

7. Hygienic Laboratory Bulletin No. 143, 1925.

the group, are reserved for separate discussion. Of the strains giving conflicting results by biochemical and serological tests, 11 are from the United States, and fairly complete histories could be obtained for them. They were all of bovine origin obtained by guinea pig inoculation with milk from infected cows. Eight of the strains were isolated from different cows in a single dairy over a period of a year. They all reacted as true "bovis" types in the dye tests, but as "melitensis" types by the agglutinin absorption tests.

TABLE 2.—*Comparison of Serological and Biochemical Classification of 447 Brucella Strains*

Serological Group / Dye Group	Number	Abortus			Melitensis		Intermediate	Rough			Abortus	Melitensis
		Bovis	Suis	Melitensis	Bovis	Melitensis	Melitensis	Bovis	Suis	Melitensis	Atypical	
Africa........	7	5		1		1						
Algeria.......	3	1				2						
Argentina.....	22	7	1		5	4		3	1	1		
Austria.......	1			1								
Canada.......	1		1									
Denmark.....	43	35	8									
England......	9	8				1						
Esthonia......	6	4			2							
France.......	16	11						3		2		
Germany.....	25	20				1					4	
Hungary......	4	2									2	
Italy.........	47	21		2	1	9	9			2		3
Malta........	6	3				2					1	
Palestine.....	2	1						1				
Russia........	10						8			2		
Sardinia.......	6					1	4			1		
Sweden.......	6	6										
Switzerland...	16	4	9				1	2				
Tunis........	6			1		2	3					
U.S.A.......	211	62	92		11	32	[1]	1	2		10	
Total......	447	190	111	5	19	55	26	10	3	8	17	3

Both the dye and absorption tests were repeated several times for each strain over a period of 4 years, and single colonies were examined. The original determinations were invariably confirmed. Two cultures of bovine origin from Esthonia and 1 strain of bovine origin originally obtained from Italy reacted in the same manner. Five cultures isolated in Argentina from cattle were classed as "bovis" types by the dye method, although they were serologically indistinguishable from true melitensis.

However, it is noteworthy that strains classed as abortus by absorption gave certain dye reactions characteristic for the melitensis type. Among these are to be mentioned 1 from Africa, 1 from Austria, 2 from Italy and 1 from Tunis. In this connection, it should be noted that the majority of the Tunisian and several of the Italian cultures finally were placed in the "intermediate" type, which serologically is very closely related to the abortus. Strikingly, all the strains which reacted in this manner are of human origin. The Austrian strain No. 426 represents the classical abortus variety as recognized by Evans.[7] This strain as well as the African and Algerian cultures behave as atypical melitensis on dyes; they grow well in thionin but are inhibited by pyronin B in a dilution of 1–200,000.

The Argentinian cultures form an interesting group. Twenty-two of them were included in this series. They had been isolated from bovine, porcine and caprine sources, and were grown, until they reached this laboratory, on a medium containing normal horse serum. They were found to correspond by dye tests, in all except one instance, to the source from which they came. The one exception was a strain of bovine origin which reacted as a melitensis. Serologically, however, they behaved as an extremely heterogeneous group. Three agglutinated spontaneously, 4 failed to agglutinate in any of the serums, even before absorption. Eight cultures of the 15 reacted serologically and biochemically according to type. However, 6 strains from bovine sources gave "bovis" dye reactions, but in the agglutinin absorption test they acted like typical melitensis. It was later found that 6 of the Argentinian cultures were thermo-agglutinable; 5 of them gave distinct clumps within 5 minutes at 90 C. The non-agglutinable strains, which were of this variety, were non-pathogenic for guinea pigs, but the serum of test animals inoculated with live cultures agglutinated the homologous strains to a fairly high titer, in fact, they clumped specifically other rough strains. It is readily appreciated that, in the serum medium upon which these cultures had been perpetuated, rough variants are easily split off. The large proportion of spontaneously agglutinable and thermo-agglutinable strains in the Argentinian collection must be attributed to the cultivation of the organisms on unsuitable mediums. Yet, it must be emphasized that the strains whose serological behavior conflicted with the biochemical reactions revealed no tendency to microbic dissociation.

Twenty of the cultures (4.7 per cent) are unclassifiable by dye reactions. Seven of these are American strains (2 of human, 1 of equine and 4 of bovine origin). They are ultra-sensitive toward all dyes. They all grow on liver slants under increased CO_2 tension, and in the control and nitrate tubes of the dye series when incubated under the same conditions. They produce H_2S, reduce nitrates without gas production and react as abortus serologically. These strains, which lend themselves to serological and H_2S classification, but not to biochemical, afford an example of the necessity of using more than one method of identification.

The other 3 American strains, which cannot be classified with certainty by dye reactions, are of porcine origin. They produce no H_2S, grow well in 1–30,000 thionin, and to some degree in 1–50,000 fuchsin. They are completely inhibited by 1–200,000 pyronin and produce gas in nitrate mediums. Serologically they belong to the abortus type.

Seven European strains, which react serologically as abortus, give confusing results in dye mediums. Six of them were isolated from cattle and 1 from a goat. They all give variable results when grown in thionin mediums. They grow, though not luxuriantly, in 1–75,000 thionin and usually, after prolonged incubation, in 1–50,000 thionin. Five of them produce H_2S. All show gas in nitrate medium, and grow in fuchsin and pyronin. Three strains of human origin, which give similar reactions in dyes, react as "melitensis" with monospecific serums. They form no gas in nitrate mediums nor do they produce H_2S. Numerous single colonies from each of the 10 cultures were also examined. In every case, they reacted in the same manner as the original strains.

Particular attention is called to the "intermediate" type. Although an antigenic variant, it is not a specific type, since by ordinary reciprocal agglutinin absorption tests it reacts as an abortus type. The usual absorbing dose of an abortus antigen removes all agglutinins from an "intermediate" type serum. A minimal dose of abortus organisms, just sufficient to remove all abortus agglutinins, leaves a small proportion of agglutinins for the homologous strain. The proportion of absorbing organisms must be very carefully adjusted in order to demonstrate these residual agglutinins (the titer never exceeds 1–40).

Even in a monospecific melitensis serum, a heavier absorbing dose of abortus antigen than was used for these tests will obscure the differences in the antigenic proportions of the abortus and "intermediate" types. The reaction is strictly quantitative. In the usual monospecific melitensis serum, however, the difference is marked. In such a serum, the "Tunis Green" type is agglutinated to approximately 25 per cent of the titer of the melitensis. A typical reaction is shown in table 3.

TABLE 3.—*Melitensis Serum*

	1–20	*1–40*	*1–80*	*1–160*	*1–320*	*Control*
80	0	0	0	0	0	0
428	++++	++++	++++	++++	++	0
Tunis Green	++++	++++	++++	++	0	0

Abortus Serum

	1–20	*1–40*	*1–80*	*1–160*	*1–320*	*Control*
80	++++	++++	++++	++++	++	0
428	0	0	0	0	0	0
Tunis Green	++++	++++	++++	++++	++	0

At the beginning of the study, the "intermediate" types were listed as a subtype of abortus. As further tests revealed more strains with similar serological affinities, they were more carefully analyzed and similarities were noticed. All the 26 strains, which reacted in this way, were classed by dye reactions and H_2S production as typical melitensis. (Only 5 strains in the entire series used for this study reacted as melitensis on dyes and as typical abortus by absorption.) Eighteen of the atypical strains were of human, 4 of bovine and 4 of caprine origin. Their geographical distribution is of interest. Sixteen of them came from the Mediterranean Basin, Italy, Sardinia and Tunis. Eight originated in Transcaucasian Russia and 1 in Switzerland. Only 1 culture of the "intermediate" was encountered in the United States, in the blood of a patient who had worked extensively with a particular Transcaucasian strain. This serologist in all probability acquired the infection from that source. It is noteworthy that no "intermediate" types were encountered in the collections which came from the northern European countries.

On the basis of Wilson and Miles'[2] theory, it is reasonable to offer the following explanation for this third type. The Brucella strains have 2 antigenic fractions—abortus and melitensis—in varying proportions. An "intermediate" type consists of an abortus type with an excess of melitensis antigen. They are probably transition forms, undergoing a gradual change in antigenic structure. That their present make-up is relatively stable, however, is proved by the fact that a Transcaucasian "intermediate" type passed through a human being without losing its characteristic serological behavior. Moreover, all the strains of this type were tested repeatedly over a period of

4 years, together with numerous single colonies from each one. Serums have been prepared from a number of typical melitensis strains, including some freshly isolated cultures. These have been absorbed with numerous abortus strains of various origins and the "intermediates" tested against them. The reactions of the group have remained remarkably constant.

This type should not be considered a definite and sharply defined antigenic unit like the 2 major types. Its existence amply confirms the complex antigenic relationship within the Brucella group. It is of interest to note that 6 strains, which are probably identical with the "intermediate" type, were observed by Wilson[8] in a study of cultures from France. Two strains with similar reactions, 1 isolated in Italy, were reported recently by Olin.[5]

THERMO-AGGLUTINATION

Because of the attention which has been given to the problem of rough variants in the Brucella group (Zdrodowski, Brenn and Voskressenski,[9] Alessandrini and Sabatucci,[10] Vercellana and Zanzucchi),[11] the entire series of strains was tested for thermo-agglutination. The method described by Pandit and Wilson[12] was followed. Forty-eight hour growths from liver agar slants were suspended in physiological saline, and placed immediately in a water-bath with a temperature of from 90–95 C. The readings were made in accordance with the technic described. Only 28 strains were found to give thermo-agglutination. Eleven were recorded as 4+ and four as 3+ reactions. The remaining strains gave partial clumping after prolonged heating. Sixteen strains could not be used for serological tests, since they spontaneously agglutinated. Strains which were thermoagglutinable acted, as a rule, as poor antigens; some failed to agglutinate in the standard serums, or sedimented so weakly that they could not be used with absorbed serums. There were, however, several strains which could be classified satisfactorily in spite of their strong thermo-agglutinability. All thermo-agglutinable strains, which were agglutinated by the monospecific serums, gave clear-cut reactions. In all cases, their serological type was the same as their biochemical one. There were 7 strains which were thus classified. Four reacted as melitensis, 1 as an abortus and 2 as "intermediates."

Of the entire series of 447 strains, only 21 or 5 per cent were too rough to be classified by means of the monospecific serums. In fact, the problem of rough dissociation was not as important in this series of studies as has been emphasized by others who worked along similar lines. This may be largely due to the fact that all the cultures in this laboratory are kept on liver hormone agar, which contains no serum or other substances usually found to produce rough dissociation. None of the strains, which have been kept for years on this medium, have shown any signs of change in antigenic structure. The strains were first tested over 4 years ago, and when reëxamined at

8. J. Hyg. **33:** 516, 1933.
9. Ann. de l'Inst. Pasteur **45:** 768, 1930.
10. Annali d'ig. **41:** 29, 1931.
11. Pathologica **18:** 247, 1926 also Boll. Soc. di biol. sper. **1:** 221, 1926.
12. J. Hyg. **32:** 45, 1932.

intervals since that time have reacted in exactly the same way. Prolonged cultivation probably has no effect on the antigenic structure of Brucellas, provided the medium is a suitable one.

USE OF THE ABSORPTION TEST TO ESTABLISH THE NATURE OF A PATIENT'S INFECTION

The absorption method may be used in the typing of a serum from patients from whom the specific organism has not been recovered, although the agglutination test indicates undulant fever. Its usefulness in this respect is naturally limited, both because of the necessity of having a serum of fairly high titer, and because of the impossibility of distinguishing between bovis and suis infections. The method followed in the laboratory is briefly as follows: Absorb 2 portions of the serum, one with a melitensis antigen, the other with an abortus; test each of the absorbed serums for agglutinins with the 2 type antigens. Uniformly good results have been obtained with serums having a titer of 1–640 or over, and the information received in this way has often been of epidemiological value. In those cases from which a Brucella was later isolated, complete reciprocal absorption tests have always confirmed the original diagnosis.

SUMMARY

By means of monospecific serums over 400 strains from 20 different countries have been classified. All the smooth cultures were easily separated into 2 main types, corresponding to the serologic "abortus-suis" and the "melitensis" types. A small subtype was observed, consisting of 26 strains, which is very similar to the abortus type in antigenic make-up. It is differentiated from the true abortus type by a greater proportion of melitensis antigen.

A comparison of the serologic findings with those obtained by means of dye reactions and H_2S production revealed conflicting results in only 5.8 per cent of the tests. All the cultures classified as "suis" type by biochemical reactions fall into the abortus type antigenically. Ten per cent of the cultures identified as "bovis" type by dye reactions are serologically indistinguishable from melitensis cultures. Forty-two per cent of these strains were isolated from a single herd of cattle in the United States. Their reaction indicates the value of systematic classification in epidemiological studies. It is suggested that certain investigators, who have obtained unsatisfactory results from serological studies, have encountered an undue proportion of such strains. Twelve per cent of the cultures, which are biochemically melitensis, are serologically identical with the abortus type. All of these are old laboratory strains of unknown origin (Austria, Italy, Africa and Tunis).

The serological classification of the Brucella strains is an indispensable part of the proper identification of the strains for epidemiological purposes. Its failure to agree with other methods of differentiation in a certain percentage of cases serves to emphasize the fallacy of relying on any one test for proper and complete identification.

THE WEIL-FELIX REACTION OF THE RABBIT IN THE DIAGNOSIS OF ROCKY MOUNTAIN SPOTTED FEVER (EASTERN TYPE)

KENNETH F. MAXCY
CHARLOTTESVILLE, VIRGINIA

For the laboratory confirmation of the diagnosis of Rocky Mountain spotted fever (exanthematic tick fever) three tests have been proposed; viz., (1) recovery of the virus from the patient's blood by inoculation of guinea pigs and its subsequent thorough study and identification, (2) a protection test carried out on guinea pigs inoculated with mixtures of passage virus and blood serum obtained from the patient during early convalescence, and (3) agglutination of the specific Proteus strains $X_{19}O$ and $X_{2}O$ by serum obtained from the patient late in the disease or during convalescence. The first two procedures mentioned involve highly specialized technics and facilities which are available in only one or two laboratories in this country. Dependence is therefore placed upon the last named procedure, namely the Weil-Felix reaction.

The specificity of this test for the typhus group of diseases has been well established and its peculiarities in relation to Rocky Mountain spotted fever studied by Spencer and Maxcy[1] and by Davis and Parker.[2] While this reaction becomes positive in a great majority of instances, occasional cases are encountered in which the specific agglutinins appear or are present in such small amounts as to leave the result in doubt. Again, it may be impossible to obtain a specimen of blood from the patient late in the course of the illness or during convalescence on account of lack of coöperation or accessibility, or on account of a fatal issue—which in the eastern United States may occur in about one in every four cases.

Having encountered these practical difficulties a procedure was sought which would yield the needed laboratory confirmation irrespective of the issue of the case and at the same time could be carried out in any well equipped diagnostic laboratory. Advantage was taken of the fact that the rabbit is susceptible to this disease and as a result of infection shows a Weil-Felix reaction just as do human beings. If rabbits could be successfully infected by inoculation with blood obtained from the patient during the early part of the illness, without first establishing the virus in guinea pigs, then the Weil-Felix observations could easily be made on this animal in the laboratory without further reference to the patient. During the past two seasons this procedure has been used on eight cases with the results which are here reported.

Received for publication, October 9, 1935.

From the Department of Preventive Medicine and Bacteriology, University of Virginia.

1. Pub. Health Rep. **45**: 440, 1930.
2. Pub. Health Rep. **47**: 1511, 1932.

TECHNICAL CONSIDERATIONS

The specific agglutination of Proteus $X_{19}O$ by the serum of rabbits two or three weeks after inoculation with Old World typhus (guinea pig passage virus) was reported by Weil and Felix in 1920.[3] Since Foot[4] had already shown that rabbits were likewise susceptible to infection with passage virus of the closely related disease—Rocky Mountain spotted fever—it was to be expected that they also would show agglutinins for the specific Proteus strains. Kuczynski[5] looked for them and found in one instance a low titer agglutination with the X_2 strain. Munter[6] had no difficulty in demonstrating agglutinins for Proteus X_{19} in the serum of rabbits inoculated with a passage strain of Rocky Mountain spotted fever virus as with typhus, but upon reinoculation found differences in the response to the two viruses which suggested that the mechanism was not identical in both diseases.

Badger and his collaborators[7] found the Weil-Felix positive for Proteus X_{19} in a dilution of 1:80 or better in six out of eight rabbits reacting to the western strain of spotted fever passage virus, but with only four out of fifteen reacting to the eastern strain. In the light of more recent work, it seems probable that their proportion of successes would have been increased had the serums been tested against X_2O as well as $X_{19}O$ and the significance of reaction in lower titers in rabbits realized.

Gordon Davis[8] has recently completely reviewed the manifestations of the Weil-Felix reaction in rabbits inoculated with passage virus of typhus-like diseases. He found that agglutinins of Proteus X_2O as well as of $X_{19}O$ appear in significant titer following injection of "spotted fever" passage virus (western type?) whereas with endemic typhus the agglutinins are highly specific for $X_{19}O$, as had been found in human infections.

In the studies here reported the antigenic suspensions were made from strains originally received from Dr. A. Felix. The cultures were repeatedly plated for purity of the "O" (non-motile) variant and absence of "H" (motile) spreading colonies before the final growth on infusion agar in Blake bottles. The resulting 0.85 per cent saline suspension was examined for absence of motility before the preservative (0.2 per cent formaldehyde) was added and the concentrated emulsion standardized for turbidity. The tendency of $X_{19}O$ cultures to revert to the "H" phase was thus carefully checked. According to Felix[9] the purity of the "O" phase is a more important consideration than is the question of whether living or killed organisms are used as antigens. Pure "O" suspensions are remarkably uniform in sensitiveness; small amounts of "H" may influence sensitiveness considerably.

Macroscopic agglutination technic was used. Serum dilutions were made

---

3. Wien. klin. Wchnschr. **33:** 423, 1920.
4. J. Med. Research **39:** 495, 1919.
5. Die Erreger des Fleck- u. Felsen-fiebers, J. Springer, Berlin, 1926.
6. Ztschr. f. Hyg. u. Infektionskr. **109:** 124, 1928.
7. Am. J. Pub. Health **23:** 19, 1933.
8. Pub. Health Rep. **50:** 404, 1935.
9. System of Bacteriology in Relation to Medicine, Medical Research Council, London, vol. 7, 1930.

in 0.5 cc. amounts beginning with 1:5; 0.5 cc. of antigen suspension was then added to each tube. Incubation was carried out at 55 C. for four hours and the racks allowed to stand in the refrigerator overnight at 4 C. before the final readings were made.

As the virus tends to disappear from the peripheral circulations during the latter part of the illness blood must be obtained from the patient before the ninth or tenth day. Clotting should be prevented by the addition of the required amount of sodium citrate in normal salt solution.

Ordinary domestic white rabbits were used in these experiments. Two or three cubic centimeters of citrated patient's blood was injected either intravenously or intraperitoneally, or both. This injection must be made within an hour or two of the time when the blood is withdrawn from the patient—and preferably at once—since the virus tends to die off rather rapidly in blood exposed to ordinary room temperatures and somewhat more slowly if kept at a low temperature.

Natural agglutinins for the specific Proteus "O" strains are not commonly encountered in the serums of domestic rabbits. In testing some thirty such animals one was found which gave a slight agglutination with X_2O in dilutions up to 1:20. Positive reactions are, however, judged upon the appearance and disappearance of specific agglutinins following the experimental inoculation.

RESULTS

In table 1 are summarized the observations on the Weil-Felix reaction of eight rabbits—each inoculated with blood from a patient in the early stages of an attack of Rocky Mountain spotted fever.

For the first five of these patients the clinical course and other laboratory findings have been reported by Dr. H. B. Mulholland.[10] Four survived and developed a positive Weil-Felix reaction toward the end of their illness. Case 7 died a few hours after admission on the seventh day. Blood obtained just before death and inoculated into guinea pigs resulted in the establishment of a passage strain. On the basis of incomplete cross immunity tests done at the National Institute of Health, U.S.P.H.S., the strain was considered to be one of "spotted fever" rather than of endemic typhus.

The three remaining cases (8, 9, 10) were children treated in the University Hospital this year. The symptoms and course were carefully observed in each instance with a complete laboratory study. Case No. 8 became afebrile in three weeks and showed a Weil-Felix reaction positive with X_2O in a dilution of 1:320 before discharge. Although the blood from case No. 9 was tested on the 10th, 18th and 28th days after onset, it failed to show agglutinins for the specific Proteus strains in significant titers at any time and was still negative when the patient went home after complete recovery. However, two guinea pigs and a rabbit were successfully infected with blood obtained on the day of admission (8th day of disease). One guinea pig developed a fever on the fifth and one on the sixth day after inoculation. Neither showed scrotal involvement at this time. They were killed and no gross

10. Virginia M. Monthly **62**: 71, 1935.

pathology found except the slightly enlarged spleen which is usual with this virus. After an incubation period of five days, the rabbit had a fever for five days and then recovered. Case No. 10 died on the eighth day of her illness with circulatory failure; an autopsy was not permitted.

TABLE 1.—*Observations on the Weil-Felix Reaction of Eight Rabbits each Inoculated Directly with Citrated Blood From Patients with Rocky Mountain Spotted Fever (Eastern Type)*

Case No.	Age	Day of Disease	Inoculation Dose Route	Weil-Felix Reaction Days After Inocula ion	Agglutinin Titer with X_2O	$X_{19}O$	K O
1	16	9th	3 cc. intravenously	4	0	0	0
			3 cc. intraperitoneally	12	0	0	0
				19	0	0	0
4	68	8th	5 cc. intravenously	3	0	0	0
			5 cc. intraperitoneally	12	0	0	0
				19	160	40	0
				33	0	0	0
7	40	7th	3 cc. intravenously.	2	0	0	0
			6 cc. intraperitoneally	11	0	320	0
				16	0	80	0
				30	0	0	0
2	14	4th	5 cc. intraperitoneally	1	0	0	0
				13	0	0	0
				20	0	0	0
3	14	4th	3 cc. intraperitoneally	1	0	0	0
				15	160	80	80
				26	80	0	10
8	15	7th	3 cc. intraperitoneally	1	0	0	0
			3 cc. intravenously	12	40	0	0
				18	20	0	0
				45	0	0	0
9	4	6th	5 cc. intraperitoneally	1	0	0	0
			3 cc. intravenously	12	0	0	0
				16	40	80	0
				18	40	80	0
10	5	7th	3 cc. intraperitoneally	1	0	0	0
			3 cc. intravenously	12	40	0	0
				18	40	0	0
				40	40	0	0

All of these cases came from the rural districts of Madison and Albemarle Counties in Piedmont Virginia. All occurred during the months when ticks are active in this section—April to July—and four gave a definite history of tick bite within a short time prior to the onset of their illness. Typhus does not appear to be endemic in this section. The clinical, epidemiological and laboratory data are, therefore, consistent in each instance with a diagnosis of Rocky Mountain spotted fever (eastern type).

Of the eight rabbits inoculated six subsequently developed specific agglutinins between the 10th and 20th days as shown in the table. Four showed higher titers for X_2 than for X_{19}. In two the titer for X_{19} was higher, and one of these failed to agglutinate X_2 even in a dilution of 1:10. In only one instance did agglutinins appear for the Kingsbury strain which has been of so much value in the diagnosis of the rural typhus of the Federated Malay States. All of the agglutinins tended to disappear from the circulation of the rabbit rather rapidly and were greatly reduced or entirely gone four to six weeks after inoculation.

Two rabbits failed to react. In one instance the blood was not obtained until the ninth day of a mild illness—probably too late to recover the virus. In the other instance through a misunderstanding the citrated blood was allowed to stand at room temperature for several hours before being injected into the rabbit. The failures were therefore explainable by technical considerations.

SUMMARY

The direct inoculation of a rabbit with citrated blood obtained from a patient early in the course of the illness and subsequent observation of this animal for the appearance of specific Proteus OX agglutinins affords a simple and useful procedure, in confirming the diagnosis of Rocky Mountain spotted fever (eastern type). It is particularly valuable where a fatal outcome would prevent these observations being made on the blood serum of the patient.

A DIFFERENTIAL STUDY OF FORTY BRUCELLA STRAINS ISOLATED IN MINNESOTA

PAUL KABLER

AND

MARGARET MacLANAHAN

MINNEAPOLIS, MINNESOTA

Numerous methods have been suggested by which the varieties of the Brucella group can be differentiated. It was the purpose of the studies reported in this paper to attempt to classify 40 strains of Brucella by use of the agglutinin absorption, the bacteriostatic action of dyes (in plate culture), and the H_2S production methods, and to record the CO_2 requirement (oxygen tension) of the various strains when originally isolated from infected material. By comparing the agreement of classification by the various methods mentioned, it was hoped that some method, or combination of methods, might be found which would prove reliable and at the same time be adaptable to the routine of a public health laboratory.

MATERIALS AND METHODS

Thirty-eight strains of Brucella which were included in this study were isolated in the Laboratories of the Minnesota Department of Health. Thirty-six of the strains were isolated from clinical undulant fever cases in man. One strain was obtained from cow's blood and one strain from a hog. Two strains were received from Dr. A. H. Sanford of the Mayo Clinic, Rochester, Minnesota, which had been isolated from clinical cases of undulant fever.

The strains of human origin were isolated either directly from a blood culture in liver broth, or from the spleens of guinea pigs which had been inoculated with a portion of the blood culture. The strains of human origin isolated at the Department of Health Laboratories were obtained from mailed-in specimens.* The broth cultures were incubated for five days at 37 C. after they reached the laboratory. At the end of five days two guinea pigs were inoculated subcutaneously, each pig receiving 2 cc. of the broth culture. At the same time four subcultures were made on special dextrose agar slants. Two of the subcultures were incubated under ordinary conditions and two in an atmosphere of 10 per cent CO_2. One guinea pig was killed and autopsied after one month, the other guinea pig was treated likewise

Received for publication, October 9, 1935.

From the Laboratories of the Minnesota Department of Health, Division of Preventable Diseases.

* One hundred cc. of liver broth are placed in a 150 cc. rubber stoppered bottle and sterilized. A lead-foil cover is placed over the stopper and crimped tightly around the neck of the bottle. The bottle is then mailed to the physician in a double, cardboard mailing container. The culture is made by drawing (sterile technic) 10 cc. of blood from the patient during a febrile attack, and adding the blood to the liver broth. The blood and broth are mixed with a rotating motion, the stopper and lead-foil cap replaced, and the bottle returned to the mailing case. The culture is then returned to the laboratory by parcel post.

at the end of six weeks. At autopsy the spleen was removed (using sterile technic), quartered, and each quarter crushed and smeared on the surface of a special dextrose agar slant. Two of the spleen cultures were incubated in air and two in an atmosphere of 10 per cent CO_2. Suspicious colonies were identified by the usual biochemical and serological methods.

The strain obtained from the cow was isolated from a blood culture using the method as described for human strains. The strain from the hog was isolated by smearing material from a suppurating vertebra on the surface of special dextrose agar slopes. The Brucella grew readily and in pure culture.

The agglutinin absorption technic employed was essentially that recommended by Francis[1] in which he used as an absorbing dose the bacterial cells in 6 cc. of antigen (25,000 P.P.M.) and 0.5 cc. of antiserum (titer 1:640) diluted with 2 cc. normal saline.

The bacteriostatic action of dyes, and the H_2S production tests were carried out after the technic of Huddleson.[2] Care was taken to prepare the mediums and the dye dilutions according to his description. The dyes used were basic fuchsin in a final dilution of about 1:30,000, thionin, 1:30,000, and pyronin, 1:200,000.

RESULTS AND DISCUSSION

By agglutinin absorption one may separate the Brucella group into two varieties; Br. abortus and Br. melitensis. The variety Br. abortus includes both Br. suis and Br. abortus (bovine). By the bacteriostatic action of dyes the Brucella can be divided into three varieties. Those strains which grow only on plates containing basic fuchsin or pyronin are designated Br. abortus. Those strains which grow only in the presence of thionin are named Br. suis, while Br. melitensis is able to grow on all three mediums.

On a favorable medium, Br. suis produces H_2S for at least six or seven days. Br. abortus produces H_2S only one or two days, and Br. melitensis does not produce an appreciable amount at any time.

Br. abortus requires an increased CO_2 atmosphere (reduced oxygen tension) for growth when originally isolated, while Br. suis and Br. melitensis will grow in either air or in an increased CO_2 atmosphere.

According to the preceding definitions the results can be easily presented in tabular form.

It is evident from the following table that there was complete agreement in the classification of 31 strains by all four methods.

It will also readily be seen that the classification by the dye plate method disagreed with that of the original oxygen requirement in only two strains M-19 and M-33. Strain M-33 was classified as Br. suis by all methods except the oxygen tension. It is possible that this discrepancy was due to an oversight of growth in the original isolation cultures when incubated in air. Strain M-19 was classified Br. melitensis by all methods except the dye plate, which placed it in Br. abortus group. Six strains, M-5, M-11, M-18, M-25, M-27 and M-29, failed to produce H_2S when grown on special liver agar. This

1. Pub. Health Rep. **46:** 2416, 1931.
2. Agric. Exper. Sta., Michigan State College. Techn. Bull. No 100, 1929.

inability to produce H_2S would have classified them as variety melitensis if no other differentiating technic had been employed. However, by the other method, strains M-11 and M-25 were classified as Br. suis, while strains M-5, M-19, M-27 and M-29 were classified Br. abortus. Thus, there was very close correlation of the classification by the dye plate method and of the classification as indicated by the original oxygen tension requirement when isolated. The percentage correlation of the classification by the H_2S production with that of other methods was not so high in our hands as that described by Huddleson.

TABLE 1.—*The Classification of Minnesota Strains of Brucella by Dye Plates, H_2S Production, Agglutinin Absorption and Original Oxygen Tension Requirements*

Strain	Dye Plates	H_2S Production	Agglutinin Absorption	Oxygen Requirement
M- 1	Br. suis	Br. suis	Br. abortus	Br. suis or Br. melitensis
M- 2	Br. suis	Br. suis	Br. abortus	Br. suis or Br. melitensis
M- 3	Br. abortus	Br. abortus	Br. abortus	Br. abortus
M- 4	Br. abortus	Br. abortus	Br. abortus	Br. abortus
M- 5	Br. abortus	Br. melitensis	Br. abortus	Br. abortus
M- 6	Br. abortus	Br. abortus	Br. abortus	Br. abortus
M- 7	Br. suis	Br. suis	Br. abortus	Br. suis or Br. melitensis
M- 8	Br. suis	Br. suis	Br. abortus	Br. suis or Br. melitensis
M- 9	Br. abortus	Br. abortus	Br. abortus	Br. abortus
M-10	Br. abortus	Br. abortus	Br. abortus	Br. abortus
M-11	Br. suis	Br. melitensis	Br. abortus	No data
M-12	Br. abortus	Br. abortus	Br. abortus	Br. abortus
M-13	Br. suis	Br. suis	Br. abortus	Br. suis or Br. melitensis
M-14	Br. abortus	Br. abortus	Br. abortus	Br. abortus
M-15	Br. suis	Br. suis	Br. abortus	No data
M-16	Br. suis	Br. suis	Br. abortus	Br. suis or Br. melitensis
M-17	Br. suis	Br. suis	Br. abortus	Br. suis or Br. melitensis
M-18	Br. abortus	Br. melitensis	Br. abortus	Br. abortus
M-19	Br. abortus	Br. melitensis	Br. melitensis	Br. suis or Br. melitensis
M-20	Br. abortus	Br. abortus	Br. abortus	Br. abortus
M-21	Br. abortus	Br. abortus	Br. abortus	Br. abortus
M-22	Br. suis	Br. suis	Br. abortus	Br. suis or Br. melitensis
M-23	Br. suis	Br. suis	Br. abortus	Br. suis or Br. melitensis
M-24	Br. suis	Br. suis	Br. abortus	Br. suis or Br. melitensis
M-25	Br. suis	Br. melitensis	Br. abortus	Br. suis or Br. melitensis
M-26	Br. suis	Br. suis	Br. abortus	Br. suis or Br. melitensis
M-27	Br. abortus	Br. melitensis	Br. abortus	Br. abortus
M-28	Br. suis	Br. suis	Br. abortus	Br. suis or Br. melitensis
M-29	Br. abortus	Br. melitensis	Br. abortus	Br. abortus
M-30	Br. suis	Br. suis	Br. abortus	Br. suis or Br. melitensis
M-31	Br. suis	Br. suis	Br. para abortus	Br. suis or Br. melitensis
M-32	Br. suis	Br. suis	Br. abortus	Br. suis or Br. melitensis
M-33	Br. suis	Br. suis	Br. abortus	Br. abortus
M-34	Br. suis	Br. suis	Br. abortus	Br. suis or Br. melitensis
M-35	Br. suis	Br. suis	Br. abortus	Br. suis or Br. melitensis
M-36	Br. suis	Br. suis	Br. abortus	Br. suis or Br. melitensis
M-37	Br. suis	Br. suis	Br. abortus	Br. suis or Br. melitensis
M-38	Br. suis	Br. suis	Br. abortus	Br. suis or Br. melitensis
M-39	Br. suis	Br. suis	Br. abortus	Br. suis or Br. melitensis
M-40	Br. suis	Br. suis	Br. abortus	Br. suis or Br. melitensis

From the number of disagreements it would seem that the ability to produce H_2S is the most variable factor included in this study and perhaps the least reliable characteristic on which to base a classification. The incidence of infection with Br. suis and Br. abortus within the various occupational groups is shown in table 2 which represents the classification as indicated by agreement of the agglutinin absorption, the dye plate methods, and the oxygen requirement of 36 strains, and by agreement of the agglutinin absorption and dye plate method for two strains, namely M-11 and M-15 for which the oxygen requirement was not known. One strain, M-31, exhibited sufficient antigenic differences to warrant its classification "para abortus" by the agglutinin absorption method; otherwise it was a typical variety suis.

M-33 (school girl of 13) and M-19 (teacher) were the two strains on which a definite classification was not made because there was disagreement of the classification as indicated by the dye plate method and the oxygen requirement for initial growth. Since the evidence supplied by these two methods seems to be more reliable and more practical, some doubt as to the exact classification of M-19 and M-33 appears to be warranted. However, M-19 is classified Br. melitensis by all methods except the dye plate, and M-33 as Br. suis except by its oxygen tension requirement. Also it is interesting to note that the strain isolated from the blood culture of the cow (M-6) was classified Br. abortus by all methods. Likewise, the strain isolated from the hog (M-2) was classified Br. suis by all methods.

TABLE 2.—*Distribution of Strains According to Occupational Groups*

Occupation	Br. suis		Br. abortus	
Farmers	M-13, M-23, M-25, M-22, M-40, M-34, M-17, M-11	8	M-9, M-21, M-4	3
Housewives			M-10, M-5, M-18	3
Packing Plant Workers	M-26, M-28, M-39, M-31, M-7, M-8, M-37, M-24, M-38, M-16, M-1	11	M-14	1
Students	M-35	1	M-27	1
Postal Clerk			M-12	1
Independent stock buyer	M-30	1		
Painter	M-32	1		
Assistant cashier			M-20	1
Truck driver	M-36	1		
Lawyer			M-29	1
Restaurant owner			M-3	1
None given		1		
	Total	24		12

Twenty-four strains of human origin fell definitely into Br. suis variety and 12 strains were Br. abortus. This ratio of Br. suis and Br. abortus as etiological agents in human infections agreed with that reported by Hardy[3] in Iowa. Two strains gave conflicting reactions, however one (M-33), appeared to be Br. suis, and one probably Br. melitensis (M-19).

Only five of the 38 human strains were isolated from female patients. Three of these strains were Br. abortus and the others were M-33, and M-19, which have previously been described.

Of the eleven strains recovered from patients doing farm labor, eight fell into the variety Br. suis and only three into the variety Br. abortus. These results might be interpreted as pointing to the hog as a more dangerous source of infection than the cow. However, it has been shown that Br. suis may produce infections in cattle, so that although a patient exhibits an infection with variety suis, it is not certain that the source of infection was swine.

Three patients constituted the housewife group from each of which an organism was isolated, corresponding to the variety Br. abortus. The packing

3. Nat. Inst. of Health Bull., No. 158, 1930.

plant workers group was the largest, embracing 12 cases from each of which a Brucella strain was isolated. A survey[4] including a part of these cases has been previously reported. Eleven of the strains were of the Br. suis varitye and only one of the variety Br. abortus. These results point to the hog as being the predominant source of infection in packing house workers, and also show the enhanced invasive power of Br. suis, that is, its ability to gain access through the abraded skin of man.

The remaining 12 sources constitute a heterologous occupational group and likewise the organisms isolated from them fell in the Br. suis or Br. abortus varieties without any particular significance.

It is well to mention the difficulties of the dye plate method of differentiation. Occasionally a batch of liver agar would reduce the dyes spontaneously, especially thionin, thereby rendering it unfit for use. This characteristic has been attributed to various substances and combinations of substances by Meyer and ZoBell.[5] They state that "Variations in peptone and protein content of the basic medium affect the toxicity of the dyes. The presence of reducing substances, such as glutathione, sulphydryl groups and respiratory pigments activate the transformation of the dye molecules. The age of the liver, the method of extraction, filtration, etc., materially influence the composition of the basic medium." However, by using fresh liver and by strict observance of directions one can readily prepare a fairly satisfactory medium. Nevertheless, it is advantageous to determine the dilution of dyes required for each lot of agar. This is accomplished by growing the standard stock strains on plates containing varying concentrations of the dyes. It is usually found that the optimum concentrations are similar to those recommended by Huddleson. With a suitable liver agar the dye plate method appeared to give valuable and fairly reliable information as to the variety of Brucella strains in question.

The H_2S production was more variable in our hands and is of less value than the dye plate method. It is possible the two methods may be used together at an advantage to the observer.

Since it seems that most of the agents of human infection in the north central United States fall into the groups Br. suis and Br. abortus, and since the agglutinin absorption method does not differentiate these two, it is of little or no value to the person seeking to classify locally isolated strains. The agglutinin absorption method is also time-consuming and necessitates considerable equipment and experience. The oxygen tension requirement of a culture when originally isolated is perhaps the most reliable single criterion as to its variety. However, this method does not differentiate Br. suis and Br. melitensis. But in this section of the United States Br. melitensis is the etiological agent so rarely that its importance is of little moment. It appears that the oxygen tension requirement, together with the bacteriostatic action of dyes on a suitable medium give a fairly accurate and reliable classification of the strain in question.

---

4. Heathman, L. S.: J. Infect. Dis. **55**: 243, 1934.
5. J. Infect. Dis. **51**: 72, 1932.

SUMMARY

Forty Minnesota strains of Brucella have been classified as follows: 25 strains of Br. suis, 13 strains of Br. abortus and 2 strains with conflicting reactions but one appeared to be Br. suis and one Br. melitensis.

The agglutinin absorption method is of little or no value in the differentiation of Brucella strains in Minnesota.

The original oxygen tension requirement together with the dye plate growth characteristics gave a fairly reliable means of differentiating the Brucella strains.

The Brucella strains isolated in Minnesota from human cases of undulant fever indicated Br. suis to be the etiological agent about twice as often as Br. abortus.

THE OBLIGATELY ANAEROBIC STREPTOCOCCI. A STUDY OF TWO STRAINS WITH SPECIAL REFERENCE TO THEIR RESISTANCE TO HEAT AND DISINFECTANTS

H. J. SEARS

AND

DOROTHY VINTON

PORTLAND, OREGON

The importance in human infection of the obligately anaerobic streptococci has been amply attested to in both the recent and earlier literature. Considering the alleged frequency of their occurrence in puerperal infection,[1] lung abscesses,[2] war wounds[3] and other suppurative and gangrenous conditions[4] it is surprising how little attention has been given by bacteriologists to a study of their detailed characteristics. Prevot[5] in 1925 has made the only serious attempt at a classification and he included only twenty seven strains in his study. He determined the relative heat resistance of some of his strains but made no investigation of their resistance to chemical disinfectants.

Of the two strains included in our study one was found in pure culture in pus aspirated from the pleural cavity of an infant of seven months suffering from empyema following lobar pneumonia. The other was isolated from the sputum of a young adult with pulmonary tuberculosis complicated with lung abscess. The two organisms were essentially identical in their cultural characteristics. Both grew readily at 37 C. but not at room temperature. Growths were obtained at the bottom of tubes of chopped beef heart broth, previously boiled to expel dissolved oxygen, and in deep shake tubes of liver agar. In the latter medium strain 1 (from the empyema case) grew to an upper limit of 8–12 mm. below the surface while strain 2 was inhibited to a depth of 12–20 mm. Colonies were visible in this medium in 24 to 48 hours, were granular, white and free from gas bubbles. A putrid odor was characteristic of the cultures on the chopped meat medium. Surface colonies were readily obtained on blood, ascites or liver infusion agar by growing under anaerobic conditions. These colonies reached their maximum size of 0.5–1.0 mm. in diameter in four or five days. Repeated attempts over a period of several months to cultivate the organisms under aerobic conditions all failed.

Received for publication, October 9, 1935.

From the Department of Bacteriology, University of Oregon Medical School.

This research was carried out with the aid of a grant from the General Education Board of the Rockfeller Foundation.

1. Schwarz, O.H., and Dieckmann, W. J.: Am. J. Obst. & Gynec. **13**: 467, 1927; Colebrook, L., and Hare, R.: J. Obst. & Gynaec. Brit. Emp. **40**: 541, 1933; Colebrook, L.: Brit. M. J. **2**: 134, 1930.
2. Bingold, K.: Virchows Arch. f. path. Anat. **232**: 22, 1921.
3. Gerard, P., and Romant: Compt. rend. Soc. de biol. **82**: 136, 1919; Cottet, J.: Compt. rend. Soc. de biol. **81**: 6, 1918.
4. Lehmann, W.: München med. Wchnschr. **73**: 233, 1926.
5. Ann. de l'Inst. Pasteur **39**: 417, 1925.

In deep tubes of chocolate agar (heated blood agar) the upper limit of growth was marked by the greenish ring described by Prevot[5] above which there usually appeared a wider zone of a pinkish color. This reaction, presumably due to hydrogen peroxide formation by the organisms in the presence of oxygen, has been described as occurring with the anaerobic bacilli by M'Leod and Gordon[6] who take the view that hydrogen peroxide formation in the absence of catalase is responsible for the failure of this class of bacilli to grow in an aerobic environment. This discoloration of chocolate agar was a noticeable feature of our strain 1 but occurred only irregularly with strain 2.

In their morphological and staining characters the two organisms differed to some extent. Strain 1 varied from 0.4 to 0.8μ in diameter and from spherical to oval in shape. It occurred in pairs and in chains of varying length. The latter often appeared in tangled masses. It exhibited definite pleomorphism, being seen frequently as bacillus-like forms having a length two or three times their thickness. Differences in size of individual cocci were prominent in the same preparation. Variations in the reaction to the gram stain were likewise noticeable. Some smears stained positively and some negatively and others showed a mixture of gram positive and negative organisms. This was true of young cultures as well as of old ones.

The second organism was generally slightly larger than No. 1, showed less variations in size and was always uniformly gram positive.

Little can be deduced from our observations regarding the pathogenicity of the two organisms for man. Strain 1 having been found as the only organism on several occasions in pus from the pleural cavity may be presumed to have had some etiological relation to the disease. The rôle of strain 2 in the pulmonary abscess cannot be estimated since it was one of several organisms in the sputum and but one sample of the latter was examined.

Two white mice inoculated subcutaneously with 0.5 cc. of a three-day meat broth culture of strain 1 developed abscesses at the site of inoculation from the pus of which the organism was recovered. Intravenous injection of three young rabbits produced neither symptoms nor lesions nor was the organism cultivatable from the blood after 48 hours. The animals were killed after 8, 8 and 12 days respectively, however, and were found to have coccidiosis. From the liver lesions of this disease the anaerobic streptococci were isolated in each case.

Organism 2 was inoculated into mice and guinea pigs intraperitoneally and into two rabbits intravenously. None of these animals showed any evidences of infection on either antemortem or postmorten examination. Coccidiosis lesions were not seen in the rabbits when killed 7 and 14 days respectively after inoculation.

RESISTANCE TO HEAT AND CHEMICAL DISINFECTANTS

We estimated the heat resistance of our organisms as follows: One tenth cc. of a three-day meat broth culture, filtered through several layers of sterile

6. J. Path. & Bact. **26**: 332, 1923.

gauze, to obviate the inclusion of particles of meat, was added to 5 cc. of 0.85 per cent NaCl solution in a wide test tube in a water bath at the desired temperature. At definite intervals a loopful of the suspension was removed and inoculated into previously boiled and cooled chopped beef heart broth tubes. The latter were incubated for three days and examined carefully for growth. Several tests of this kind were made employing temperatures ranging from 60 to 80 C. Both strains by this method showed themselves surprisingly resistant to heat. Both yielded viable organisms after one hour (the longest period of exposure used) at 60 C. and after one half hour at 80 C.

Investigation of the resistance of our organisms to disinfectants was limited to the testing of a few substances in common use for tissue disinfection. Our first tests were carried out on the principle of the Hygienic Laboratory method for phenol coëfficient determination. To various aqueous dilutions of the disinfectant in wide test tubes held at 20 C. was added 0.1 cc. of a filtered meat broth culture of the organism. A 4 mm. loopful was removed from each tube at intervals of 2½ minutes over a period of 15 minutes and inoculated to tubes of beef heart broth. Growth or absence of growth in the latter after three days' incubation was accepted as indicating the presence of viable organisms or complete sterilization, respectively. Table 1 gives

TABLE 1.—*Killing Power of Phenol for Anaerobic Streptococcus No. 1*

Dilution of phenol	Presence or Absence of Growth After Periods of Exposure in Minutes					
	2½	5	7½	10	12½	15
1–50	0	0	0	0	0	0
1–60	+	+	0	0	0	0
1–70	+	+	+	+	0	0
1–80	+	+	+	+	+	+
1–90	+	+	+	+	+	+

TABLE 2.—*Sterilizing Effect of Various Disinfectants on Anaerobic Streptococcus No. 1*

Disinfectant	Range of the five dilutions tested	Highest dilution killing in 2½ minutes	Highest dilution killing in 15 minutes
Hexyl-resorcinol	1–1000 to 1–8000	1–1000	1–2000
Merthiolate	1–1000 to 1–4000	None	1–1000
Metaphen	1–500 to 1–2000	None	1–500
Crystal violet	1–50 to 1–200	None	None
Mercurochrome	1–50 to 1–200	None	None
Acriflavine	1–50 to 1–200	None	None

the detailed results by this method with chemically pure phenol which was used as a basis of comparison. Table 2 is a summary of the results of the tests with the other substances using our strain 1.

It is obvious that this streptococcus possesses a high degree of resistance to a number of substances which might be expected to have a high bactericidal power for gram positive non-spore forming cocci. However, qualitative determinations of survival periods may be misleading in judging of the practical efficiency of a disinfectant since their exact values are determined largely by purely arbitrary conditions of experiment. For example, the time required for complete sterilization of a suspension of organisms may be increased or decreased readily by changing the number of organisms in the original suspension. The sterilization of a bacterial suspension by any method is not a sudden but a gradual process. The rate at which the organisms are killed seems to proceed according to a definite law, that governing the rate of monomolecular chemical reactions. Since complete sterilization of a body cavity or a tissue surface can rarely be accomplished by the use of a disinfectant it would seem that this rate of killing would be a better in vitro index of the efficiency of a bactericidal substance than the time required to kill all organisms in an arbitrarily chosen suspension.

This rate was determined for our anaerobic streptococci using a single dilution of each of the disinfectants. The method was as follows: Five cc. of the disinfectant dilution were placed in a water bath at 20 C. and inoculated with 0.1 cc. of a three day broth culture. At intervals 0.1 cc. of the fluid was

TABLE 3.—*The Rate of Killing of Anaerobic Streptococcus, Strain 1, by Various Disinfectants in Aqueous Solution*

Time of Exposure Minutes	Number of Surviving Organisms in Thousands				
	Phenol	Hexyl-Resorcinol 1–1000	Merthiolate 1–1000	Mercurochrome, 2%	Crystal Violet 2%
0*	1200*	1200*	1350*	1350*	1200*
1	712	1100	1200	410	1100
2	700	910	912	560	1000
3	682	712	886	260	408
4	650	650	710	270	236
5	552	548	748	240	206
6	343	343	660	250	196
8	182	182	624	177	104
10	206	192	602	371	102
15	202	162	448	160	81
20	118	108	320	109	40
25	82	46	288	123	13
30	16	26	196	110	11
35	15	15	101	89	8
40	9	10	92	130	2
45	16	16	41	41	3
50	11	11	18	60	1
55	9	9	11	64	—
60	12	12	10	31	—

* On account of the rapidity with which the bacteria were killed after exposure to the solution the count at zero time was made on a separate suspension using water as the suspending agent instead of the disinfectant. These figures are therefore only approximations.

removed, suitable dilutions were made in NaCl solution and 0.1 cc. portions of each dilution were plated in duplicate on liver infusion agar. The plates were incubated in an anaerobic jar for three days. Colony counts on these plates gave data from which we calculated the number of organisms surviving each interval of exposure to the disinfectant. Table 3 summarizes the results of these tests. The figures reported are the average counts on the two plates. It is obvious from the inconsistencies in the counts that considerable allowance must be made for errors due to the limitations of the method. The significance of the results are clearly shown, however, in figure 1 in which the data on strain 1 is presented graphically. It is obvious that all of the disinfectants except phenol exert a marked killing action from the beginning of contact with the organisms, which action proceeds rapidly until one half to three fourths of the bacteria are killed before a noticeable slowing occurs. The cause of the apparently low bactericidal power of the substances tested by the first method is seen in the high resistance of a very small percentage of the organisms in the suspension rather than in a general insusceptibility of the strain. In the case of phenol, if we ignore the count at zero time (see footnote to table 3) a definite lag in killing action is observed lasting for four

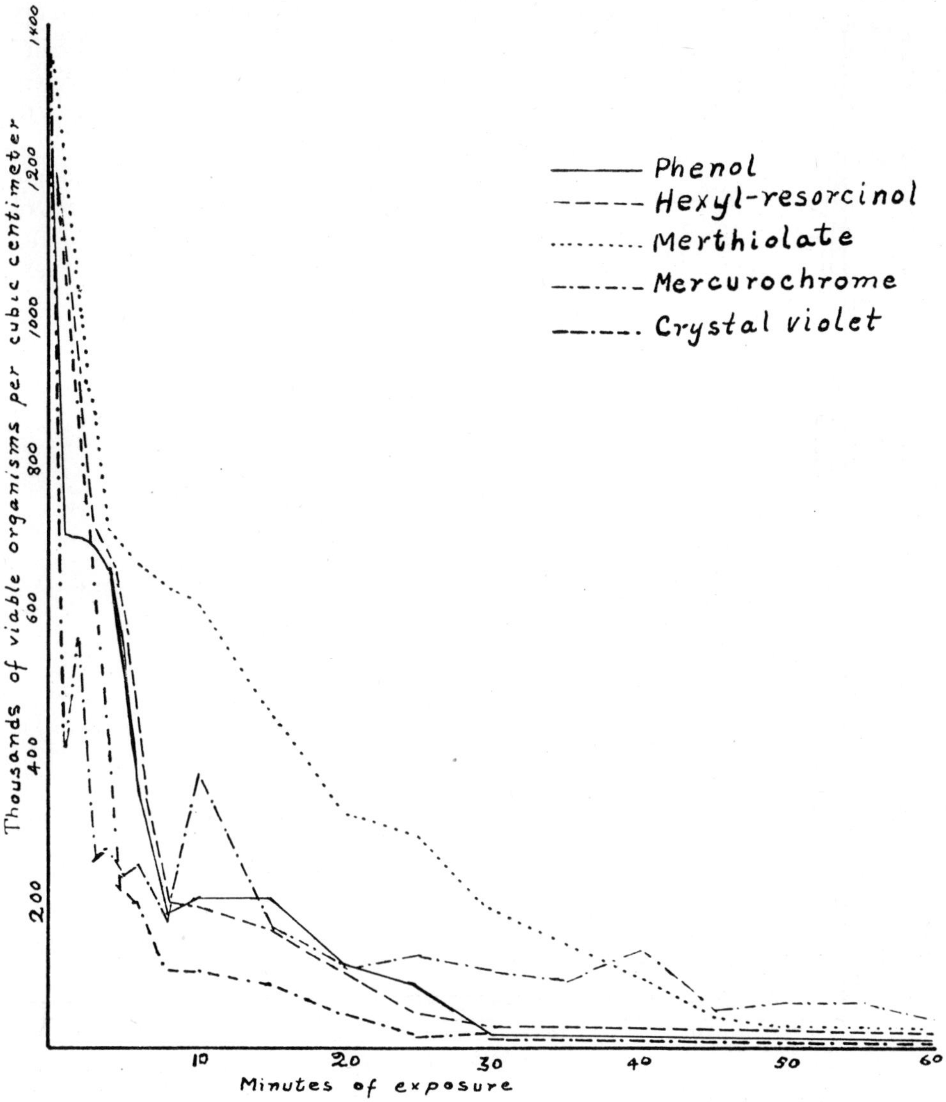

Fig. 1.—Rate of killing of anaerobic streptococcus, strain 1, by phenol 1:100, hexyl-resorcinol 1:1000, merthiolate 1:1000, mercurochrome 1:50 and crystal violet 1:50.

minutes. After this time the curve shows a sharp downward trend comparable with those of the other substances. This lag period seems to be characteristic of phenol, having been described by Chick[7] for Staphylococcus aureus.

7. J. Hyg. **10:** 237, 1910.

Experiments were also carried out to determine the rate of death due to heat. The organisms were exposed in water to temperatures of 50, 60, 70 and 80 C. and counts of the survivors made at intervals. The data from these experiments with strain 1 are shown graphically in figure 2.

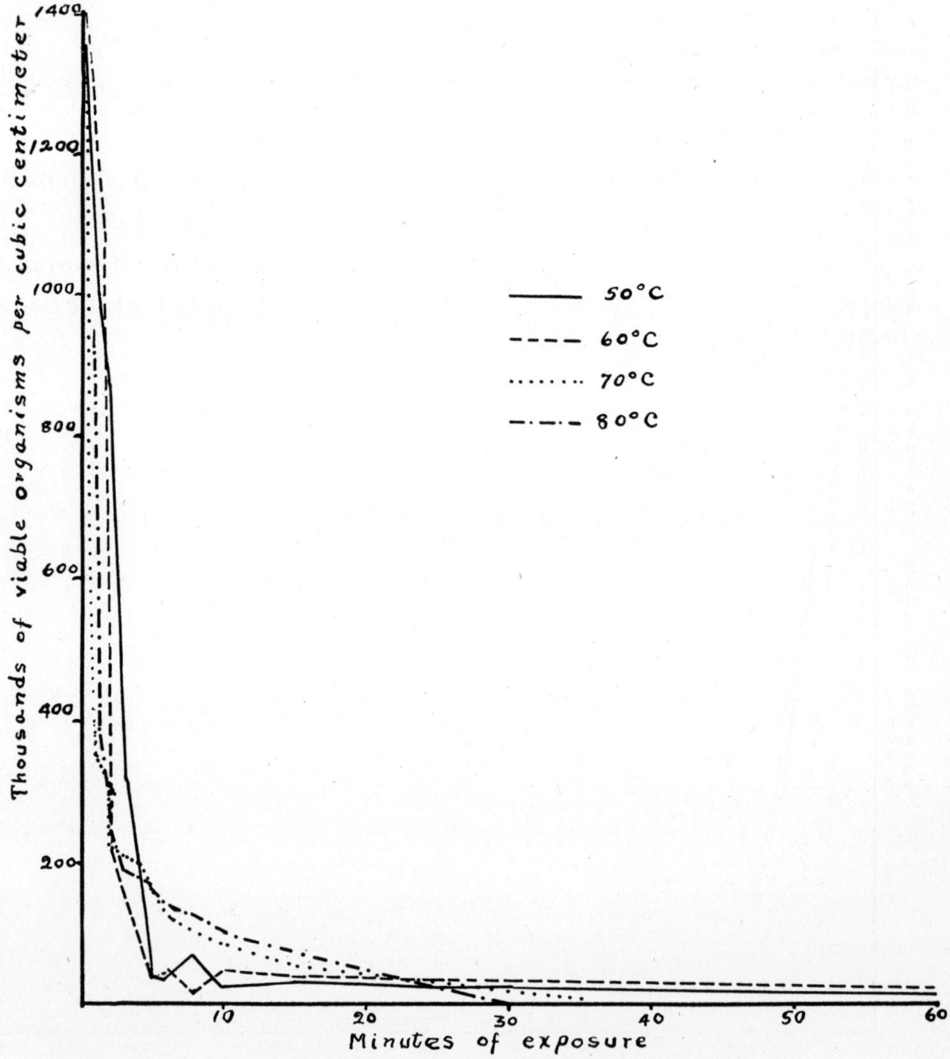

Fig. 2.—The rate of killing of anaerobic streptococcus, strain 1, by exposure in water to temperatures of 50, 60, 70 and 80 C.

Organism 2 gave results both with heat and with the chemical disinfectants that were practically the same as those for 1.

It is clear from these results that, though cultures of the two strains of anaerobic streptococci employed in our experiments usually contain individual organisms that resist the action of heat and disinfectants to a high degree, the great majority of the organisms in the cultures are killed quickly by these agencies.

SUMMARY

Two strains of obligately anaerobic streptococci isolated from morbid lesions in man are described with respect to their morphology, cultural characters and pathogenesis for laboratory animals.

A special study is reported of the resistance of these organisms to heat and chemical disinfectants. Phenol 1 per cent, mercurochrome 2 per cent, crystal violet 2 per cent, hexyl-resorcinol 1–1000 and merthiolate 1–1000 all show rapid killing of most of the cocci in suspensions but permit the survival of some individuals for long periods. Temperatures of 55, 60, 70 and 80 C. reveal similar characteristics of these streptococci killing the majority of individuals in three or four minutes but failing to kill some by exposures of one half to one hour. The differences in the rate of killing by the four temperatures used seem to be confined to the last ten per cent. Of the above mentioned disinfectant dilutions merthiolate 1–1000 seemed to be the least effective in these in vitro tests.

TRENDS IN THE PREVALENCE OF DIPHTHERIA

ESCHSCHOLTZIA L. LUCIA

AND

HILDA F. WELKE

SAN FRANCISCO

During the past forty years, countless publications relating to the prevention and treatment of diphtheria have been contributed to medical and public health literature. Before Von Behring's publication of 1893,[1] in which he first presented evidence of the effectiveness of antitoxin in the treatment of human cases, relatively little was written about the disease. In the years which followed, reports on the use of antitoxin were many and the interest thus stimulated has been maintained up to the present time. Complete epidemiological data are lacking, however, despite the importance of the morbidity and mortality from diphtheria among children. Because of this incompleteness of available statistics, it is impossible to determine how much of the downward trend of diphtheria mortality and morbidity has been due to the use of serum therapy and active immunization, and how much has been due to changes in population, environment, and in the disease itself. For this reason, studies of the mortality and morbidity rates should extend as far back into the nineteenth century as possible. Something of the extent of the dissemination of the disease during inter-epidemic periods should be known. It has been recognized that the use of antitoxin was introduced as a therapy when the mortality from diphtheria was naturally declining and it is therefore assumed that the rate of decline would not have been so rapid, had not antitoxin been used.

The proof of the effectiveness of active immunization against morbidity from the infection is even more difficult to present. The statistics which are available are not sufficiently specific to show whether or not active immunization has caused a decline in morbidity. As in the case of mortality from diphtheria, advantage is being taken of a falling market.

If the effectiveness of prophylactic or therapeutic treatment is to be evaluated quantitatively, it is necessary to make comparisons between two populations which are in every respect similar (as to the distribution of age, possibilities of contact, over-crowding, etc.), except that in one, the treatment is withheld while in the other, all persons at risk to the infection have an equal opportunity for such treatment. It becomes apparent immediately that such comparisons are impossible because where human beings are concerned the number of variables whether environmental or individual, which react upon them and their immunities and susceptibilities are legion. The

---

Submitted for publication, September 18, 1935.

From the Department of Hygiene, University of California, Berkeley, and the Department of Public Health, San Francisco, Calif.

1. Deutsche med. Wchnschr. **19:** 392, 1893.

only epidemiological procedure which may be used is to compare the morbidity and mortality data in widely separated cities or countries. When this is done, similarities in trends over a period of fifty years are striking in spite of differences in reporting, in medical care, in public health procedure and in proportion of child population. The common tendency to a lowered mortality or morbidity seems to be best explained on the basis of the cyclic periodicity of the disease.[2] The two medical procedures, passive and active immunization, can hardly be held responsible for the almost universal decline of diphtheria.

If it could be shown that the number of cases and deaths depends upon the proportion of known susceptibles in the population under twenty years of age, the effectiveness of active immunization could be evaluated in any community. Glenny[3] concluded that if there were many naturally Schick negative persons in a population, artificial immunization of Schick positive persons would be more successful than if the reservoir of susceptibles (Schick positives) were large. Dudley[4] has been able to confirm this opinion by analyzing the statistics of a controlled school population in Greenwich, England. He began his Schick investigations in 1921, and in 1922 published a paper in which it was shown that the Schick immunity of groups of boys was directly proportional to the risk of contact with diphtheria cases. Dudley has followed his populations through the intervening years and because artificial active immunization was begun in 1928, he has been able to make enlightening comparisons of a "before and after" nature. His conception of the importance of latent infection and latent immunity as influencing the successful immunization of a population possibly explains the gratifying results obtained, for example, in New York City, with toxin-antitoxin and toxoid. When artificial active immunization is superimposed on a high level of natural latent immunity, a large population of immune and partially immune persons should result. It does not necessarily follow that the same proportion of successful immunizations will result in other communities where conditions of natural latent immunity may be entirely different because of a paucity of cases of recognized or unrecognized diphtheria. The prevention of diphtheria by active immunization may prove to be ineffectual, not because the method is at fault, but because immunization procedures should have been modified to meet local requirements in terms of the known reservoir of susceptibles and the history of diphtheria prevalence.

By Schick testing population groups representative of various ages, a fair idea of the amount of natural immunity could be obtained. Then also, the age specific morbidity and mortality rates would give some indication of the prevalence of the disease. However, public health administrators and persons interested in campaigns for the active immunization of children

2. Friedberger, E.: Diphtherieepidemien der letzten Jahre, das Heilserum und die Schutzimpfung, Berlin, Urban & Schwarzenberg, 1931.

3. J. Hyg. **24:** 301, 1925.

4. Dudley, S. F., May, P. M., and O'Flynn, J. A.: Active Immunization Against Diphtheria, Medical Research Council Special Report Series, No. 195, London, His Majesty's Stationery Office, 1934.

rarely make a preliminary study because to them the process of immunization seems of paramount importance. In the Recommended Procedures for Diphtheria Immunization as suggested by the sub-committee on Evaluation of Administrative Practices of the Committee on Administrative Procedures of the American Public Health Association[5] it has been stated that "Except for epidemiological purposes and to determine the immunizing effectiveness of a preparation not previously used, there is no particular value in routine Schick testing infants or children between 6 months and 6 years of age, either before or after the use of the single dose of alum precipitated toxoid. In only such children of 6 years of age or over, and adults as have been proved to be susceptible to diphtheria by development of a positive Schick reaction, should active immunization be undertaken, and in these a Schick test should regularly be made 6 months after the completion of the inoculation, whatever the preparation which has been used, to determine whether they have by that time become immune." It should be noted that the members of the Committee realized the necessity of Schick testing all persons over 6 years of age before active immunization is begun.

By perusing the Monthly Epidemiological Report of the Health Section, League of Nations, March–April 1934[6] it is seen that the trend of diphtheria morbidity rates for the total population has been upward in most European countries during the years 1923–1933. The trend has been downward in the United States, Denmark, Sweden, Norway, and New Zealand. If active immunization is responsible for this downward trend in the United States as a whole because of the immunization campaigns carried on in a limited number of communities and states, it must be assumed that the same relative amount of active immunization must also have been carried on in the other countries which have experienced a similar decline in morbidity. It becomes obvious that there may be other factors of much greater importance which may assist in the increase or decrease of diphtheria incidence, for instance the relative reduction in child population. A tabled comparison of the relative reduction in child population in New York City and San Francisco follows:

	Per Cent of Total Population	
	1900	1930
New York City (under 15 years)	31	24
San Francisco (1–9 years)	14	8

In other words the population of the ages susceptible to diphtheria is being proportionately reduced. With the increasing unfavorable conditions for dissemination of the infection because of a relatively decreased reservoir of susceptibles, natural active immunity will probably also decrease and it is not unlikely that the incidence of diphtheria with its attendant deaths will rise again. Unfortunately the burden of proof of effectiveness of control falls on health officials and physicians who may find themselves in a difficult

5. Am. J. Pub. Health **25:** 712, 1935.
6. Epidemiol. Rep., League of Nations **13:** 49, 1934.

position because the available data concerning the populations which they have immunized are not complete.

It was therefore decided to obtain as much information as could be found for a given city which would be useful in the study of diphtheria prevalence. San Francisco was chosen because it is a large western city, old enough to have at least some vital data which extend back to the nineteenth century. The population has been well established for a number of decades and has not been greatly affected by migrations. The following data were obtained:

1. Total population, census enumerations, 1860 to 1930.
2. Population by age groups, census enumerations, 1860, 1890 to 1930.
3. Total deaths by age groups, municipal reports, 1866–67 to 1901–02; 1902 to 1933, health department reports, mortality reports, United States census.
4. Deaths from diphtheria by age groups, 1866–67 to 1933.
5. Total cases of diphtheria, San Francisco Health Department, 1906–1933.
6. Cases of diphtheria by age groups, 1922–33.
7. Immunizations done by health department, 1925–30.

The following rates were calculated from the above data:

1. Crude death rate for diphtheria, 1866–67 to 1933.
2. Death rates for diphtheria for the age groups, 1–4, 5–9, 1–19; 1866–67 to 1933.
3. Proportionate mortality rates for diphtheria for the age groups: 1–4, 5–9, 10–19, 1–19; 1866–67 to 1933.
4. Crude morbidity rates for diphtheria, 1906 to 1933.
5. Morbidity rates for diphtheria for age groups: 1–4, 5–9, 1–19; 1922 to 1933.
6. Per cent of population ages 1 to 19 immunized, 1925 to 1930.
7. Fatality rates for diphtheria, 1906 to 1933.
8. Fatality rates for diphtheria for the age groups 1–4, 5–9, 10–19, 1922 to 1933.

For purposes of comparison, the morbidity and mortality rates for Providence, Rhode Island[7] were calculated and plotted. This New England city was chosen because, although the population is somewhat smaller than that of San Francisco, an efficient immunization campaign has been in progress for a number of years. Death rates for diphtheria were calculated also for the State of Rhode Island for the period 1860–1929.

Huber[8] in an excellent publication on the control of communicable disease prevalent in Massachusetts, presented charts of the proportionate mortality rates for diphtheria in various age groups. The figures were retabled from the charts for the age groups 1–4 (1887–1923), and 5–9 (1849–1923) and extended to 1929 from the Annual Mortality Reports, United States Bureau of the Census.

---

7. Forty-eighth Annual Report of the Superintendent of Health of the City of Providence, 1930.

8. Boston M. & S. J. **195:** 87, 1926.

It was intended that international comparisons should likewise be made, but time did not permit. It is hoped that further investigations will be possible.

DISCUSSION

Mortality and morbidity.—The trend of mortality from diphtheria in San Francisco is compared with that of Providence, Rhode Island (figure 1). The deaths included in these rates are those which were reported as being caused by diphtheria or croup. Before discussing the comparison of the two curves, it perhaps would be well to review a few of the significant dates in the history of diphtheria. Klebs first described the organism in 1875; his findings were confirmed by Loeffler in 1884. Roux and Yersin discovered the toxin

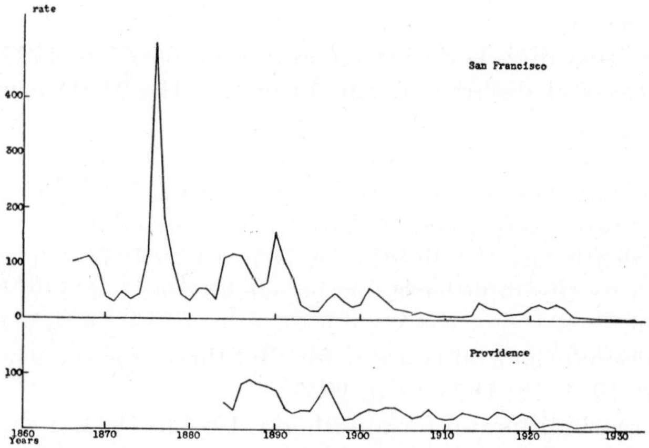

Fig. 1.—Death rates for diphtheria per 100,000 population in San Francisco and Providence, Rhode Island.

in 1888. Von Behring first reported the use of antitoxin for treatment of human cases of diphtheria in 1893, but it was not until 1895–96 that this biologic was assumed to be generally used for treatment of cases and for the passive immunization of contacts. Von Behring introduced toxin-antitoxin for use in active immunization in 1913; Park and Zingher almost immediately thereafter began to use it in New York City. These dates should be kept in mind in order to appreciate the full significance of the movement of diphtheria.

It must also be pointed out that an epidemic occurred in San Francisco during the period 1875–78. Before that time, the extent of mortality was very similar to that which occurred immediately after the epidemic. The death rate from diphtheria began its downward course a second time after the peak year of 1890.

In looking over the reports of the San Francisco Health Department it was found that antitoxin was not referred to in the fiscal report of 1893–94 nor in that of 1894–95. In the report of the city bacteriologist dated July 1, 1896, it was stated that San Francisco had been remarkably free from the "dread scourge of infancy" but that there was a sufficient number of cases to warrant the use of culture swabs. It was mentioned that the New York City Laboratory was producing antitoxin. It is usually difficult to estimate the extent to which a new procedure is adopted by the medical profession but a quotation from a "Report on Diphtheria Antitoxine" by J. H. Davisson,[9] a member of the California State Board of Health, may be apropos: "Prior to January 1895 little diphtheria antitoxine was used in California.

"It was an innovation in medicine . . . a new and unfamiliar remedy which, for the most part, was imported from Germany and France, as it was not prepared for the trade, except in New York in small quantities. . . .

"It was also a matter of commerce and, often, speculation . . . being sold at fabulous prices without any sort of security against dangers or failures due to circumstances mentioned. . . ."

These "circumstances" were extremes of temperature, decomposition, imitations, etc. In January 1895 the California State Board of Health[10] prepared a bill asking for an appropriation of $6,000 with which to proceed in the establishment of a department of bacteriology in the State University, where antitoxin could be prepared or procured under the direction of the State Board of Health. It was later found cheaper to purchase the product from reliable laboratories than to produce it under state supervision. California thus provided for free distribution of antitoxin for at least one biennium. The first order to purchase the biologic was in April 1895, when the Secretary was instructed to obtain $125 worth of Roux antitoxin and a like amount of Behring antitoxin. Later in the same month $250 worth of an American product was purchased, and after June of the same year, a new supply was purchased each month. The instructions were to use an average dose of 1,000 units (Behring standard). Doses were to be repeated every 12 to 24 hours until 6,000 units were given to a single case. The injections were to be given under the skin. The antitoxin was said to be more effective if given early in the disease.

It is clearly indicated that the use of antitoxin disseminated more slowly than is usually believed to be true. Therefore, the tremendous fall in diphtheria mortality which occurred in the nineties can not be attributed entirely to the use of antitoxin.

Returning now to a consideration of conditions in San Francisco, it was found that during the epidemic of 1897, the Health Department purchased 295,000 units of antitoxin and distributed it among physicians, for use in the treatment of patients unable to pay for the biologic. One hundred forty-four cases were treated. The physicians co-operated by returning to the health authorities complete histories. These are reported in full.[11] The fatality rate among the treated cases was 7.5 per cent. The total number of units in approximately 78 per cent of the cases ranged between 500 to 3,000.

The rates for Providence do not extend as far back as those for San Francisco, but in figure 2, where the comparison is made between San

9. Fourteenth Biennial Report of the State Board of Health of California, p. 269, 1896.

10. Fourteenth Biennial Report of the State Board of Health of California, p. 12, 1895.

11. Report of the Health Officer; Municipal Report of the Board of Supervisors of San Francisco **2:** 28, 1897–98.

Francisco and Rhode Island, the similarities in general trend become more apparent. The last high peak in mortality in Providence was reached in 1896, in Rhode Island in 1895, and the corresponding peak in San Francisco in 1897. There was, however, a higher peak in the last named city in 1901.

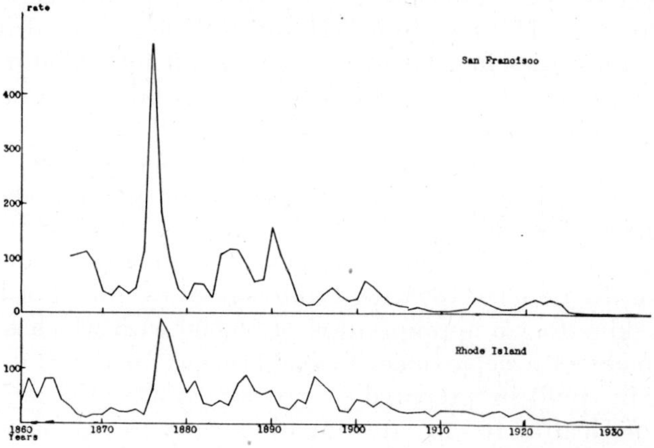

Fig. 2.—Death rates for diphtheria per 100,000 population in San Francisco and the State of Rhode Island.

Figure 3 shows that in Providence, in spite of great fluctuations in morbidity rate, the corresponding mortality rates have remained low and have proportionately fluctuated less. The same may be said of San Francisco, although the scale used in figure 4 makes this truth less apparent.

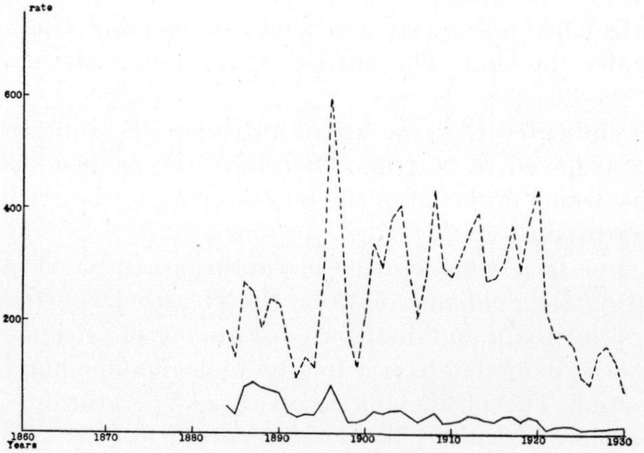

Fig. 3.—Death and case rates for diphtheria per 100,000 population in Providence, Rhode Island.

Death rate——— Morbidity rate ---------

The next three charts (figures 5, 6, 7) present the mortality and morbidity rates in San Francisco for specific age groups (1–4, 5–9, 1–19). Unfortunately the data were not available for the calculation of age specific morbidity rates prior to 1922. These three charts show that the 1–4 age group consistently has the highest mortality rate but that since 1893, it has not participated to the same relative extent. The 5–9 age group is now its close second in mortality rate and exceeds the preschool group in morbidity. Figure 7 shows the combined effects of the preschool and school populations. This specific death

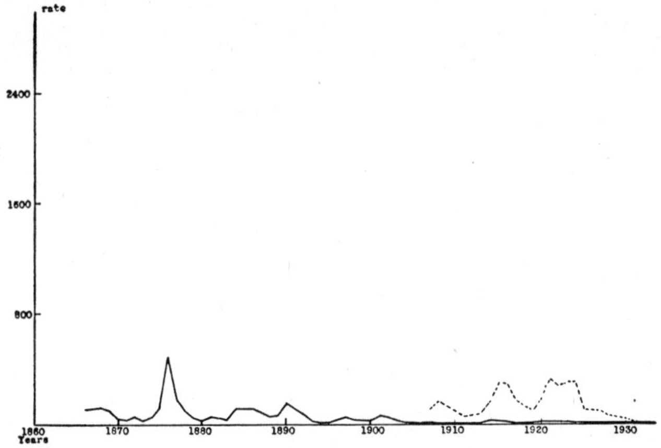

Fig. 4.—Death and case rates for diphtheria per 100,000 population in San Francisco.
Death rate——— Morbidity rate---------

rate should be compared with the total diphtheria death rate (figure 4). The two charts are on the same scale (as are also figures 5 and 6). A comparison of the charts illustrates the futility of using crude death rates for a disease which for the most part strikes only a small and very definite portion of the population.

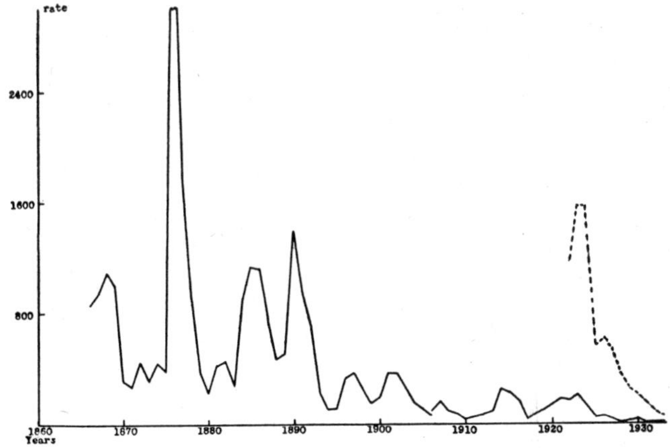

Fig. 5.—Death and case rates for diphtheria per 100,000 population aged 1–4 years in San Francisco.
Death rate——— Morbidity rate---------

Proportionate mortality.—It is usually customary to obtain a death rate by basing it on the population at risk of death. The proportionate mortality rate for diphtheria may also be calculated by ratioing the number of diphtheria deaths to the total number of deaths occurring in a specific age group.

This eliminates changes which have taken place in the general death rate. It is an accepted fact that great improvement has been made in life expectation, primarily because of the reduction in the infant mortality rate and in the number of deaths among children. Of the total deaths in the age groups 1–4,

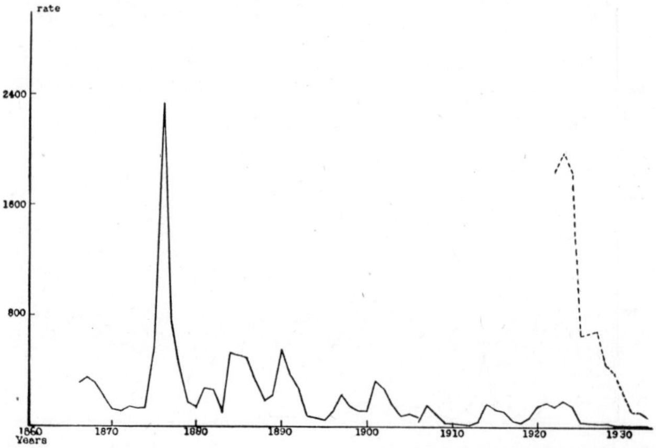

Fig. 6.—Death and case rates for diphtheria per 100,000 population aged 5–9 years in San Francisco.

Death rate——— Morbidity rate---------

5–9, 10–19, how many are caused each year by diphtheria? The age specific proportionate mortality rates for diphtheria in San Francisco have been plotted (figures 8, 9, 10). As late as 1923, approximately 20 per cent died

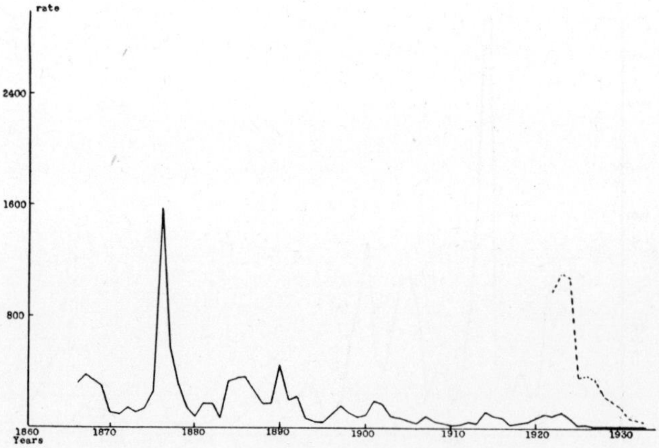

Fig. 7.—Death and case rates for diphtheria per 100,000 population aged 1–19 years in San Francisco.

Death rate——— Morbidity rate---------

from diphtheria in the 1–4 age group, and even in 1933, 6 per cent of the deaths were from this cause.

In the age group 5–9, diphtheria has been even more important as a cause of death than in the earlier age group. The risk of dying from any cause is now low for children of early school age; however, in the period from 1920–24, diphtheria was annually the cause of death in from 33 to 42 per cent of all deaths occurring in this age group. Even in the age group 10–19 years the proportionate mortality hovered around 10 per cent.

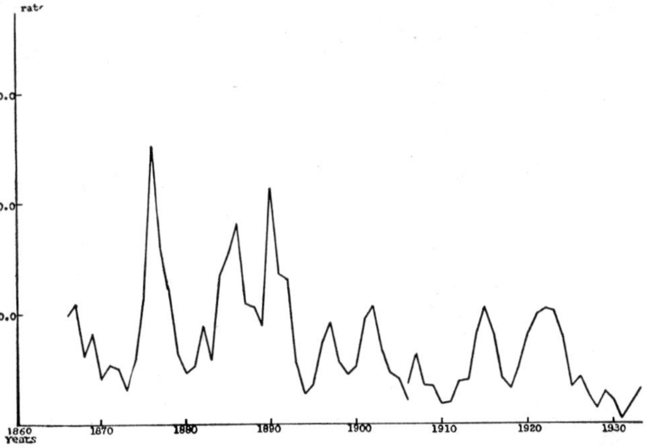

Fig. 8.—Proportionate mortality rates for diphtheria per 100 total deaths among persons aged 1–4 years in San Francisco.

There do not seem to be definite trends downward in proportionate mortality of diphtheria except perhaps in the age group 1–4. The other two curves are very irregular and saw-toothed over the entire period of years (1866–67 to 1933).

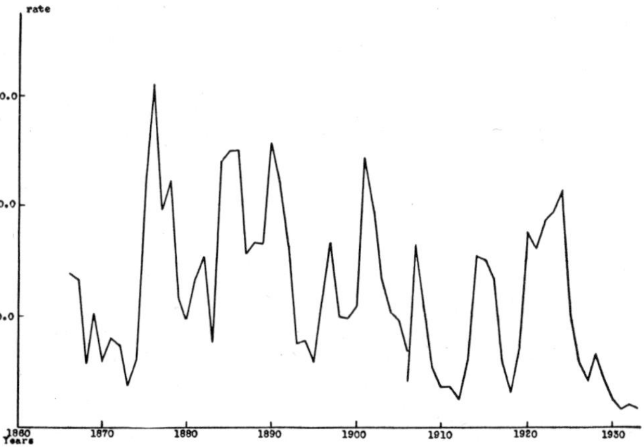

Fig. 9.—Proportionate mortality rate for diphtheria per 100 total deaths among persons aged 5–9 years in San Francisco.

The proportionate mortality rates for the age groups 1–4 and 5–9 for diphtheria in Massachusetts have been plotted for comparison (Huber[8]) (figure 11). There is little similarity in trends of proportionate diphtheria mortality rates in San Francisco and Massachusetts. There has been some flattening out but the trend seems to be downward in the Massachusetts curves. This is not the case in San Francisco. The striking resemblance lies in the fact that diphtheria in both communities is more important as a cause of death in the 5–9 age group.

In San Francisco since 1925, there has been a drop in proportionate mortality in all age groups investigated. This, of course, may be due to an

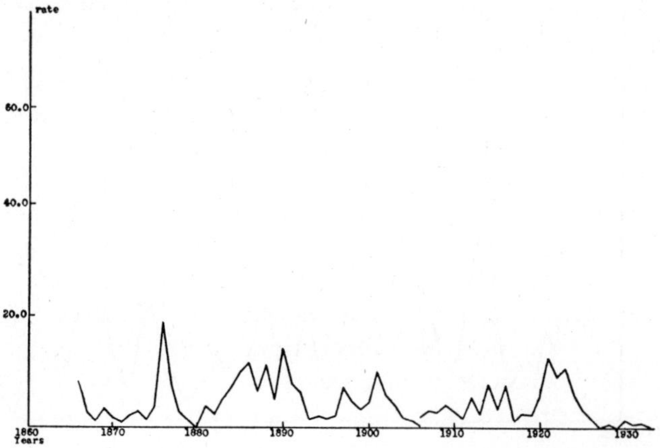

Fig. 10.—Proportionate mortality rates for diphtheria per 100 total deaths among persons aged 10–19 years in San Francisco.

increase in another cause of death which might fictitiously lower the diphtheria rate in relation to a higher total number of deaths. Such is not the case, however, because the total number of deaths has been decreasing in all age groups.

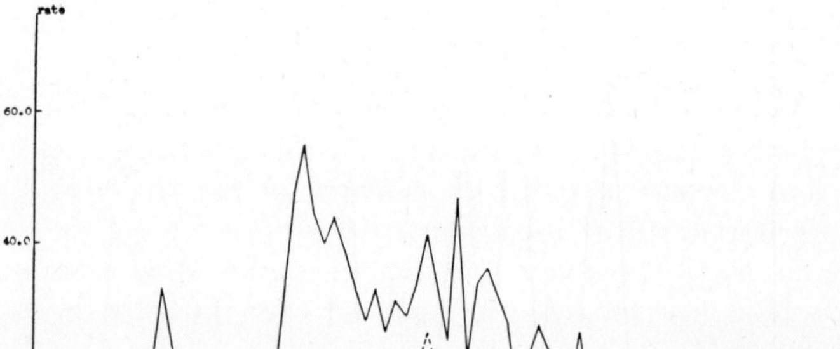

Fig. 11.—Proportionate mortality rates for diphtheria per 100 total deaths among persons aged 1–4 and 5–9 years of age in Massachusetts.

1–4 age group--------- 5–9 age group———

Fatality.—The fatality rates for the same age groups have been calculated, but it was considered unnecessary to plot them for the short period (1922–33), especially since the mortality and morbidity rates have already been shown (figures 4, 5, 6, 7). The morbidity rate in the 1–4 age group has dropped so low that the fatality rate rose to 29 per cent in 1933. The fatality rate in the 5–9 age group remained unchanged, and dropped to zero in the 10–19 age group.

Immunization.—The last comparison will be made between Providence, Rhode Island, and San Francisco, California, with regard to the great decrease in morbidity rate which has obtained in both cities. Providence has been carrying on systematic immunization for a number of years through its immunization clinics. In the Forty-Eighth Annual Report of the Superintendent of Health (1930), the routine of the work of immunization is presented. Statistics of the number of Schick tests performed are given and the reactions to the test; whether the test was given before or after immunization, the age groups of the children immunized, etc. The statistical summary presents the figures for the number of immunes (not immunized) in the preschool, school and adult population. It is proper to include those who are Schick negative without artificial protection. Health authorities should be interested in, not how many immunizations are done in a given period of time, but whether or not there is a reserve of immunes natural or artificial, in the usually susceptible age groups. This point is not generally sufficiently emphasized.

Diphtheria morbidity and mortality have gone down in both cities (Providence, Rhode Island, and San Francisco, California), one in which an active campaign of immunization has been going on for some time and where it is possible to make an estimate of the number of immunes in the population, and the other in which some immunization has been done, but where there is no record of the extent of the immune population. The question arises: Will the morbidity rate from diphtheria rise in San Francisco and not in Providence?

SUMMARY

The statistical evidence presented indicates that the decrease in mortality from diphtheria which occurred in the last decade of the 19th century and in the first decade of the 20th century in San Francisco can not be necessarily attributed to the use of antitoxin.

Age specific death rates and proportionate mortality rates indicate that children of school age have been most affected by diphtheria as a fatal disease, since 1900.

In the absence of records it can not be properly stated that the decrease in morbidity from diphtheria in San Francisco can be ascribed to a program of prevention.

It is evident that the drop in mortality and morbidity rates in the absence of an extensive official program of immunization, is probably due to a large latent, immune population in San Francisco.

The present low endemicity of the disease may tend to build up a large reservoir of susceptibles.

A program of immunization should be undertaken which will make data available concerning the extent of the reservoir of Schick susceptibles and which will build up a reserve of immunes in the susceptible age groups. Such a program would provide for Schick tests both before and after immunization, unless only children under 6 years of age were inoculated.

STAPHYLOCOCCUS FOOD POISONING

REPORT OF A SMALL MILK-BORNE EPIDEMIC

HOWARD J. SHAUGHNESSY
AND
THOMAS C. GRUBB
SPRINGFIELD

The majority of staphylococcus food poisoning epidemics appear to have resulted from the consumption of cream-filled pastry or similar bakery products which have been improperly handled. Up to the present time we are aware of only two previous reports of food poisoning epidemics caused by the consumption of milk contaminated with staphylococci. In 1914 Barber[1] reported a small milk-borne epidemic in the Philippine Islands and Crabtree and Litterer[2] in 1934 described their investigation of a milk-borne epidemic in which 242 cases occurred. Tanner and Ramsey[3] reported gastro-intestinal disturbances occurring in laboratory workers who drank some milk experimentally inoculated with a particular micrococcus. The purpose of this report is to describe another milk-borne epidemic of food poisoning in which staphylococci isolated from the milk were shown to produce an enterotoxin capable of causing vomiting in monkeys and humans.

HISTORY OF THE EPIDEMIC

Early in July 1935 the Illinois Department of Public Health was notified of a small epidemic of food poisoning occurring on a farm in the southern part of the State. Investigation of this epidemic revealed the following facts. The farmer and three members of his family had each suffered several attacks of gastro-intestinal disturbance at desultory periods during the past year. Shortly before the Department was notified of the epidemic some milk and home made ice cream were taken to a neighboring house where several of the people who consumed the milk or ice cream developed typical symptoms of food poisoning. Without having knowledge of this, the farmer's wife served home made ice cream and cake to twenty members of a missionary society being entertained in her home, and fourteen of the members complained of epigastric pains, nausea, vomiting, and diarrhea within three or four hours. A son who had been away from the farm for a considerable time drank some milk and cream shortly after his return home and later developed the typical food poisoning syndrome. By this time the family suspected that the milk was the cause of their trouble and stopped using it altogether. Since that time no gastro-intestinal disturbances have occurred.

Received for publication, September 19, 1935.

From the Division of Laboratories, Illinois State Department of Public Health

1. Philippine J. S. (Trop. Med. B) 9: 515, 1914.
2. Am. J. Pub. Health **24:** 1116, 1934.
3. Am. J. M. Sc. **184:** 80, 1932.

In all of the above cases nausea, cramps, vomiting and diarrhea developed approximately four hours after consuming the milk or ice cream. The victims rapidly recovered and no deaths occurred. The epidemiological evidence rather conclusively implicated the milk and ice cream as the vehicles of a toxic organism or substance and the incubation period, as pointed out by Jordan,[4] suggested that staphylococci rather than any members of the Salmonella group were the specific etiologic agents.

MILK SUPPLY

The milk was supplied by three cows which appeared healthy and had not previously shown any signs of illness. The milking was done by a small boy who had no history of sore throat, intestinal troubles or infection of his fingers. The milk was air cooled and consumed raw usually two to three hours after milking. However, in several instances it appeared that milk consumed or made into ice cream shortly after being drawn was capable of causing food poisoning. While the barn where the cows were kept was in a filthy condition, the milk was apparently handled with some appreciation for sanitary practices. The milk from each of the cows was normal in appearance and flavor but a positive bromthymol blue test was obtained on one quarter of each cow, suggesting that mastitis or garget was present in all of the cows. Composite samples and samples of milk from the quarters showing a positive bromthymol blue test were collected aseptically, immediately placed in an iced container, and transported to the State Laboratories by automobile. The time interval from the collection of the samples until they were examined was approximately eight hours.

LABORATORY EXAMINATION OF MILK, BLOOD AND FECES

The laboratory examination of the milk samples consisted of streaking on blood agar, Endo agar, a quantitative plating on nutrient agar and a direct microscopic examination. The total counts of the various samples ranged from 890 to 19,500 colonies per cc., all of which contained white or yellow staphylococci. The blood agar plates contained only hemolytic and non-hemolytic staphylococci, though a few green-producing streptococci were found in one of the samples. While the majority of the samples showed no growth on Endo medium, two of the samples contained short, gram negative, non-sporulating and non-lactose splitting bacilli, the biochemical characteristics of which indicated that they were not members of the typhoid, dysentery or Salmonella groups. The direct microscopic examination revealed an abnormally large number of leucocytes in the samples drawn from the quarters showing a positive brom thymol blue test. No long chain streptococci were seen either in the original samples or in those incubated 24 hours at 37 C. A rough, yellow staphylococcus, a green-producing streptococcus and several hemolytic and non-hemolytic smooth, white and yellow staphylococcus colonies were transplanted to sheep blood agar slants and subsequently transferred at intervals of three to five days after suitable incubation.

4. J. A. M. A. **97**: 1704, 1931.

Fecal specimens from the farmer and three members of his family were plated on Endo and Wilson and Blair mediums, but no members of the typhoid, dysentery or Salmonella groups were found. Samples of blood were also drawn from these people but no agglutinins for S. enteritidis, S. suipestifer, S. aertrycke, S. paradysenteriae Hiss Y or S. paradysenteriae sonnei were found in their serums. Cultures of these blood samples in veal infusion broth were sterile.

FEEDING EXPERIMENTS

Experiments were undertaken to determine if any of the isolated staphylococci or streptococcus strains were capable of producing an enterotoxin. The technic of Woolpert and Dack[5] was closely followed, which in brief consists of growing the organisms in a semi-solid medium in an atmosphere of 20 to 25 per cent carbon dioxide and feeding the sterile Berkefeld filtrate of these cultures to Macacus rhesus monkeys by stomach tube. In the case of green-producing streptococcus the above technic was modified by the addition of five per cent sheep blood to the medium as recommended by Jordan and Burrows[6] in their work with a similar organism.

Filtrates were prepared from one rough, yellow, non-hemolytic strain; three smooth, white, non-hemolytic strains; one smooth, yellow, non-hemolytic strain; two smooth, white, hemolytic strains of staphylococci and one smooth, green-producing streptococcus strain. From 25 to 40 cc. (10 to 20 cc. per kilogram weight of the monkey) of each filtrate were fed by stomach tube to adult Macacus rhesus monkeys. Also from 2 to 5 cc. (0.9 to 2.0 cc. per kilogram weight of the monkey) of each filtrate were injected intravenously into monkeys. The results were entirely negative with all but one strain of a smooth, white, hemolytic staphylococcus which was isolated from the composite sample of milk from all quarters of all of the cows. The filtrate from this strain produced vomiting in monkeys from one hour and forty-five minutes to one hour and fifty-five minutes after from 25 to 40 cc. had been fed. Five cc. of this filtrate injected intravenously caused a monkey to vomit within one hour and forty minutes. A human volunteer drank one cc. of this filtrate in a glass of milk (250 cc.) at breakfast and exactly four hours later vertigo, nausea, cramps, vomiting and diarrhea occurred, lasting for a period of three to four hours.

At the conclusion of these experiments a large batch of filtrate was prepared from the one strain which had caused vomiting and 40 cc. were fed to each of the monkeys used in the above experiments. This dose did not cause vomiting in the majority of the animals, indicating that most of them were not susceptible to the enterotoxin. It is therefore possible that some of the other strains of staphylococci isolated from the milk were capable of producing a toxic filtrate but their potential toxigenicity was not disclosed because insusceptible animals were used. It is also possible that some of the strains isolated would have been found to be toxin-producers if all of the

---

5. J. Infect. Dis. **52:** 6, 1933.
6. J. Infect. Dis. **55:** 363, 1934.

filtrates had been tested on humans, since Jordan and Burrows[7] have pointed out that humans are far more susceptible to staphylococcus enterotoxin than monkeys. However, for the purposes of this investigation it was sufficient to demonstrate the presence of at least one strain of staphylococci in the incriminated milk which was able to produce an enterotoxin. Since the susceptibility of monkeys to staphylococcus enterotoxin is so uncertain, we would strongly recommend that in work of this type preliminary feeding experiments with a known toxic filtrate should be made before testing the toxigenicity of a suspected organism.

All of the milk samples were pooled and incubated four hours at room temperature (85 F.). A plate count made at this time showed that the milk contained millions (too many to count on 1:100,000 dilution plates) of staphylococci per cc. Thirty cc. of this pooled sample were fed to each of two monkeys, but no vomiting resulted. When the known toxic filtrate was later fed to all of the monkeys it was found that the two animals used in this experiment were insusceptible to the enterotoxin and therefore no conclusions concerning the presence or absence of an enterotoxin in the pooled milk sample can be drawn.

FERMENTATION AND SEROLOGICAL REACTIONS OF ISOLATED STRAINS

Although Stritar and Jordan[8] concluded that food poisoning strains of staphylococci do not possess any uniform and characteristic fermentation reactions, it was considered of interest to determine the sugar reactions of the seven staphylococcus and the one green-producing streptococcus strains isolated from the milk. The staphylococci were grown in nutrient broth containing 0.5 per cent of the various sugars and the streptococcus in veal infusion broth containing the same concentration of sugars. Phenol red was the indicator and all tubes were incubated at 37 C. for seven days. The majority of the strains fermented dextrose, mannite, sucrose and lactose, and did not attack arabinose, rhamnose or xylose.

The only strain found to produce the food poison did not show any differences in its fermentation reactions from the reactions obtained with several other strains not producing the poison. However, since it has just been pointed out that many of the monkeys were insusceptible to the enterotoxin and thus there may have been other toxigenic strains besides the one found, there is no valid basis for attempting to correlate the fermentation reactions of the various strains with the results of the feeding experiments. The results of the fermentation tests at least agree with the statement of Stritar and Jordan[8] that, "all proved food poisoning strains ferment both lactose and mannitol."

Jordan and Burrows[7] have recently found that the ability to produce an enterotoxin may be restored to certain food poisoning organisms which have lost this power by serial transfers on starch agar. In view of this finding we were curious to learn if food poisoning organisms could be differentiated by

7. J. Infect. Dis. **57**: 121, 1935.
8. J. Infect. Dis. **56**: 1, 1935.

their ability to attack starch. All of the staphylococcus and streptococcus strains isolated from the milk were streaked on one per cent starch veal infusion agar plates and incubated aerobically and in a 25 per cent carbon dioxide atmosphere for 48 hours at 37 C. However, when the plates were flooded with Lugol's iodine solution there was no evidence that the starch had been hydrolyzed.

Barber[1] found that a month after the last of his five attacks of food poisoning his serum contained agglutinins in a dilution of from 1:50 to 1:80 for the specific staphylococcus food poisoning strain, while his serum never agglutinated the other isolated strain of staphylococcus, which did not produce an enterotoxin, in a dilution higher than 1:40. We therefore felt it of considerable interest to determine whether the blood of the farmer and the three members of his family contained specific agglutinins for the staphylococcus strain which had been shown to produce a toxic filtrate. The results of the agglutination tests with the serums of the four people were entirely negative, indicating that either the strain used as the antigen was not the one that caused the poisoning, or that the ingestion of toxic substances did not cause the production of agglutinating antibodies. It would have been desirable to test the agglutinating power of the serums against the other staphylococcus and streptococcus strains isolated from the milk, but not sufficient serum remained after testing them for dysentery and Salmonella agglutinins as described above.

COMMENT

Dolman[9] has recently stated that staphylococcus food poisoning is probably of little epidemic importance since these organisms only produce an appreciable amount of a gastro-intestinal irritant under such artificial laboratory conditions as a semi-solid medium and in an atmosphere containing a high carbon dioxide content—an environment which Dolman finds difficult to imagine in foodstuffs contaminated with staphylococci. We cannot concur with this view since cream-filled pastry is certainly an ideal semi-solid medium and practically nothing is known about the carbon dioxide content of this and similar foodstuffs contaminated with various growing organisms. The artificial laboratory conditions used to demonstrate the toxigenic potentialities of staphylococci are necessary to exalt the toxicity or increase the quantity of the poison so that experimental animals—which this and other reports (Jordan and Burrows[7]) have amply demonstrated are far less susceptible than humans—may be used to test the toxigenicity of suspected food poisoning organisms. The recent method devised by Jordan and Burrows[7] to restore the toxigenicity of food poisoning organisms which have lost their power to produce an enterotoxin, gives the bacteriologist still another valuable method of finding the causative organism in foods incriminated in outbreaks of food poisoning.

Up to the present time several outstanding workers (Hucker,[10] Rosell[11])

9. J. Infect. Dis. 55: 172, 1934.
10. Proc. 26th Ann. Conv. Internat. Assoc. Milk Dlrs., p. 175, 1933.
11. Proc. 26th Ann. Conv. Internat. Assoc. Milk. Dlrs., p. 185, 1933.

in the field of dairy science have steadfastly maintained that while milk from a cow with a streptococcus mastitis or garget is undesirable for human consumption from the aesthetic point of view, it will not cause any human disease or illness. However, Breed[12] and Brooks[13] have cited at least six epidemics of food poisoning in New York State due to the drinking of raw milk from cows with a streptococcus mastitis. Although udder infections due to staphylococci appear to be comparatively rare, the epidemics reported by Barber,[1] Crabtree and Litterer[2] and ourselves indicate that milk from a cow with a staphylococcus mastitis is equally as dangerous as milk from a cow with mastitis caused by streptococci.

As far as we know, this report is the first to show the successful repetition of the monkey feeding experiments with staphylococcus filtrates carried out by the Chicago workers. The incubation periods preceding vomiting after the monkeys have been fed or intravenously injected with the toxic filtrates agree remarkably well with those reported by the Chicago investigators.

SUMMARY

The investigation of a small epidemic of food poisoning involving some 25 persons is described in which there was little doubt that the consumption of raw milk from cows with a staphylococcus mastitis was the cause of the poisoning. The most convincing circumstantial evidence thus far recorded that ice cream may also serve as a vehicle for enterotoxic substances produced by staphylococci is indicated by this investigation. A hemolytic staphylococcus of the albus variety was isolated from the incriminated milk which, under suitable laboratory cultivation, produced a toxic substance capable of causing vomiting in monkeys and man. It appears probable, therefore, that the cause of the food poisoning was the consumption of milk or ice cream containing a gastro-intestinal irritant elaborated by one and perhaps other strains of staphylococci isolated from the milk. It seems possible that if the recently described technical methods for determining the ability of micro-organisms to produce an enterotoxin are utilized on streptococci and staphylococci from infected udders, mastitis milk may not appear so innocuous as formerly supposed.

12. Proc. 23rd Ann. Conv. Internat. Assoc. Milk Dlrs., p. 63, 1930.
13. J. Prev. Med. **6**: 111, 1932.

THE FATE OF PHAGOCYTIZED ACIDFAST BACTERIA AS DETERMINED BY THE SINGLE CELL METHOD

I. POLYMORPHONUCLEAR LEUCOCYTES

MARION HOTOPP

AND

MORTON C. KAHN

NEW YORK CITY

The purpose of the present communication is to discuss the fate of certain acidfast bacteria when phagocytized by polymorphonuclear leucocytes. The early outpouring of polymorphonuclear leucocytes following the injection of different strains of tubercle bacilli is well known.[1] This phenomenon occurs independently of the area inoculated and recurs as often as organisms are injected. The later stimulation of monocytes, epithelioid cells and clasmatocytes is characteristic of infection with mycobacteria. All these phagocytic cells engulf tubercle bacilli with remarkable rapidity.

It has been difficult to determine the fate of the acidfast bacillus once engulfed because of the slow growth characteristic of members of this group of bacteria. Furthermore, investigators disagree concerning the presence or absence of degenerative changes in the stained engulfed organisms. Sabin re-reported the presence of acidfast débris in clasmatocytes in vivo.[2] She interprets this as possible evidence of fragmentation of ingested tubercle bacilli by these cells.

Borquist[3] did not observe any fragmentation of ingested tubercle bacilli by clasmatocytes in her in vitro preparations. Workers who obtained lytic action upon tubercle bacilli by phagocytes other than clasmatocytes, obtained their cells by stimulation with various types of oil. The inadvisability of this procedure for studies of this kind is discussed in a later paragraph.

It appeared to us that more definite information concerning the fate of acidfast bacilli within phagocytic cells could be obtained. Whether or not the organisms were viable might be demonstrated if cells which had harbored these bacteria for a known length of time could be isolated and transplanted to favorable mediums. The micro-droplet single cell technic applied by one of us[4] to the study of bacteria, seemed admirably suited to this purpose. Since polymorphonuclear leucocytes are the first to respond to the introduction of acidfast organisms, it seemed most logical to begin by investigating

---

Submitted for publication, October 8, 1935.

From the Department of Public Health and Preventive Medicine, Cornell University Medical College.

This study is part of group investigation being carried on in conjunction with the Medical Research Committee, National Tuberculosis Association.

1. Metchnikoff, E.: Immunity in Infective Diseases, translated by G. F. Binnie, Cambridge University Press, 1905; Long, E. R., Vorwald, A. J., and Holley, S.: Am. J. Path. **7**: 555, 1931; Long, E. R., Vorwald, A. J., and Donaldson, L.: Arch. Path. **12**: 956, 1931.

2. Sabin, F. R., and Doan, C. A.: J. Exper. Med. **46**: 627, 1927.

3. Borquist, M., and Rowe, C.: Am. Rev. Tuberc. **24**: 172, 1931.

4. Kahn, M. C.: Am. Rev. Tuberc. **20**: 150, 1929.

their action. The guinea pig was used as the source of phagocytic cells because of its susceptibility to the human strain of tubercle bacillus. Preliminary work was done using the Mycobacterium marinum isolated from an iguana by Aronson[5] because of its rapid growth. Later experiments have been performed in vivo with the H-37 Saranac Laboratory strain of human tubercle bacillus, and as a contrast to these a study of a non-acidfast organism, the Bacillus subtilis was made.

TECHNIC

The polymorphonuclear leucocytes used in this experiment were obtained by injecting aleuronat into the peritoneum of normal guinea pigs. Each injection consisted of 0.5 grams of aleuronat sterilized by boiling in 10 cc. of Locke's solution. Two injections made five hours apart were found most suitable for our purposes. The pig was sacrificed by a blow at the base of the neck 18 to 24 hours after injection, and the peritoneum opened under sterile precaution. The exudate was mixed with 1 cc. of Ringer's solution containing 0.05 per cent of heparin to prevent clotting. It was then withdrawn and transferred to three tubes, for the purpose of vital staining.

These tubes were previously prepared by depositing two small drops of a saturated alcoholic solution of neutral red and allowing the alcohol to evaporate. The dye was re-dissolved in a drop of Ringer's solution just before the exudate was added. This ensured even distribution of the dye to the cells.

Wright stained films of the exudate were also made at the beginning of each experiment to determine the percentage and type of polymorphonuclear leucocytes present—80 to 95 per cent of the cells were found to be eosinophils, the rest lymphocytes and large mononuclear cells. If a differential count of the mononuclear cells was desired, a supra-vital neutral red preparation was made employing the technic described by Sabin,[6] and her criteria for identification of cell types was followed.

After withdrawal of the exudate, every guinea pig was carefully autopsied to rule out the presence of tuberculosis or other infection. Varying amounts of bacilli in Ringer's-heparin solution were added to the tubes containing cell exudate and only cultures that were at their optimum growth period were used. Most strains of tubercle bacilli were phagocytized spontaneously,[7] exposure to serum was therefore, unnecessary for the strains employed. The best concentration for our purpose was 1 to 3 organisms for every phagocytic cell as determined by a modified Ziehl-Neelsen stain. The percentage of cells engulfing bacilli was too small if fewer bacteria were present, and with larger numbers the cells ingested too many and became fragile. This interfered with the removal of free bacteria from the droplets. It also might possibly have interfered with the digestion of the bacteria, and was therefore avoided.

The Ziehl-Neelsen technic was modified by limiting the acid alcohol wash to 2 seconds—to include both acidfast and non-acidfast organisms in the count. Methylene blue was applied only 15 seconds so that the bacteria were not obscured by overstaining of the leucocytes. The exudate containing

5. Nat. Tuberc. A. Tr. **27:** 184, 1931.

6. Bull. Johns Hopkins Hosp. **34:** 277, 1923.

7. Lucke, B., Strumia, M., Mudd, S., McCutcheon, M., and Mudd, B. H.: J. Immunol. **24:** 455, 1933.

the leucocytes and micro-organisms was incubated for 24 to 48 hours with frequent gentle machine shakings to ensure adequate distribution. Samples were withdrawn and examined at intervals. A Ziehl-Neelsen stain was made of each sample and the percentage of leucocytes containing engulfed bacteria and the average number of those engulfed were charted.

The single cell method was employed for the purpose of manipulating the leucocytes. A line of micro-droplets of exudate containing leucocytes and engulfed bacilli was deposited upon the under surface of an especially prepared cover slip,[4] using a relatively coarse micro-pipette. A second pipette was used to take up a portion of the leucocytes from these droplets. Large clumps of cells and débris that would clog the tip of the pipette were avoided. The leucocytes in the second pipette were then deposited into smaller droplets at right angles to the first line of droplets. The diameter of the micro-drops was not greater than $1\frac{1}{2}$ times the diameter of the oil immersion field. A very fine bacterial micro-pipette was then used to remove all cells except the polymorphonuclear leucocytes. This was done before the neutral red faded, because of the repeated addition and removal of sterile Ringer's heparin solution necessary to this manipulation. The pipette was cleared frequently by rubbing the tip across the surface of the cover slip in an area removed from the line of drops thus treated. After the tip was cleared, several droplets were blown from the micro-pipette until 1 or 2 were obtained which were free of all débris. In the same manner, clumps and free tubercle bacilli were then removed. Any cells which obscured other cell borders were also discarded. The depth of fluid in the drop was adjusted so that the lower surface of the deepest portion came well within the focus of the oil immersion lens. Ten to 12 drops were prepared in this manner. The slide upon which the cover slip is mounted was then removed from the moist chamber, sealed with vaseline and the preparation examined under oil. Any free bacilli or particles suggesting micro-organisms were charted; the slide was returned to the moist chamber and the charted particles removed. The slide was then rechecked under oil.

After returning the slide to the moist chamber, a very fine micro-pipette containing sterile Ringer's heparin solution was used to withdraw fluid from a drop checked under oil. Care was taken to remove no leucocytes. A larger micro-droplet was then made of this fluid at a free space on the cover-slip to make absolutely sure that no micro-organisms were overlooked. The first drop was then filled with the sterile fluid to protect the leucocytes from drying. This procedure was repeated with all drops in which no unengulfed bacilli were visible under oil. The drops containing only fluid, that is to say those in which no bacteria could be demonstrated by the oil immersion lense, were collected with a micro-pipette and planted on Petroff egg slants as an additional check of the absence of free organisms. These will be referred to hereafter as "fluid" controls.

The leucocytes which had been freed of all unphagocytized bacteria were taken up with a fresh micro-pipette and planted on Petroff's egg medium. For the sake of brevity, these are designated as "washed" leucocytes. Drops of the original exudate containing free bacilli and leucocytes were taken up and transferred to egg slants in amounts containing not more than two times the number of organisms in the "washed" leucocyte slants. This was done to control the viability of the organisms which had been exposed to the leucocyte-containing exudate.

Engulfed mycobacteria in living leucocytes can rarely be distinguished from the surrounding cell as they do not take up neutral red and they possess the same refractive index as the cell protoplasm. It was often observed that a cell, which apparently contained no tubercle bacilli, would suddenly display as many as 8 or 10 when injured with the pipette.

It was necessary to insure the presence of engulfed organisms in those leucocytes which were to be planted on egg medium whatever the chance distribution. Only in this way could clear cut results be obtained. Therefore, a large number of cells were utilized for each experiment. Bacteria-exudate mixtures containing a relatively high percentage of leucocytes which had engulfed organisms were employed. When 10 or more per cent of leucocytes contained micro-organisms, 100 to 200 washed cells were planted on each Petroff egg slant. Two hundred or more washed cells were planted when 8 to 10 per cent of the leucocytes contained bacteria. No preparations showing less than 8 per cent of leucocytes with engulfed bacteria were used.

As already stated, preliminary work was done using the Mycobacterium marinum isolated from an iguana by Aronson[5] because of its rapid growth. The bacilli were grown on Petroff's gentian violet egg medium. Only cultures under 10 days old were used.

EXPERIMENTAL

Ten experiments were performed. For each one, the peritoneal exudate from a freshly prepared normal guinea pig was incubated in vitro with iguana tubercle bacilli at 37 C.

The leucocytes put out into micro-droplets after 24 hours incubation were practically all viable as revealed by pseudopod formation, whereas after 48 hours about 75 per cent showed signs of degeneration.

The phagocytic cells ceased engulfing bacteria after the first five hours. Ziehl-Neelsen stains of bacteria-exudate mixtures incubated for 4 or 5 hours and for 24 hours, showed nearly the same proportion of engulfing leucocytes and the same number of organisms engulfed for each mixture. No change suggestive of lytic action was observed in any of the stains.

For each guinea pig employed, 2 to 5 Petroff slants were planted with at least 100 washed leucocytes in each. In all, 38 slants each containing at least 100 leucocytes that had been freed of all unphagocytized bacteria were planted. Of these 32 showed good growth—6 showed no growth after a period of at least two months. All plants made after 3, 4, 5, 5½, 18, 20, 24 and 48 hours incubation gave rise to luxuriant growth. The six showing no growth were all in the 1 to 2½ hour incubation group and were from exudates containing a low percentage of engulfed organisms. Possibly, due to insufficient shaking, the engulfing leucocytes were not evenly distributed throughout the exudate. Eleven control tubes were inoculated with 24 hour broth cultures of iguana tubercle bacilli and 11 controls were planted with free bacilli in leucocytic exudate. All of these showed growth within two weeks. Ten slants were planted with fluid from drops in which no free bacteria were observed but contained washed leucocytes. No growth was observed in any of these after a period of two months or more. From this, it is evident that iguana tubercle bacilli may remain in living leucocytes from 20 to 45 hours as a minimum without losing their ability to multiply.

One experiment was made with the iguana tubercle bacillus incubated in vivo with polymorphonuclear leucocytes. The organisms were injected intraperitoneally into a guinea pig which had previously been prepared with aleuronat. After the bacteria had remained in the peritoneum 18 hours, the pig was killed and the exudate subjected to the technic described above. The results were entirely comparable to those of the experiments in vitro.

EXPERIMENT WITH HUMAN TUBERCLE BACILLUS

This experiment was repeated, using the H-37 strain of tubercle bacillus and incubating it with peritoneal exudate in vivo. Large quantities of a fine suspension of tubercle bacilli in Locke's solution were injected into the peritoneum. In four experiments, the guinea pigs were prepared with aleuronat prior to the injection of organisms. In six, the H-37 strain was given in two injections, 4 hours apart, without previous preparation. Heavy suspensions of the bacteria in 5 cc. amounts were used because of the enormous number taken up by the omentum.

The guinea pigs were sacrificed 18 to 24 hours after the bacilli were injected. The Ziehl-Neelsen stains showed that 10 to 40 per cent of the leucocytes contained phagocytized acidfast organisms. The phagocytes rarely engulfed more than 2 or 3 bacteria. "Free bacilli" controls and "fluid" controls were made, and 2 slants containing from 100 to 200 leucocytes freed of all unengulfed bacteria were planted for each experiment. Ten experiments were performed. None of the 19 slants inoculated with washed leucocytes containing these organisms gave rise to growth after 12 weeks of incubation. Of the 10 control cultures inoculated with approximately similar numbers free bacteria, nine gave rise to growth and one dried up. The fluid taken from 10 drops containing phagocytized but no free organisms, as far as could be determined by oil immersion, was also planted upon 10 slants of Petroff medium with negative results as regards growth after 12 weeks of incubation.

USE OF OIL

We then attempted to determine whether the presence of oil so altered the relationship of the acidfast bacillus to the leucocyte as to make its use undesirable in the study of lytic action. Iguana tubercle bacilli were exposed to olive oil and to mineral oil for periods of 24 and 48 hours. In both cases, the action was similar. The brilliant orange color of the iguana bacillus culture was transferred to the oil. The growth became white. Transplants were made directly to egg slants. The organisms exposed 24 hours grew luxuriantly. Those exposed 48 hours showed a very feeble growth.

The bacteria were centrifuged gently in a Hopkins tube, as much oil as possible removed, and the bacilli resuspended in Ringer's solution. It was not possible to remove every trace of oil.

These organisms were incubated with leucocytes-containing exudate. After 4 to 5 hours, Ziehl-Neelsen stains showed marked fading of the bacilli both within the leucocytes and in the surrounding medium. Very little change was noted in similarly stained organisms exposed to oil before the addition of exudate.

When the H-37 strain was treated similarly, the same marked increase in fading in the Ziehl-Neelsen stains was observed.

Four experiments were made using the micro-droplet technic. Iguana tubercle bacilli were exposed to olive oil for 24 hours and freed of as much oil as possible in the manner described. They were incubated with the leucocytic exudate in vitro for 18 to 24 hours. The usual controls were made. Two slants each containing at least 200 "washed" leucocytes were planted for each experiment. No growth occurred after six weeks of incubation either in the tubes into which the washed leucocytes containing the micro-organisms were inoculated or in those containing the control substance. These changes indicate the inadvisability of using oil in the stimulation of phagocytic cells when the action of the leucocyte upon the engulfed organism is of importance.

B. SUBTILIS

To demonstrate the action of polymorphonuclear leucocytes upon a species of non-acidfast bacteria as a further control, the subtilis bacillus was subjected to the same procedure as already described. Ten experiments were made—four in vivo, six in vitro. In vivo: The bacteria were promptly engulfed and there was no multiplication of free organisms, although 5 cc. of a very heavy suspension of B. subtilis was injected. The bacilli were allowed to remain in the peritoneum for 18 to 24 hours before the pig was killed. Examination of the Gram-stained exudate showed that many organisms were engulfed and that they had become ragged and were reduced to a series of fine particles. In the supravital neutral red stain, the phagocytized bacteria rapidly took up the neutral red dye and assumed a purplish color. The leucocytes were put into micro-droplets and freed of undesired cells and unengulfed organisms as described above. Each of two 5 per cent serum agar slants were planted with 100 to 200 "washed" leucocytes for each experiment. The usual controls were made of free bacilli in exudate and of fluid from droplets that had been checked under oil to ensure the absence of extraneous organisms. The eight slants of "washed" leucocytes engulfing subtilis bacilli in vivo showed no growth after a period of three weeks, although three control tubes containing free organisms in exudate showed good growth in 24 hours. One control slant never showed growth. There were no free bacilli detectable in the Gram stain of this exudate although 20 per cent of the leucocytes had engulfed organisms and the average number engulfed was 3. Four transplants of fluid from drops which were shown to be free of extraneous organisms when examined under oil showed no growth after three weeks.

In the six experiments in vitro, difficulties were encountered because of the slow rate of phagocytosis and the rapid rate of multiplication of the free organisms under these conditions. It was impossible to obtain more than 10 to 15 per cent of phagocytizing leucocytes. In an effort to increase phagocytosis, the bacilli were subjected to 1:4 dilution of horse serum for $\frac{1}{2}$ hour before they were added to the exudate. This caused prompt agglutination of the bacilli but did not retard their rate of growth in broth. Although phagocytosis was increased markedly, the use of horse serum was discarded because of the complicating factor of agglutination.

Normal human serum caused no agglutination of the subtilis bacillus. The cells phagocytizing bacilli increased to 20 to 30 per cent with its use and the organisms were engulfed relatively soon after inoculation. If a very small initial inoculation was used, multiplication could be reduced sufficiently to render the exudate suitable for our purposes. In three experiments, normal human serum was added—in three no serum was added. The results were identical, viz., no growth obtained. The six controls of free subtilis bacilli in exudate showed markedly luxuriant growth. The six controls of fluid from droplets from which all extraneous bacteria had been removed showed no growth. The 12 agar slants containing at least 150 to 200 "washed" leucocytes never exhibited growth, although the presence of sufficient engulfed organisms was evident because of their neutral red staining. The slants were incubated for 2 weeks or more.

It can be assumed therefore that the action of the leucocytes upon the engulfed organisms was similar in vivo and in vitro and whether or not the bacteria were exposed to serum.

DISCUSSION

From these observations, made with the single cell technic, it would appear that the polymorphonuclear leucocytes of guinea pigs are not capable of destroying a rapidly growing mycobacterium such as M. marinum in spite of the fact that such leucocytes engulf bacteria avidly. The bacteria may remain within the living cell for one or two days and suffer no apparent injury. With the H-37 strain of human tubercle bacillus, however, the polymorphonuclear leucocytes seem able to combat them effectively, at least under our experimental conditions.

Further studies are under way to determine the fate of tubercle bacilli in other types of cells, using the same method, and also to investigate whether any difference exists between the reaction of leucocytes in normal guinea pigs and of those previously infected with tubercle bacilli. The observation of the action of oil upon these acidfast organisms would seem to open up a field of speculation as to whether or not substances should be employed for the purpose of calling out various types of cells which may alter the organisms so that the reaction of leucocytes to them is changed. Suitable controls should first be made before such substances are employed.

SUMMARY

The micro-droplet single cell method was applied to the study of phagocytized bacteria.

The viability of Mycobacterium marinum was not affected by its presence within the living polymorphonuclear leucocyte in vitro for a minimum of 20 to 45 hours, while the viability of the H-37 strain of human Mycobacterium tuberculosis seemed to be definitely affected.

There was no growth of B. subtilis after being engulfed by leucocytes in vivo or in vitro.

The presence of olive and of mineral oil was found to be detrimental to the growth of the human and iguana strains of tubercle bacilli.

THE RACIAL INCIDENCE OF POLIOMYELITIS IN THE UNITED STATES WITH SPECIAL REFERENCE TO THE NEGRO

PAUL H. HARMON

CHICAGO

The extensive study of poliomyelitis in this country during the past two decades has furnished data from which many epidemiological investigations have been made. However, there has never been an adequate survey of the incidence of this disease among racial groups. A few opinions have been expressed concerning its prevalence in the colored race in certain localized epidemics. In New York[1] in 1907, there were but 2 cases reported in the colored race in a total of 752 cases, an absolute incidence only one-seventh that in the white race. Francis[2] reported an epidemic in Texas in 1913 where but 19 of 143 cases were in negroes. The case fatality rate in the latter group was 36.8 as compared with 6.4 in the white group. In the great epidemic of 1916 in New York[3] the total case rate for all ages among negroes was reported as 241 for 100,000 of population while in the white race this rate was 383. In a report of the Detroit epidemic of 1924, Watkins and McKenzie[4] state that of a total of 300 cases, there were but 5 in negroes, although this latter group made up one-twelfth of the population. Crouch[5] in a report of the 1927 epidemic in Fort Worth, Texas, failed to find a single case in the colored population, while there were 58 in the white populace. The United States census[6] reported the comparative mortality rates from poliomyelitis for certain southern states for the decade of 1914 to 1923. From these averages no clear conclusion could be drawn.

From the above sources, which are but local impressions, there is an indication that the disease is relatively infrequent in the colored race. We have been unable to find recorded statistics concerning the incidence of the disease among orientals in this country which would be of interest in view of the supposed rarity of epidemic poliomyelitis in China.[7] In order to answer these questions, we have obtained data upon the incidence and fatality of poliomyelitis from eight southern states and from two large northern cities where there is a large negro population, and from the Pacific Coast states that have the largest number of orientals in their population.[8]

Submitted for publication, October 22, 1935.

From the Department of Surgery, University of Chicago.

1. Wells, M. W.: in "Poliomyelitis." International Committee for the Study of Infantile Paralysis, Baltimore, Williams & Wilkins Company, 1932, p. 417.
2. Pub. Health Rep. **28:** 1693, 1913.
3. Department of Health, New York City: The Epidemic of Poliomyelitis in New York City in 1916, 1917, p. 367.
4. Ann. Clin. Med. **4:** 149, 1925.
5. Texas State J. Med. **23:** 414, 1927.
6. U. S. Census Bureau: Mortality Statistics, 1923.
7. Zia, S. H.: Nat. M. J. China **16:** 135, 1930.
8. For these data we are indebted to the State Health Departments of Maryland, Virginia, Tennessee, North Carolina, South Carolina, Alabama, Louisiana, Mississippi, California, Oregon, and Washington, and to the City Health Departments of Chicago and New York.

For the purposes of analysis, the statistical material presented in the accompanying tables is divided into two sections, determined by the presence of epidemic fluctuations of the disease. In the southern section of the country, there have been almost no epidemics of acute poliomyelitis.[1,9] On the other hand, the yearly case rate for that section is comparable with that in interepidemic years in the northern and central sections where well defined epidemic fluctuations[10–12] occur. In the first group we have included the states of North Carolina, South Carolina, Alabama, Louisiana, Tennessee and Mississippi (tables 1 to 6). To represent the second section, data is available from Maryland and Virginia and from the cities of Chicago and New York (tables 7 to 10). Data, segregated by race, are available from the city of New York only for the epidemic years of 1916, 1931 and 1933.

TABLE 1.—*Cases and Deaths—Poliomyelitis*
White and Colored
North Carolina—1916–1932

Year	No. of Cases		Case Rate		No. of Deaths		Death rate		Case Fatality Rate	
	White	Colored	White	Colored	White	Colored	White	Colored	White	Colored
1916	*	*	*	*	28	12	1.7	1.6		
1917	*	*	*	*	27	10	1.6	1.3		
1918	*	*	*	*	11	10	0.6	1.3		
1919	*	*	*	*	16	2	0.9	0.3		
1920	*	*	*	*	13	2	0.7	0.3		
1921	*	*	*	*	13	4	0.7	0.5		
1922	*	*	*	*	7	1	0.4	0.1		
1923	*	*	*	*	3	3	0.2	0.4		
1924	*	*	*	*	10	8	0.5	1.0		
1925	*	*	*	*	24	3	1.2	0.4		
1926	*	*	*	*	34	15	1.7	1.8		
1927	21	3	1.0	0.4	12	8	0.6	1.0	57.2	37.5
1928	42	9	2.0	1.1	18	7	0.9	0.8	42.8	77.8
1929	121	12	5.7	1.4	17	4	0.8	0.5	14.0	33.3
1930	75	16	3.3	1.7	17	7	0.8	0.8	22.7	43.7
1931	89	14	3.9	1.5	20	6	0.9	0.6	22.5	42.8
1932	43	9	1.9	0.9	14	1	0.6	0.1	32.6	11.1

By reference to tables 1, 3 and 6, it can be seen that the incidence as represented in case rates for 100,000 of population among the negroes, exceeds that in the white race two to four times with but few exceptions. The rate for negroes is approximately the same as that for the white race in 4 of 33 instances in these three tables. In no case does the incidence in the colored race exceed that in the white race. The most complete and impressive record is given for the state of Mississippi (table 6), a population unit where the negroes and whites are about equal. In these same tables the death rates among the colored and white populations are similar. This fact implies that poliomyelitis is a more fatal disease in the colored population (see case fatality rates, tables 1 to 6).

In communities where epidemics of the disease are manifest (tables 7 to 9), the same general trend is seen of a relatively low case rate among negroes

---

9. Doull, J. A.: Am. J. Hyg. **8:** 633, 1928.

10. Lavinder, C. H., Freeman, A. W., and Frost, W. H.: Pub. Health Bull. No. 91, 1918; Forsbeck, F. C., and Luther, E. H.: New England J. Med. **203:** 1115, 1930; United States Public Health Service, The Prevalence of Notifiable Diseases, Pub. Health Rep. Supp.

11. Limper, M. A.: Thelander, K. E., and Shaw, E. G.: J. Prev. Med. **5:** 475, 1931; Harmon, P. H.: Am. J. Dis. Child. **47:** 1216, 1934.

12. Personal Communication from J. M. Stevens, Supervising Morbidity Statistician, State of California, Department of Health.

with a high case fatality rate. Variations from the trends are more marked in epidemic years. For instance, in 1916 in Maryland, and in 1930 in Chicago, the incidence in the colored race exceeds that for the white race. The sig-

TABLE 2.—*Deaths and Death Rates—Poliomyelitis*
White and Colored
South Carolina—1915–1929

Year	No. of Deaths		Death Rate	
	White	Colored	White	Colored
1915	15	15	1.9	1.8
1916	10	7	1.3	0.8
1917	9	9	1.1	1.0
1918	10	8	1.2	0.9
1919	6	6	0.7	0.7
1920	9	8	1.0	0.9
1921	7	9	0.8	1.0
1922	8	7	1.0	0.8
1923	2	7	0.2	0.8
1924	25	13	2.7	1.5
1925	13	6	1.4	0.7
1926	13	14	1.4	1.6
1927	7	10	0.7	1.1
1928	10	7	1.1	0.9
1929	7	10	0.7	1.3

TABLE 3.—*Cases and Deaths—Poliomyelitis*
White and Colored
Alabama—1924–1932

Year	No. of Cases		Case Rate		No. of Deaths		Death Rate		Case Fatality Rate	
	White	Colored	White	Colored	White	Colored	White	Colored	White	Colored
1924	16	17	1.0	0.8	15	2	1.7	0.2	93.7	28.6
1925	60	15	3.7	1.7	18	4	1.1	0.5	30.0	26.7
1926	24	13	1.5	1.5	12	12	0.7	1.3	50.0	92.3
1927	24	6	1.5	0.7	16	8	1.0	0.9	66.6	
1928	44	14	2.8	1.5	13	9	0.5	1.0	28.3	64.3
1929	47	11	2.8	1.2	19	8	1.1	0.9	40.4	72.7
1930	55	12	3.2	1.3	17	5	1.0	0.5	30.9	41.7
1931	37	20	2.1	2.1	11	13	0.6	1.4	29.7	65.0
1932	29	6	1.7	0.6	7	0	0.4	0.0	24.1	0.0

TABLE 4.—*Deaths and Death Rates—Poliomyelitis*
Louisiana—1918–1932

Year	No. of Deaths		Death Rate	
	White	Colored	White	Colored
1918	11	1	0.9	1.0
1919	7	2	0.6	0.3
1920	5	4	0.5	0.6
1921	2	0	0.2	0.0
1922	5	1	0.4	0.1
1923	6	3	0.5	0.4
1924	5	6	0.4	0.9
1925	14	1	1.2	0.1
1926	8	6	0.7	0.9
1927	19	19	1.5	1.8
1928	9	11	0.7	1.6
1929	6	6	0.5	0.8
1930	28	17	2.2	2.6
1931	16	3	1.3	0.5
1932	6	4	0.5	0.6

nificance of this fact will be indicated in a later section (see page 336). In the city of New York, data for both the white and colored races are available for only a few epidemic years (table 10). The general tendency to a higher case fatality rate is again seen.

TABLE 5.—*Deaths and Death Rates—Poliomyelitis*
White and Colored
Tennessee—1917–1931

Year	No. of Deaths		Death Rate	
	White	Colored	White	Colored
1917	25	6	1.4	1.3
1918	27	7	1.5	1.5
1919	16	7	0.9	1.6
1920	13	7	0.7	1.6
1921	23	9	1.2	2.0
1922	16	4	0.8	0.9
1923	20	7	1.0	1.6
1924	24	3	1.2	0.7
1925	31	5	1.6	1.2
1926	24	2	1.2	0.5
1927	32	5	1.6	1.2
1928	30	8	1.4	1.8
1929	30	2	1.2	0.4
1930	22	3	1.0	0.6
1931	21	3	1.0	0.6
1932	14	2	0.6	0.9

TABLE 6.—*Cases and Deaths—Poliomyelitis*
White and Colored
Mississippi—1915–1931

Year	No. of Cases		Case Rate		No. of Deaths		Death Rate		Case Fatality Rate	
	White	Colored	White	Colored	White	Colored	White	Colored	White	Colored
1915	35	20	4.0	2.1	0	3	0.0	0.4	0.0	15.0
1916	160	107	18.6	11.4	14	17	1.6	1.9	8.8	15.9
1917	32	24	3.7	2.5	4	5	0.5	0.6	12.5	20.9
1918	28	29	3.2	3.1	3	6	0.4	0.7	10.7	20.7
1919	48	28	5.6	3.0	9	10	1.0	1.2	18.7	35.7
1920	36	30	4.2	3.2	7	3	0.8	0.4	19.9	10.0
1921	33	16	3.9	1.7	8	3	0.9	0.4	24.2	18.7
1922	19	2	2.2	0.2	5	10	0.6	1.2	26.3	
1923	32	11	3.8	1.2	6	8	0.7	0.9	18.7	72.8
1924	19	6	2.2	0.6	9	5	1.0	0.6	47.3	83.3
1925	37	10	4.4	1.0	13	6	1.5	0.7	35.1	60.0
1926	38	11	4.5	1.2	16	9	1.9	1.0	42.1	81.8
1927	45	11	4.8	1.3	14	6	1.5	0.6	30.5	54.5
1928	41	18	4.4	2.1	13	5	1.5	0.5	31.7	27.8
1929	18	10	1.9	1.2	6	9	0.6	1.0	33.3	90.0
1930	33	12	3.5	1.4	3	10	0.3	1.1	9.1	83.3
1931	38	14	4.0	1.7	8	4	0.9	0.4	21.2	29.6
1932	26	8	2.5	0.8	10	7	1.0	0.7	38.4	87.4

TABLE 7.—*Cases and Deaths—White and Colored*
From Poliomyelitis
Maryland—1916–1932

Year	No. of Cases		Case Rate		No. of Deaths		Death Rate		Case Fatality Rate	
	White	Colored	White	Colored	White	Colored	White	Colored	White	Colored
1916	285	68	24.8	28.4	86	25	7.5	10.4	30.2	36.8
1917	80	9	6.9	3.7	13	4	1.1	1.7	16.2	44.4
1918	—	—	—	—	15	3	1.3	1.2	—	—
1919	—	—	—	—	33	4	2.7	1.6	—	—
1920	41	6	3.4	2.4	7	6	0.6	2.4	17.1	100.0
1921	196	25	15.9	10.2	33	4	2.9	1.6	16.8	16.0
1922	32	7	2.6	2.9	9	5	0.7	2.0	28.2	71.5
1923	22	5	1.7	2.0	4	3	0.3	1.2	18.2	60.0
1924	170	22	13.4	8.8	15	3	1.2	1.2	8.8	13.6
1925	40	10	3.1	4.0	8	6	0.6	2.4	20.0	60.0
1926	40	6	3.0	2.3	8	5	0.6	2.0	20.0	8.3
1927	27	4	2.0	1.6	6	1	0.4	0.4	22.2	25.0
1928	279	10	20.3	3.9	23	4	1.7	1.6	8.2	40.0
1929	19	2	1.5	0.8	3	1	0.2	0.4	15.8	50.0
1930	41	2	3.0	0.8	6	1	0.4	0.4	14.6	50.0
1931	36	14	2.4	5.2	7	3	0.5	1.1	19.4	20.7
1932	34	1	2.4	0.3	5	1	0.4	0.4	14.7	100.0

Since it is known that the age incidence of this disease is an important factor influencing fatality rates,[10,11] we have re-examined the only specific data available upon this question. The report of the epidemic of 1916 in the city of New York[3] shows a similar age incidence of the disease in both racial

TABLE 8.—*Cases and Deaths—Poliomyelitis*
Virginia—1915–1932

Year	No. of Cases	Case Rate	No. of Deaths			Death Rates			Case Fat. Rate
			Total	White	Colored	Total	White	Colored	Total Only
1915	241	11.1	37	21	16	1.7	1.5	2.3	15.3
1916	330	14.9	68	57	11	3.1	3.8	1.6	20.6
1917	267	11.9	68	54	14	3.0	3.9	2.1	25.6
1918	82	3.6	31	22	9	1.4	1.4	1.3	36.6
1919	143	6.2	39	30	9	1.7	1.9	1.4	27.3
1920	72	3.1	25	19	6	1.1	1.2	0.9	34.8
1921	134	5.7	28	20	8	1.2	1.3	1.2	20.1
1922	78	3.3	25	20	5	1.1	1.3	0.7	32.1
1923	147	6.3	27	17	0	1.2	1.1	0.0	18.4
1924	127	5.4	27	13	14	1.1	0.8	2.0	21.3
1925	94	3.9	29	20	9	1.2	1.2	1.3	30.8
1926	67	2.8	27	21	6	1.1	1.2	0.9	40.3
1927	71	2.9	33	24	9	1.4	1.4	1.3	46.5
1928	97	4.0	31	23	8	1.3	1.3	1.2	31.9
1929	325	13.4	36	29	7	1.5	1.7	1.0	11.1
1930	119	4.9	21	13	8	0.9	0.8	1.2	17.6
1931	68	2.8	16	10	6	0.6	0.5	1.0	23.6
1932	43	1.7	19	18	1	0.8	1.0	0.2	44.2

TABLE 9.—*Cases and Deaths—Poliomyelitis*
White and Colored
City of Chicago—1916–1932

Year	No. of Cases		Case Rate		No. of Deaths		Death Rate		Case Fatality Rate	
	White	Colored	White	Colored	White	Colored	White	Colored	White	Colored
1916	282	5	11.6	5.7	49	0	2.0	0.0	17.4	0.0
1917	554	6	22.4	6.3	182	4	7.5	4.2	32.6	66.6
1918	97	0	3.9	0.0	24	1	0.9	1.0	24.8	
1919	108	1	4.2	0.9	17	0	0.7	0.0	15.7	
1920	78	0	3.0	0.0	8	0	0.3	0.0	10.6	0.0
1921	134	1	5.0	0.8	31	0	1.1	0.0	23.5	
1922	*	*	*	*	15	0	0.6	0.0	30.6	*
1923	*	*	*	*	4	0	0.2	0.0	4.7	*
1924	*	*	*	*	2	0	0.1	0.0	3.0	*
1925	*	*	*	*	6	1	0.2	0.7	10.6	*
1926	*	*	*	*	3	0	0.1	0.0	10.7	*
1927	145	3	5.0	1.9	19	1	0.7	0.6	13.3	33.3
1928	23	2	0.8	1.0	8	0	0.3	0.0	34.1	0.0
1929	28	0	0.9	0.0	8	0	0.3	0.0	28.6	0.0
1930	173	18	5.6	7.9	17	3	0.5	1.3	9.9	16.7
1931	161	9	4.9	3.7	22	1	0.7	0.4	13.7	11.1
1932	48	1	1.5	0.4	9	0	0.3	0.0	18.8	0.0

TABLE 10.—*Cases and Deaths—Poliomyelitis*
White and Colored
New York—1916, 1931, 1933

Year	No. of Cases		Case Rate		No. of Deaths		Death Rate		Case Fatality Rate	
	White	Colored	White	Colored	White	Colored	White	Colored	White	Colored
1916	8805	109	170.9	107.5	2372	34	46.2	33.6	26.9	31.2
1931	4073	75	61.9	22.9	482	12	7.3	3.6	11.8	16.0
1933	812	19	12.3	5.8	88	2	1.3	0.6	10.8	10.5

groups with similarly a greater incidence of the disease in the colored group than in the white group.

In the states of Oregon and Washington where there is a population of 31,600 orientals, or one for every 80 whites, there have been but three deaths reported among orientals from poliomyelitis during the ten years 1922 to

1932, while during the same period there were but 487 deaths in the white population. More detailed information is available for the Bay region about San Francisco.[12] In the 1930 epidemic in that city, 234 cases were reported. Of these, 10 were among orientals (44 per 100,000), while the remaining 224 cases in the non-oriental group gave a slightly lower case rate (36.6 per 100,000). In six counties about San Francisco Bay, a total of 1,024 cases of poliomyelitis were reported during the twelve year period of 1920 to 1933. These last data indicate a more widespread dissemination of and susceptibility to the disease among the orientals of California than in the two other states.

DISCUSSION

That the incidence of poliomyelitis in the colored population of several localities is one-half to onc-fourth that of the white population is shown by the data presented above. The same general trend is shown in each of the ten localities studied. Exceptions to the trend are shown during certain epidemic years in Maryland and in the city of Chicago. These would argue in favor of the decreased incidence in the colored race being due to lessened opportunity for infection rather than to a genuine racial immunity. Although the difficulty that the negro presents to statisticians is real, data obtained in recent years, which are probably more accurate, are similar to that of former years. They show a definitely increased case fatality rate among negroes as compared with that among whites. This raises the question of error resulting from non-reporting of mild cases among negroes. Since the same trends appear in recent years when community consciousness to poliomyelitis has been aroused, such potential error is probably not great.

That there is no oriental insusceptibility of the disease seems to be indicated in the data presented from California. Among orientals in theii native country, there is an insignificant amount of clinical poliomyelitis,[7] while individual immunity to the disease, as measured by the virus neutralization test, appears to be as widespread as it is in this country,[13] where clinical poliomyelitis is prevalent. As far as can be learned from the meager statistical data existent upon the incidence of the disease among orientals in this country, poliomyelitis is not as prevalent as among whites in the same locality. This incidence is probably determined by the opportunity for contact infection rather than to any real racial immunity.

CONCLUSIONS

The incidence of poliomyelitis in whites in both southern and northern localities is from two to four times that in negroes, according to the data herein assembled. Mortality rates per 100,000 of population are practically identical. Thus, case fatality rates among negroes exceed those of the white races. There is apparently a lessened incidence of the disease among orientals as compared with whites in the same area but this does not seem to be due to racial insusceptibility. It is possible that opportunity for contact infection is the determining factor in the data reported.

---

13. Jungeblut, C. W.: J. Immunol. **24:** 157, 1933; Lenette, E. H., and Hudson, N. P.: Proc. Soc. Exper. Biol. and Med. **30:** 449, 1933.

PULLORUM DISEASE IN TURKEYS

E. P. JOHNSON

AND

G. W. ANDERSON

BLACKSBURG, VA.

INTRODUCTION

During the past ten years occasional reports have occurred in the literature relative to pullorum disease in turkeys. The isolation of Salmonella pullorum from the tissues of turkeys has been reported on few occasions. These findings are not only of scientific interest, but they have stimulated investigators in various parts of the country to attempt to determine the importance of the disease in turkeys, as well as the effects of such foci of infection upon the programs in vogue at present for the eradication of pullorum disease in domestic fowls. Within the past few years certain laboratories have conducted agglutination tests with blood serums from quite a large number of turkeys, and have found positive reactions, although in low dilutions in many cases.

In this paper we will report two rather extensive outbreaks in which the death of a large number of poults was due to S. pullorum infection. The significance of low-titer agglutination reactions with serums from birds harboring non-pathogenic organisms will also be discussed.

REVIEW OF LITERATURE

Hewitt[1] 1928 observed pullorum infection in turkey poults that were hatched in an incubator that had been used for hatching chicken eggs. According to Tittsler,[2] Dalling, Mason and Gordon[3] 1929 reported the isolation of S. pullorum from a six-weeks-old turkey in England. The poult had been allowed to run with chicks from the time of hatching, which led these workers to consider the chicks as the source of infection. Brunett[4] 1930 reported the isolation of S. pullorum from the ovaries of mature turkeys. De Volt and Gow[5] 1930 described the lesions in a young turkey affected with pullorum disease as hepatitis and enteritis. The liver is described as being enlarged and streaked with alternate bands of congestion and degeneration. Tittsler[2] 1932 reported the isolation of an organism from young turkeys which gave all the reactions which characterize S. pullorum. In 1933, in a paper before the sixth annual conference of laboratory workers in pullorum

---

Received for publication, October 26, 1935.

From the Department of Biology, Virginia Agricultural Experiment Station.

1. Cornell Vet. **18:** 272, 1928.
2. Poultry Sc. **11:** 78, 1932.
3. Vet. Rec. **9:** 41, 1929.
4. Poultry Sc. **9:** 356, 1930.
5. Cornell Vet. **20:** 398, 1930.

disease control at Dover, Delaware, one of us (Johnson) reported that he had isolated S. pullorum from the heart blood of a four-day-old poult, and also from the atrophied testicles of a mature turkey.

REPORT OF TWO OUTBREAKS

The owners brought to the laboratory several week-old poults that were in a moribund condition. We were informed that the poults began to die at three days of age. In one flock this continued until the twelfth day, when all but one had died in the flock of 116 birds. The course of the disease in the second flock was similar as to duration, but only 46 poults died of the 140 in the flock. The two lots of poults came from incubators located in different towns, that had been used for hatching turkey eggs for two successive previous hatches. The affected flocks were located about five miles apart. The symptoms described by the owners, as well as those we observed, were as follows: droopiness, a tendency for the poults to crowd, white diarrhea only in a few, continued peeping noise or cries, loss of appetite, and finally, toppling over to die in a few hours.

GROSS LESIONS

The lesions observed at autopsy were quite similar in both groups. The most constant was slight duodenitis with occasional petechia in duodenal mucosae. The livers were invariably enlarged, light-brown, or nearly cream colored, with occasional hemorrhagic streaks on the surfaces. Unabsorbed yolk was a constant feature, even in the poults that died at ten days of age. The lungs were usually free from gross lesions. Only an occasional bird was found to have slight congestion of these organs. This feature seemed to be the only thing to differ at all from the lesions usually found in chicks dying from pullorum disease.

BACTERIOLOGIC FINDINGS

Smears from hearts, livers and yolks of affected poults on meat infusion agar, and on liver infusion agar with brilliant green added, resulted in growth of an organism in practically pure form which resembled S. pullorum. On examination we found this to be a Gram negative, non-motile short rod, which in carbohydrate mediums produced acid and gas in dextrose, mannite, arabinose, galactose, levulose, mannose, rhamnose, and xylose. It produced neither acid nor gas in sucrose, dulcitol, lactose, maltose, dextrine, inosite, inulin, raffinose, salicin, and sorbite. It was agglutinated with known positive pullorum serum in a dilution beyond 1:1200. With known negative pullorum serum, it did not react.

BREEDING FLOCKS ON AFFECTED FARMS

The breeding flock on the farm that sustained the heavier loss consisted of eight females and two males. These birds all appeared healthy, but on an agglutination test of this flock one female was found to give a positive reaction in a dilution beyond 1:400 with a stock culture of S. pullorum as antigen, and similarly with the organism recovered from the poults. This bird was brought to the laboratory for examination. On autopsy slight edema was found about the heart, and also an ovary typical of pullorum disease in chickens. Numerous ova were dark, angular in shape, and of a cheesy consistency. Our bacteriologic examinations of this material also revealed an organism identical with the one recovered from the poults.

The breeding flock on the second farm consisted of 27 females and three males. The agglutination test on the serums of these revealed only one reactor. This likewise, gave complete agglutination with S. pullorum in a dilution beyond 1:400, as well as with the organism recovered from the poults. On autopsy of this bird no lesions were found with the exception of two slightly discolored ova in the ovary. On streaking agar plates with these tissues, growth resulted which was typical of S. pullorum, but a contaminating spreader prevented us from making complete identification of this organism.

TRANSMISSION TO CHICKS

The pathogenicity of the organisms recovered from the two groups of poults was tested by feeding 0.5 cc. of a 24-hour culture in saline suspension to chicks. The chicks that were used for this purpose were three days of age at the time of feeding, and came from blood tested stock. Of the six chicks that were fed organisms isolated from poults where the greater losses were manifested, one died on the fifth day following feeding. This chick was typical of pullorum disease, and the causative organism was recovered in pure culture from various organs. One other became visibly sick on the eighth day and was killed. In this bird there were no marked lesions except retained yolk. S. pullorum, however, was recovered from the heart and yolk. The four remaining chicks showed no marked symptoms, but were killed on the 14th day, and S. pullorum was recovered from two of these.

Of six similar chicks fed the organism recovered from the poults where the lesser outbreak occurred, one died on the sixth day, and the organism was recovered. The other five were killed on the 14th day, and the organism was recovered from one chick. Of the 12 control chicks kept under similar conditions, no losses occurred. Two were killed on the 14th day and examined bacteriologically. S. pullorum was not found.

AGGLUTINATION TESTS FOR PULLORUM DISEASE IN TURKEYS

Quite separate from the two outbreaks of pullorum disease in turkeys which is reported, we were interested in attempting to determine the significance, if any, of low-titer agglutination reactions with turkey serums and S. pullorum as antigen. This question is worthy of an answer based upon experimental procedure, since our testing laboratories are finding a large number of samples of turkey serums that agglutinate S. pullorum antigen in low dilutions, e.g., 1:25. In most of these flocks there is no history of marked loss among poults nor other manifestations of pullorum disease. Our experimental procedure consisted of using 14 mature turkeys whose blood serums agglutinated S. pullorum antigen in a dilution of 1:25. Thirteen of these were females, and one was a male. Eggs from these birds were collected and hatched in a small chick incubator from which 33 poults were obtained. These were raised in sanitary wire cages until several weeks old. None of these developed symptoms of pullorum disease. From two poults that were so weak that they were scarcely able to stand after being freed from the shell, we recovered an organism in pure culture from heart, liver and yolk. This organism will be designated as P_1 and its characteristics described.

An identical organism was isolated from the heart and liver of one of the adult females at the time of autopsy.

CULTURAL AND MORPHOLOGICAL CHARACTERISTICS OF P_1

On meat infusion agar P_1 grows as small, discrete opaque colonies. It stains readily with aniline dyes, and was found to be a Gram positive, motile diplo-bacillus. It produces acid but no gas in dextrose, mannite and sucrose at 37 C. for 48 hours. Dextrose and mannite are changed in 24 hours. With dulcitol it does not react, but acid is produced in lactose in 72–96 hours. It was found to be non-pathogenic for chicks and poults.

AGGLUTINATION REACTIONS OF P_1 AND S. PULLORUM

Since P_1 was isolated in pure culture from dead turkey poults, it was thought advisable to study the agglutinability of the adult turkey serum toward this organism. Suspensions of P_1 and S. pullorum were standarized to MacFarland's nephelometer tube 1, and to p_H 8.2–8.4. The dilutions of serum-antigen mixtures were 1:25, 1:50, 1:100, and 1:200. Our tests on the 14 adult turkeys reveal complete agglutination with the serums of 5 of these in dilutions of 1:100 when P_1 was used as antigen. With S. pullorum as antigen the serum from none of these gave complete agglutination in a dilution above 1:25. Agglutination was considered to be complete when there was distinct clumping of the antigen and the liquid above the agglutinated particles remained clear.

DISCUSSION AND CONCLUSIONS

The subject of pullorum disease in unusual hosts is worthy of special consideration, since no program for the establishment of pullorum disease-free flocks of poultry would be effective without due emphasis on these sources of infection. The two outbreaks of the disease herin reported impress us vividly with the seriousness of this infection in poults. From the previous reports in the literature, the mortality among poults affected with pullorum disease has been less marked. Certain investigators have even expressed doubt as to the pathogenicity of S. pullorum for turkeys. The outbreaks herein described should tend to remove all doubt as regards the seriousness of pullorum disease in poults. The question remains, however, as to whether the infection in these outbreaks came from the incubators used in hatching the eggs, or from the female in each flock affected with the disease.

Since two previous hatches of turkey eggs in these incubators had resulted in no disease among the poults raised in these groups, the evidence points clearly to the transmission of S. pullorum through the eggs of the affected female in each group. The fact that nearly 100 per cent mortality resulted in one flock does not discredit this view, as it is well known that a few affected individuals can easily spread the infection to a large number in a short time.

No information could be obtained to satisfactorily explain the source of the infection in the affected females in either flock.

The results of the agglutination tests run on these flocks, as well as the data obtained on tests of other flocks, give us information which we believe is important from the standpoint of removing breeders that would be potentially dangerous on the basis of the agglutination test. Our tests gave complete agglutination in dilutions beyond 1:400 with serums from the females that on autopsy had lesions of the disease, and from which S. pullorum was recovered. On the other hand, from poults obtained from the 14 turkeys whose serums gave only positive reactions in dilutions of 1:25, and in which there were no recognizable lesions on autopsy, nor S. pullorum recovered, we isolated an organism described as P_1. In running agglutination tests with this organism as antigen, we found that the serums of these birds agglutinated P_1 in higher dilutions than they did S. pullorum. These facts indicate that there is marked cross agglutination with this non-pathogenic organism which might on the basis of the test, lead to the removal of outstanding breeders that harbor non-pathogenic organisms. From these results the question arises as to what dilution with complete agglutination should constitute the basis for the removal of dangerous breeders. The information yielded from this work indicates that a titer above 1:50 would be necessary to locate birds harboring S. pullorum.

THE BLOOD p_H OF LEUKOTIC FOWLS AND THE FILTERABILITY OF THE LEUKOSIS AGENT

E. P. JOHNSON

AND

W. B. BELL

BLACKSBURG, VA.

No tests are known at present to be entirely satisfactory for the recognition of early cases of leukosis in fowls. Examinations of blood smears and making frequent blood counts give considerable information regarding blood dyscrasias, but these methods are tedious and the results are frequently difficult to interpret accurately. The experiments on blood p_H determinations herein recorded were carried out to see if by this method early changes might be detected whereby affected birds might be recognized and removed from the flock.

The term leukosis is used in this paper to designate the various expressions of the disease-complex as described by Johnson.[1] This includes the erythro, myeloid and lymphoid forms. The latter is frequently spoken of as lymphomatosis and fowl paralysis.

DETERMINATION OF p_H

The material used for blood p_H determinations consists of 50 normal and 35 leukotic fowls. The colorimetric method outlined by Cullen[2] was used throughout this work. This requires only a small amount of blood, and the determinations could be run more rapidly and without errors, since the errors due to loss of CO_2, dilution of plasma, variations in temperature, and the Donnan equilibrium effects are avoided in this technic. The blood was collected from the wing vein in a syringe containing heparin to prevent clotting. All readings were made at 20 C., and at 40 C. The latter approximates the body temperature of the fowl. A La Motte blood p_H outfit containing all the necessary standard solutions and pipettes was used.

A survey of the literature revealed only one reference to the p_H of normal fowl's blood, reported by Des Ligneris.[3] Accordingly, we first made determinations on the blood of 50 mature fowls selected without regard to sex or breed.

The blood p_H of leukotic fowls was established from determinations on the blood of fowls received in the laboratory for diagnosis, and from those on the blood of birds in which the disease had been produced experimentally. These results are given in table 1.

The average blood p_H of normal fowls was found to be 7.56 at 40 C. At 20 C. it was found to be 7.60, which shows the effect of temperature on p_H determinations. Since 40 C. is the approximate normal temperature of domestic fowls, our readings indicate fairly accurately the actual p_H of the blood in fowls. To avoid the loss of CO_2, the blood was drawn from the wing vein into an oiled syringe containing heparin, and immediately transferred

Received for publication, November 12, 1935.

From the Department of Biology, Virginia Agricultural Experiment Station.

Aided by a grant from the Virginia Academy of Science.

1. Virginia Agric. Exper. Sta. Tech. Bull. **56:** 1, 1934.
2. J. Biol. Chem. **52:** 501, 1922.
3. Brit. J. Exper. Path. **13:** 189, 1932.

to a vial containing oil, so that the plasma was kept beneath oil at all times during the determinations.

From table 1 it is noted that the average blood p_H of leukotic fowls is 7.57 at 40 C. Since our procedure was identical in the two groups, we must conclude that the effects of the leukosis agent on blood p_H is not sufficient to be of diagnostic value.

TABLE 1.—*Blood p_H of Leukotic Fowls*

Bird No.	p_H 20 C.	p_H 40 C.	p_H Diff.	Bird No.	p_H 20 C.	p_H 40 C.	p_H Diff.
1	7.60	7.55	.05	19	7.59*	7.55	..
2	7.60	7.55	.05	20	7.65	7.60	.05
3	7.67	7.63*	..	21	7.65	7.60	.05
4	7.55	7.53	.02	22	7.58	7.53	.05
5	7.55	7.60	.05	23	7.58	7.55	.03
6	7.50	7.47	.03	24	7.58	7.53	.05
7	7.55	7.52	.03	25	7.60	7.57	.03
8	7.60	7.57	.03	26	7.60	7.57	.03
9	7.65	7.60	.05	27	7.60	7.55	.05
10	7.58	7.56	.02	28	7.63	7.58	.05
11	7.53	7.49*	..	29	7.60*	7.56	..
12	7.65	7.60	.05	30	7.64*	7.60	..
13	7.45	7.41*	..	31	7.60	7.58	.02
14	7.53	7.49*	..	32	7.63	7.60	.03
15	7.55	7.50	.05	33	7.65	7.63	.02
16	7.70	7.65	.05	34	7.70	7.65	.05
17	7.65	7.62	.03	35	7.70	7.65	.05
18	7.60	7.55	.05				

Average p_H at 20 C. 7.61
Average p_H at 40 C. 7.57
Average difference 0.04
* Calculated by using average difference.

It is of interest to note in this connection that determinations were made on the blood of birds with all the various forms of leukosis, and in no case was the blood p_H sufficiently altered to classify the different forms of the disease on this basis.

FILTRATION EXPERIMENTS

The filtration experiments were undertaken with the hope of determining the approximate size of the causative agent, and to further test the conclusions drawn by Johnson,[1] that the various expressions of the disease are due to a single filtrable agent, and that the various forms may occur singly, or in combination.

The material used for the filtration experiments consisted of 24 birds injected with the various filtrates, and 24 controls. Suitable tissues from all birds were fixed in Helly's fluid, and sections were stained with the azure-eosin combination of Giemsa. Two sets of filters were used. One set, prepared from collodion solutions, was made by dissolving 6 gms. of pyroxylin in 100 gms. of alcohol-ether mixture. Membranes of varying porosities were obtained by varying the proportion of alcohol to ether. The membranes were designated according to the alcohol-ether mixture, i.e., a 50–50 membrane was made from a collodion solution containing 50 parts of alcohol by weight. Three such solutions were prepared, from which membranes were obtained as follows:

Solution	Membranes prepared
a. 6 gms. pyroxylin (DuPont) 50 gms. alcohol (95%) 50 gms. ether	50–50
b. 6 gms. pyroxylin 40 gms. alcohol 60 gms. ether	40–60
c. 6 gms. pyroxylin 30 gms. alcohol 70 gms. ether	30–70

The other set of membranes used was obtained from Schleicher and Schull Company. These are designated according to the content of nitro-cellulose in the collodion impregnating the membrane. The permeability of these filters depends upon their density, i.e., the percentage content of nitro-cellulose in the acid collodion of the filter. One and one-half, 3, 4.5, and 6% filters were used. Of these standard filters, the 4½% membrane will generally prevent the passage of hemoglobin from a 1% solution.

GRADING OF MEMBRANES

A Seitz filtration apparatus was used to hold the membranes during filtration. The membranes were placed in this apparatus in place of the regular filter disc, and supported by two Whatman's No. 1 filter papers. The flask was connected to a water pump (A. H. Thomas Co. No. 5303), and subjected to a vacuum of 27 inches of mercury as indicated by a gauge. After sterilization of the membranes and flasks, colloid suspensions and organisms of known particle size were subjected to filtration through the membranes, in order to determine the size of the particles that would be retained by the membranes. The presence of organisms in the filtrates was determined by inoculation of small amounts of the filtrates into liver infusion broth, and on liver infusion agar. The presence of the colloid particles in the filtrates was determined by comparing the filtrates with the original material. Only suspensions that possessed color were used in order to be able to detect their presence in the filtrates. A concentration of approximately 1% was used throughout the process of grading the membranes. The results of these determinations are given in table 2.

TABLE 2.—*Filterability of Materials of Known Size Through Collodion Membranes*

Materials Filtered	Approximate Diameter in Millimicrons	Collodion Membranes			S. & S. Co. Membranes			
		50–50	40–60	30–70	1.5%	3%	4.5%	6%
Salmonella pullorum	1000–1500	R	R	R	R	R	R	R
Prussian blue	400	R	R	R	R	R	R	R
Ferric oxide hydrosol	100	P*	P*	P*	P	P	P*	R
Congo red	40	P	P	P*	P	P	P	P*
Litmus	2	P	P	P	P	P	P	P

* Concentration Decreased.
R = retained.
P = passed.

Salmonella pullorum and Prussian blue, with approximate size of 1,000 to 1,500 and 400 millimicrons respectively, are retained by all membranes. The ferric oxide hydrosol, Congo red and litmus, with sizes of approximately 100, 40, and 2 millimicrons respectively, pass the membranes. Ferric oxide hydrosol is decreased in concentration after passing all membranes, being decreased more by the 30–70 membrane than the 40–60 or the 50–50 membranes. Congo red is decreased in concentration only when passed through the 30–70 membrane. Litmus passes all membranes freely.

These results indicate that the 50–50 membrane will retain particles of approximately 400 millimicrons in size, pass most particles of approximately 100 millimicrons in size, and that it will pass completely particles of approximately 40 millimicrons in size. This membrane, therefore, will hold back particles that have a size between the limits of 100 and 400 millimicrons.

The 40–60 and the 30–70 membranes show practically the same thing. The 30–70 membrane, however, holds back ferric oxide hydrosol to a greater extent than either of the other membranes and this membrane holds back Congo red to a certain extent, whereas the 50–50 and the 40–60 membranes pass completely this material. The size of the particles held back by the 30–70 membrane, therefore, is somewhat smaller than that of those held back by the 40–60 or 50–50 membranes.

DETECTION OF LEAKS IN MEMBRANES

After the saline solution containing the agent had been filtered through the collodion membranes a suspension of Salmonella pullorum, corresponding in density to MacFarland Nephelometer tube 1, was tried for filterability, and the filtrates collected in sterile flasks. The filtrates were cultured in liver infusion broth and on liver infusion agar. If no growth appeared after incubation of these cultures at 37 C. for 48 hours the membranes were considered to have been free from microscopic leaks during the filtration of the tissue extract.

MATERIALS FILTERED

The heart, liver, and spleen, from diseased birds were ground in a mortar with sterile physiological salt solution. This material was then filtered through gauze and finally through Whatman's filter paper No. 1, to remove as many of the large particles as possible. This solution, in a few cases, was then filtered through Berkefeld N filters, while in others it was centrifuged before subjecting it to filtration through the collodion membranes.

The material used was obtained from two birds that showed typical lesions.

1.—A Barred Plymouth Rock pullet received in the laboratory for diagnosis. The bird was weak, emaciated and scarcely able to stand. The autopsy revealed a greatly enlarged liver with large areas of white tumor-like tissue throughout the organ; the radius marrow was hyperplastic and gelatinous. The differential blood count revealed 4 granulocytes with eosinophilic rods, 4 with eosinophilic round granules, no basophils, 1 monocyte, 21 lymphocytes, 11 hemocytoblasts, and 51 myelocytes. Microscopic examination of the tissues fixed in Helly's fluid, and stained with the azure-eosin combination of Giemsa revealed enormous areas of hemocytoblasts and myelocytes at the peripheries of large areas of necroses in the liver. The case was diagnosed as myeloid leukosis.

2.—This bird was from the experimental group. The bird was weak and droopy. Autopsy revealed the liver to be greatly enlarged and studded with numerous white glistening areas. The radius marrow was very hyperplastic and gelatinous. The differential blood count revealed: 11 granulocytes with eosinophilic rods, 1 granulocyte with eosinophilic round granules, 1 basophil, 2 monocytes, 73 hemocytoblasts, and 1 myelocyte. Microscopic examination of the tissues revealed marked areas of hemocytoblasts and granulocytes about vessels in the liver, and marked infiltration of hemocytoblasts in the sciatic nerve. The case was diagnosed as hemocytoblastosis.

STERILITY OF FILTRATES

All filtrates used for injecting purposes were checked for sterility by inoculating liver infusion broth and liver infusion agar. These cultures were incubated at 37 C. for 48 hours, after which, if no growth was present, the filtrates were injected into the chicks. In those cases where the filtrates were not sterile the material was refiltered and checked a second time for sterility before it was used for inoculation of the chicks. It was observed that when the filtrates from the membranes were not sterile the membranes were found to have microscopic leaks when the checks for leaks were made.

BIRDS INJECTED

The birds used in these experiments were hatched in the laboratory from eggs secured from a flock of White Leghorns, in which the disease has not been known to occur for the last five years. The chicks were placed into sterile wire cages as soon after hatching as possible, and were injected when approximately a week old. The injected chicks were then put into separate cages and kept in a separate room from the chicks kept as controls. Two attendants cared for the birds, one for each of the groups. The cages were cleaned once a week or oftener, and the rooms were washed several times during the experiment. The rooms were screened and well ventilated, and kept at a temperature that was confortable for the birds at all times. The birds were kept until they developed symptoms of leukosis or until it was thought that they had had sufficient time to show symptoms.

FILTRATION THROUGH MEMBRANES OBTAINED FROM SCHLEICHER AND SCHULL COMPANY

The procedure followed was the same as that described in series 1. Table 2 gives the results. Preliminary filtrations were run to determine the proper vacuum to use. It was found that the 3, 4.5, and 6% membranes would withstand a vacuum of 27 inches of mercury, whereas the 1.5% membrane would work best if a vacuum of only eight inches of mercury were used. Higher vacuums injured the membranes. The results given in table 2 show that Salmonella pullorum and Prussian blue, with approximate sizes of 1,000 to 1,500 and 400 millimicrons respectively, are retained by all membranes used. Ferric oxide hydrosol, with an approximate size of 100 millimicrons, is slightly retained by the 4.5% membrane and completely retained by the 6% membrane. Congo red is passed completely by the 1.5, 3, and 4.5% membranes, but is held back partially by the 6% membrane. Litmus is completely passed by all the membranes.

These results indicate that the 1.5 and the 3% membranes will prevent the passage of particles that lie between the range of 100 and 400 millimicrons in size. The 4.5% membrane will slightly retain particles of 100 millimicrons in size, therefore this membrane will completely hold back particles that are slightly larger than 100 millimicrons, and particles that are smaller than those which will pass the 1.5 and the 3% membranes. The 6% membrane will partially retain particles that are approximately 40 millimicrons in size, therefore the particles completely retained are slightly larger, being in the range between 40 and 100 millimicrons.

MATERIALS FILTERED

The material filtered in this series was prepared as described in the first series. The check was made for leaks in the filters and for sterility of the filtrates before the injections into the birds were made.

The material filtered in this series was taken from a case of leukosis that had been produced experimentally.

3.—This bird was a White Leghorn female that had received intramuscularly 0.5 cc. of filtrate from a 50–50 membrane. Approximately 4½ months after receiving the injection the bird showed typical paralysis of the left wing and the right leg. The sciatic nerve, upon autopsy was found to be enlarged and the radius marrow was found to be hyperplastic. The differential blood count revealed: 14 granulocytes with eosinophilic rods, 2 granulocytes with eosinophilic round granules, no basophils, no monocytes, 66 lymphocytes, 17 hemocytoblasts, and 1 myelocyte. Microscopic examination of the tissues revealed infiltrations of hemocytoblasts around the vessels in the liver and spleen and in the sheath surrounding the sciatic nerve. The radius marrow was active with hemocytoblasts in predominance. Diagnosis, hemocytoblastosis.

BIRDS INJECTED

The birds injected in this series came from the same source and were handled by exactly the same methods as described for series 1. Tables 3 and 4 give the results with the various filtrates.

TABLE 3.—*Filterability of Leukosis Agent Through Collodion Membranes*

Bird No.	Type of Disease Affecting Donor	Membrane Filtered Through	Results
221	Myeloid Leukosis	50–50	Hemocytoblastosis
209	Myeloid Leukosis	50–50	Negative
254	Hemocytoblastosis	50–50	Negative
281	Hemocytoblastosis	50–50	Lymphomatosis and Myeloid Leukosis
291	Myeloid Leukosis	40–60	Negative
239	Myeloid Leukosis	40–60	Hemocytoblastosis
283	Hemocytoblastosis	40–60	Lymphomatosis and Hemocytoblastosis
570	Hemocytoblastosis	40–60	Drowned
227	Myeloid Leukosis	30–70	Negative
267	Myeloid Leukosis	30–70	Hemocytoblastosis
258	Hemocytoblastosis	30–70	Myeloid Leukosis and Hemocytoblastosis
218	Hemocytoblastosis	30–70	Hemocytoblastosis

TABLE 4.—*Filterability of Leukosis Agent Through Membranes From Carl Schleicher and Schull Company*

Bird No.	Type of Disease Affecting Donor	Membrane Filtered Through	Results
201	Hemocytoblastosis	1.5%	Died (Intercurrent Infection)
285	"	1.5%	Hemocytoblastosis
256	"	1.5%	Hemocytoblastosis
180	"	3.0%	Hemocytoblastosis
284	"	3.0%	Intercurrent Infection
278	"	3.0%	Hemocytoblastosis and Myeloid Leukosis
204	"	4.5%	Negative
113	"	4.5%	Negative
264	"	4.5%	Negative
109	"	6.0%	Negative
299	"	6.0%	Hemocytoblastosis
295	"	6.0%	Negative

DISCUSSION

The filtration experiments herein recorded furnish conclusive evidence that the leukosis agent is filtrable through collodion membranes that hold back Salmonella pullorum. This is in direct agreement with the results obtained by Furth and Miller.[4] All of our experimental birds were kept in sanitary metal cages with raised wire floors in screened rooms, and were found to be free from intestinal parasites. Moreover, our inoculating material was examined to make sure that it was free from microscopic organisms before any injections were made into birds. Our transmissions, therefore, with these bacteria-free filtrates to parasite-free birds, give no support to the claims that leukosis is due to bacteria and intestinal parasites.

The collodion membranes prepared in our laboratory were made according to the method described by Eggerth[5] and were found to be quite satisfactory for this work. We realize, however, that the filtration of blood and other tissue extracts may be influenced by many factors that are difficult to control. According to Bland[6] adsorption is reduced to a minimum when collodion membranes are used in filtration work. From the work of Elford and Andrewes[7] with filtration of phage through collodion membranes graded according to Elford's technic,[8] it is apparent that this material behaves when filtered very much the same as colloids in that there is an initial phase during which the adsorbing capacity of the membrane becomes saturated, followed by filtration of the phage through the equilibrated membrane.

From an examination of our results with injections of the filtrates, it may be noted that various forms of leukosis developed regardless of the form had by the donor of the inoculating material. This further supports the view that a single filtrable agent is responsible for the various expressions of the disease. In this work we did not encounter a case of erythroleukosis. This may be explained on the basis of early cases. All birds were killed and autopsied as soon as we were sure that the disease was developing. From our earlier work with this disease it appears that the erythro form is a later stage. On the other hand the hemocytoblastosis, which is the earliest stage, and involves chiefly the polyvalent stem cell, may develop into the other forms as the disease progresses, or combinations of the various forms may occur, as shown in this work.

Moreover, a separation of two or more filtrable agents did not occur with the filters used in these experiments. The wide range of 100 to 400 millimicrons might seem too great for such purpose, but since lymphoid and myeloid forms of the disease occurred from material passing filters of identical pore size within these limits, it appears that a separation of such agents on the basis of size did not take place.

The results obtained with the 6% membrane appear misleading in that one bird developed leukosis. Further study of this case has convinced us that

4. J. Exper. Med. **55:** 479, 1932.
5. J. Biol. Chem. **48:** 203, 1921.
6. Brit. J. Exper. Path. **9:** 283, 1928.
7. Brit. J. Exper. Path. **13:** 446, 1932.
8. Brit. J. Exper. Path. **10:** 126, 1929.

it was of spontaneous origin. This bird was killed and autopsied only two months after being injected with the filtrate. On autopsy it was found to have a greatly enlarged liver, weighing 250 gms. The incubation periods were much longer with all the other birds, varying from 4 to 6 months. However, no case of leukosis developed in our control birds which were all autopsied and studied thoroughly at the close of the experiments. This work shows clearly that the particle size of the agent is less than 400 millimicrons, and probably greater than 100 millimicrons.

SUMMARY

The average blood p_H of 50 normal fowls was found to be 7.56, and that of 35 leukotic fowls 7.57. This slight difference in blood p_H is concluded to be insufficient for the identification of leukotic birds on this basis.

Our filtration experiments give no support to the claims that leukosis is due to bacteria, or to intestinal parasites. These results, on the other hand, demonstrate quite clearly that the causative agent of the various forms of leukosis is filtrable through membranes that retain S. pullorum, which has dimensions of 1,000–1,500 millimicrons.

A separation of two or more filtrable agents, on the basis of particle size, as factors in the etiology of the various forms of leukosis, was impossible with the filters used in these experiments.

These results, therefore, are in accord with the view that a single filtrable agent is responsible for the various forms of the disease. From these results it may be concluded that the particle size of the leukosis agent lies between the limits of 400 and 100 millimicrons, or possibly less.

GENERAL INDEX

Acidfast organisms, dissociation of, 247
Actinomycosis, pathogenesis of, 115
Anderson, G. W.: Pullorum disease in turkeys, 337
Applebaum, Martha: The effect of bile on the bacteriophage phenomenon, 195

Bacteria, acidfast, fate of phagocytized, 324
acidfast, dissociation of, 247
carbohydrate utilization by, 234
effects of ozone on, 204
growth stimulating factors for, 28, 121
Bacteriophage phenomenon, the effect of bile on the, 195
Bacteriophages, "prezone" of certain, 215
Beard, Paul: Growth stimulating factors for microorganisms, 28
Bell, W. B.: The blood p_H of leukotic fowls and the filterability of the leukosis agent, 342
Berry, George P.: Psittacosis: A review of the literature on the lesions of the central nervous system with a report of a case, 129
Bonynge, C. W.: The demonstration of capsules about hemolytic streptococci with India ink or azo blue, 5
Broadhurst, Jean: Cytoplasmic inclusion bodies in the human throat, 134
Brucella group, serologic classification of, 280
Brucella strains, differential study of forty, isolated in Minnesota, 293
Brucella, extraction of a precipitable substance from, 45
Buggs, C. W.: Properties of homogenized herpes virus, 98
Burrows, William: Oxidation-reduction potentials in Salmonella cultures; II. Characteristic potentials produced by members of the suipestifer and enteritidis groups, 259
Butt, E. M.: The demonstration of capsules about hemolytic streptococci with India ink or azo blue, 5

Carbohydrate utilization, quantitative determinations of by bacteria, comparison with acid-indicator methods, 234
Castles, Ruth: Experimental meningococcal infection in the mouse, 263
Clawson, B. J.: The destruction of tubercle bacilli, within phagocytes in vitro, 64
Cod liver oil, peroxides in irradiated, 185
Cohn, M. L.: Vaccination against tuberculosis—a comparative study in man and animals, 158
Corper, H. J.: Vaccination against tuberculosis—a comparative study in man and animals, 158
Cross, E.: Growth stimulating factors for micro-organisms, 28

Damerow, A. P.: Vaccination against tuberculosis—a comparative study in man and animals, 158
Diphtheria, trends in the prevalence of, 306
Diplococcus morbillorum, 1

Edwards, Philip R.: Fermentative varieties of Salmonella aertrycke, 225
Endocarditis, relationship of strains of green streptococci to subacute bacterial, 230
Eyre, Sarah: The antigenic similarity of two strains of non-capsulated, methemoglobin-producing organisms to type XXIX pneumococcus, 190

Fabian, F. W.: Dissociation of Saccharomyces acerissacchari Fabian and Hall and Pichia alcoholophila Klöcker, 165
Food poisoning, staphylococcus, a small milk-borne epidemic of, 318
Finkle, Isadore I: Studies on bacterial nutrition; II. The distribution of a growth stimulating factor in animal and plant tissues, 121
Fox, Herbert: The relationship of strains of green streptococci to the clinical character of subacute bacterial endocarditis, 230

Gelatin, note on the liquefaction of by Salmonella, type Dar-es-Salaam, 128
Green, R. G.: Properties of homogenized herpes virus, 98
Grubb, Thomas C.: Staphylococcus food poisoning; report of a small milk-borne epidemic, 318

Hadley, Philip B.: Note on the spontaneous contamination of a bacterial culture by an organism resembling Hartmanella castellanii, 23
Harmon, Paul H.: The racial incidence of poliomyelitis in the United States with special reference to the Negro, 331
Hartmanella castellanii, note on the spontaneous contamination of a bacterial culture by an organism resembling, 23
Herpes virus, properties of homogenized, 98
Hotopp, Marion: The fate of phagocytized acidfast bacteria as determined by the single cell method; I. Polymorphonuclear leukocytes, 324
Hudson, N. Paul: Failure to infect monkeys with poliomyelitis virus through isolated intestinal loops, 10

Inclusion bodies, cytoplasmic in the human throat, 134
Inflammation, invasiveness and virulence in relation to resistance, 81

Johan, Bela: Rural typhoid fever, 70
Johnson, E. P.: The blood p_H of leukotic fowls and the filterability of the leukosis agent, 342
Pullorum disease in turkeys, 337
Jordan, Edwin O.: Oxidation-reduction potentials in salmonella cultures; II. Characteristic potentials produced by members of the suipestifer and enteritidis groups, 259
Note on the liquefaction of gelatin by Salmonella, type Dar-es-Salaam, 128
Joyce, R. L.: Demonstration of capsules about hemolytic streptococci with India ink or azo blue, 5
Jungeblut, Claus W.: On the mechanism of immunity in experimental poliomyelitis, 150

Kabler, Paul: A differential study of forty Brucella strains isolated in Minnesota, 293
Kahn, Morton C.: The fate of phagocytized acidfast bacteria as determined by the single cell method; I. Polymorphonuclear leukocytes, 324
Kendall, Arthur Isaac: The effects of ozone upon certain bacteria and their respective phages; studies in bacterial metabolism, CV, 204
Observations upon the "prezone" of certain bacteriophages; studies in bacterial metabolism, CVI, 215
Koser, Stewart A.: Studies on bacterial nutrition; II. The distribution of a growth stimulating factor in animal and plant tissues, 121

Landau, A.: Dissociation of two unusual acidfast organisms isolated from human sources, 247
Lennette, Edwin H.: Failure to infect monkeys with poliomyelitis virus through isolated intestinal loops, 10
Leukotic fowls, the blood p_H of, and the filterability of the leukosis agent, 342
Liming, Rosamond M.: Cytoplasmic inclusion bodies in the human throat, 134
Lord, Frederick T.: The pathogenesis of actinomycosis; recovery of actinomyces-like organisms from the normal mouth, 115
Lucia, Eschscholtzia L.: Trends in the prevalence of diphtheria, 306

MacLanahan, Margaret: A differential study of forty Brucella strains isolated in Minnesota, 293
MacLean, Margaret Estelle: Cytoplasmic inclusion bodies in the human throat, 134
Mastitis, streptococci from bovine, 105
Maxcy, Kenneth F.: The Weil-Felix reaction of the rabbit in the diagnosis of Rocky Mountain spotted fever (Eastern type), 288
Meningococcus infection, experimental, in the mouse, 263

Menkin, Valy: Studies on inflammation. XI. Invasiveness and virulence in relation to resistance, 81
Meyer, K. F.: The serologic classification of the Brucella group, 280
Mice, salivary gland disease of, 59
Miller, C. Phillip: Experimental meningococcal infection in the mouse, 263
Montu, Elizabeth: Comparative observations on streptococci from human gastro-intestinal ulcerations and from bovine mastitis, 105

Nutrition: Studies on bacterial, II. The distribution of a growth stimulating factor in animal and plant tissues, 121

Opsonins for Diplococcus morbillorum, 1
Opsonins for Streptococcus scarlatinae, 1
Ozone, effects of, upon certain bacteria and their respective phages, 204

Patterson, Marjorie, B.: The effect of bile on the bacteriophage phenomenon, 195
Peroxides, bactericidal effect of, in irradiated cod liver oil, 185
Pichia alcoholophila Klöcker, dissociation of Saccharomyces aceris-sacchari Fabian and Hall and, 165
Pneumococcus, antigenic similarity of two strains of non-capsulated, methmoglobin-producing organisms to type XXIX, 190
Poliomyelitis, failure to infect monkeys through isolated intestinal loops, 10
mechanism of immunity in experimental, 150
racial incidence of in the United States with special reference to the Negro, 331
Psittacosis; review of the literature on lesions of the central nervous system with report of a case, 129
Pullorum disease in turkeys, 337

Reiter, Dorothy O.: Studies on the extraction of a precipitable substance from genus Brucella, 45
Rettger, Leo F.: Variation of Salmonella pullorum, 172
Rocky Mountain spotted fever (Eastern type), Weil-Felix reaction of rabbit in diagnosis of, 288

Saccharomyces aceris-sacchari Fabian and Hall, dissociation of, and Pichia alcoholphila Klöcker, 165
Sahyun, Melville: Growth stimulating factors for micro-organisms, 28
Salivary gland disease of mice, 59
Salmonella aertrycke, fermentative varieties of, 225
Salmonella cultures, oxidation-reduction potentials in; characteristic potentials produced by members of the suipestifer and enteritidis groups, 259
Salmonella pullorum, variation of, 172
Saunders, Felix: Studies on bacterial nutrition; II. The distribution of a growth stimulating factor in animal and plant tissues, 121
Schultz, E. W.: Growth stimulating factors for micro-organisms, 28
Sears, H. J.: The obligatie, anaerobic streptococci a study of two strains with special reference to their resistance to heat and disinfectants, 299
Serum, opsonins for Diplococcus morbillorum and for Streptococcus scarlatinae in convalescent measles serum, convalescent scarlet fever serum and placental extract, 1
Shaughnessy, Howard J.: Staphylococcus food poisoning; report of a small milk-borne epidemic, 318
Shinn, Lawrence E.: Note on the spontaneous contamination of a bacterial culture by an organism resembling Hartmanella castellanii, 23
Snow, J.: Growth stimulating factors for micro-organisms, 28
Spoelstra, Raymond C.: Studies on bacterial nutrition; II. The distribution of a growth stimulating factor in animal and plant tissues, 121
Sprunt, Douglas H.: Psittacosis; review of the literature on the lesions of the central nervous system with a report of a case, 129
Staphylococcus food poisoning; small milk-borne epidemic of, 318
Steenken, W. Jr.: Dissociation of two unusual acidfast organisms isolated from human sources, 247
Stevens, Franklin A.: The bactericidal effect of peroxides in irradiated cod liver oil, 185
Stovall, W. D.: The antigenic similarity of two strains of non-capsulated, methemoglobin-producing organisms to type XXIX pneumococcus, 190
Streptococci anaerobic, two strains with reference to resistance to heat and disinfectants, 299
capsules about hemolytic, 5
effect of dissociation of, on fibrinolytic and anticlotting activity, 92
from human gastro-intestinal ulcerations and bovine mastitis, 105
green, in endocarditis, 230
hemolytic, demonstration of capsules about, with India ink or azo blue, 5
obligate anaerobic, 299
Streptococcus scarlatinae, 1

Taylor, Inez: Cytoplasmic inclusion bodies in the human throat, 134
Thompson, Juanita: Salivary gland disease of mice, 59
Torrey, John C.: Comparative observations on streptococci from human gastro-intestinal ulcerations and from bovine mastitis, 105
Trevett, Laurence D.: The pathogenesis of actinomycosis; recovery of actinomyces-like organisms from the normal mouth, 115
Tubercle bacilli, destruction of, within phagocytes in vitro, 64
Tuberculosis, vaccination against, in man and animals, 158
Tunnicliff, Ruth: Effect of dissociation of streptococci on their fibrinolytic and anticlotting activity, 92
Opsonins for Diplococcus morbillorum and for Streptococcus scarlatinae in convalescent measles serum, convalescent scarlet fever serum and placental extract, 1
Typhoid fever, rural, 70

Van Roekel, H.: Variation of Salmonella pullorum, 172
Veazie, Lyle: The serologic classification of the Brucella group, 280
Vidal, C. B.: Vaccination against tuberculosis—a comparative study in man and animals, 158
Vinton, Dorothy: The obligate anaerobic streptococci a study of two strains with special reference to their resistance to heat and disinfectants, 299

Walker, Arthur William: Observations upon the "prezone" of certain bacteriophages; studies in bacterial metabolism, CVI, 215
The effects of ozone upon certain bacteria and their respective phages; studies in bacterial metabolism, CV, 204
Wedum, A. G.: Quantitative determinations of carbohydrate utilization by bacteria, comparison with acid-indicator methods, 234
Weil-Felix reaction in Rocky Mountain spotted fever, 288
Welke, Hilda F.: Trends in the prevalence of diphtheria, 306
Wickerham, L. J.: Dissociation of Saccharomyces aceris-sacchari Fabian and Hall and Pichia alcoholophila Klöcker, 165